T0303895

Randomized Phase II Cancer Clinical Trials

Chapman & Hall/CRC Biostatistics Series

Editor-in-Chief

Shein-Chung Chow, Ph.D.

Professor
Department of Biostatistics and Bioinformatics
Duke University School of Medicine
Durham, North Carolina

Series Editors

Byron Jones
Biometrical Fellow
Statistical Methodology
Integrated Information Sciences
Novartis Pharma AG
Basel, Switzerland

Jen-pei Liu
Professor
Division of Biometry
Department of Agronomy
National Taiwan University
Taipei, Taiwan

Karl E. Peace
Georgia Cancer Coalition
Distinguished Cancer Scholar
Senior Research Scientist and
Professor of Biostatistics
Jiann-Ping Hsu College of Public Health
Georgia Southern University
Statesboro, Georgia

Bruce W. Turnbull
Professor
School of Operations Research
and Industrial Engineering
Cornell University
Ithaca, New York

Chapman & Hall/CRC Biostatistics Series

Chapman & Hall/CRC Biostatistics Series

Randomized Phase II Cancer Clinical Trials

Sin-Ho Jung

Duke University
Durham, North Carolina, USA

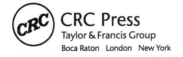

CRC Press
Taylor & Francis Group
Boca Raton London New York

CRC Press is an imprint of the
Taylor & Francis Group, an **informa** business

A CHAPMAN & HALL BOOK

CRC Press
Taylor & Francis Group
6000 Broken Sound Parkway NW, Suite 300
Boca Raton, FL 33487-2742

Printed on acid-free paper
Version Date: 20130315

International Standard Book Number-13: 978-1-4398-7185-0 (Hardback)

Visit the Taylor & Francis Web site at
http://www.taylorandfrancis.com

and the CRC Press Web site at
http://www.crcpress.com

Contents

Preface

A clinical trial is an important research tool in the evaluation of the efficacy and safety of cancer therapies. Cancer therapies include anticancer drugs, gene therapy, surgical procedure, radiation therapy, and combinations of these. An experimental therapy is evaluated through three phases of cancer clinical trials. A phase I trial has the objective of selecting the appropriate dose level of an experimental therapy (mostly an anticancer drug) to be used for further investigation. Once a dose level is chosen, the experimental therapy is tested through a small phase II trial requiring 50 to 100 patients. An experimental therapy that is shown to have a promising activity in phase II is evaluated by a large-scale phase III trial compared to a current standard therapy. Since evaluation of an experimental therapy through these clinical trials is limited to a specific type of disease, a single experimental therapy may go through multiple phase II and III trials for different disease types, especially when it is shown to be very efficacious from earlier trials.

If a new cancer therapy is shown to be inefficacious from a phase II trial, it is very likely that no phase III trials will be conducted for further evaluation. In this sense, phase II trials are called screening trials. Among the three phases of cancer trials, phase II trials usually comprise the largest volume of cancer research activity for individual cancer centers and cooperative cancer trial groups. In order to expedite the conduct of phase II trials, a traditional phase II trial has been designed as a single-arm trial to treat all the patients using the experimental therapy to be compared with a historical control. This simple phase II trial design has resulted in many issues, including increased false positivity of phase II trial results and many negative phase III trials. Pointing out these issues, many oncologists and biostatisticians began to propose to use a randomized phase II trial to compare an experimental therapy with a prospective control therapy.

It is critical to use accurate statistical methods for designing and analyzing phase II trials. Because of the small sample sizes, exact statistical methods have been used for phase II clinical trials. This book is intended to provide diverse statistical design and analysis methods for randomized phase II trials in oncology. Since a large part of methodologies for randomized phase II trials stems from those of single-arm phase II trials and many phase II cancer clinical trials still use single-arm designs, we also review the statistical methods for single-arm phase II trials in Chapters 1 to 5. This book will be useful for cancer clinicians as well as biostatisticians.

Chapter 1

Introduction

Cancer clinical trials investigate the efficacy and toxicity of experimental cancer therapies. Through a phase I trial, we determine an appropriate dose level for treating humans based on the information collected from preclinical animal studies. In a phase I trial, the most popular primary clinical outcome is toxicity. Usually, for an anticancer chemotherapy, both the efficacy and toxicity increase as the dose level increases. We choose a dose with a tolerable toxicity level for further investigation of the therapy.

Once a dose level is determined from a phase I trial, we assess the drug's anticancer activity through phase II clinical trials. Phase II clinical trials have the objective of screening out inefficacious experimental therapies before they proceed to further investigation through large-scale phase III trials. In order to expedite this process, a conventional phase II trial is designed as a single-arm trial to treat patients with the experimental therapy only. In this case, the efficacy of the experimental therapy is compared with that of a historical control. The most popular primary endpoint of phase II cancer clinical trials is tumor response, which is measured by the change in tumor size before and during treatment. For a solid tumor, if the index tumor shrinks to half or less compared to the baseline, we call it a partial response. If the tumor disappears during treatment, then we call it a complete response. Overall response is defined as a partial or complete response.

If an experimental therapy is shown to have anticancer activity through a phase II trial, we proceed to a phase III trial to compare its efficacy with that of a standard therapy using a confirmatory endpoint such as overall survival. Unlike conventional single-arm phase II trials, a phase III trial randomizes the patients between an experimental therapy and a standard therapy, a *control*. The ultimate goal of cancer therapies is to extend the lifetime of cancer patients. In this sense, we usually choose overall survival time, defined as the time period between registration and death from any cause, as our primary efficacy endpoint. While a single-arm phase II trial requires around 50 patients, a phase III trial usually requires hundreds, or possibly thousands, of patients for proper evaluation of an experimental therapy.

Phase II trials generally require a shorter study period than phase III trials. Consequently, phase II trials have small sample sizes, so that exact statistical methods are preferable to asymptotic methods for their design and analysis. Various exact methods have been published for phase II trials with binary outcomes (e.g., tumor response). For survival outcomes (e.g., progression-free survival or time to recurrence), however, we have to use an asymptotic method due to lack of exact methods. Furthermore, phase II trials use a surrogate outcome (such as tumor response, or progression-free survival) rather than a confirmatory endpoint, such as overall survival, which requires a longer follow-up time. As another effort to lower the sample size of phase II trials, we may compromise-type I error rate and power, such as a one-sided alpha of 5% to 20% and a power of 80% to 90%, compared to two-sided alpha of 5% and a power of 90% or higher in phase III trials.

Usually, the historical control data for a single-arm phase II trial come from a previous study, frequently a previous phase II trial. The patient populations for different phase II trials are often quite heterogeneous, so that the distributions of patient characteristics for a new single-arm phase II trial are quite different from those of the prior trial which provides the historical control. Furthermore, as in most phase II trials, a historical control study may have a small sample size, so that the estimated response rate will have a large variance. In designing a new single-arm phase II trial, however, we often treat the estimated response rate from a previous trial as the true parameter value. Even if all the conditions are comparable between a new single-arm trial and a previous study giving the historical control data for the new study, regarding the response rate for the historical control as a parameter can drastically increase the type I error rate in testing. The methods of response assessment may be different between a historical control study and the current trial.

Because of these and other reasons, the traditional single-arm phase II trial designs lead to a high failure rate of phase III trials, see, for example, Djulbegovic et al. (2008). Wrong trial designs and selection of endpoints of phase II trials lead to failure of phase III clinical trials as well. For example, endpoints utilized for cytotoxic compounds may not be appropriate in the development of newer targeted, cytostatic therapeutic agents. Randomized phase II trials with a prospective control resolve these shortcomings of traditional single-arm phase II trials.

In this book, we review design and analysis methods of single-arm phase II trials (Chapters 2–5) and investigate methods for randomized phase II trials (Chapters 6–10). In Chapter 11, we discuss some statistical methods that can be used for both single-arm and randomized phase II cancer clinical trials. Although we discuss the statistical methods for phase II cancer clinical trials, they can be used for phase II trials for other diseases with some minor modification. Some methods can be used for phase III cancer clinical trials.

References

Djulbegovic, B., Kumar, A., Soares, H.P., Hozo, I., Bepler, G., Clarke, M., Bennett, C.L. (2008). New cancer treatment successes identified in phase 3 randomized controlled trials conducted by the National Cancer Institute–Sponsored Cooperative Oncology Groups, 1955 to 2006. *Archives of Internal Medicine*, 168 (6), 632–642.

Chapter 2

Single-Arm Phase II Trial Designs

Traditionally, phase II cancer clinical trials have single-arm designs using over-all response as the primary endpoint. In a traditional single-arm phase II trial, patients are treated by only an experimental therapy. At the end of such a trial, the efficacy of the experimental therapy is evaluated compared to that of a preselected historical control, which is usually chosen among the current standard therapies for the study population. In this chapter, we review some optimal designs for single-arm phase II clinical trials.

2.1 Single-Stage Designs

For ethical reasons, most phase II clinical trials are conducted through two stages. If the accrual rate is very fast, however, we may use a single-stage design.

Suppose that we want to investigate an experimental therapy for a patient population. Let p denote the response rate of the experimental therapy, and p_0 denote the response rate of a selected historical control therapy to which the experimental therapy will be compared.

In order to test the hypotheses $H_0 : p \leq p_0$ vs. $H_1 : p > p_0$, we treat n patients with the experimental therapy. Let X denote the number of respon-ders among n patients. We reject the experimental therapy if $X \leq a$ for a rejection value a. Assuming the patient responses are independent and iden-tically distributed, X is a binomial random variable with n independent trials and probability of success p, denoted as $B(n, p)$. For a response rate p, the probability of rejecting the therapy (or failing to reject H_0) is $P(X \leq a|p) = B(a|n, p)$, where $B(x|n, p) = \sum_{i=0}^{x} b(i|n, p)$ and $b(x|n, p) = \binom{n}{x} p^x (1 - p)^{n-x}$ are the cumulative distribution function and the probability mass function of $B(n, p)$.

For a specified type I error rate α^*, the rejection value a is chosen as the smallest integer a satisfying

$$\alpha \equiv 1 - B(a|n, p_0) \leq \alpha^*.$$

Suppose that we consider the experimental therapy to have promising anti-cancer activity if its response rate is $p_1(> p_0)$ or higher. Then, for $H_1 : p = p_1$, the one-stage design specified by (n, a) has a power of

$$1 - \beta = 1 - B(a|n, p_1).$$

The design of a single-stage phase II trial with a type I error rate not exceeding α^* and a power of at least $1 - \beta^*$ proceeds as follows.

2.1.1 Design of Single-Stage Phase II Trial

1. Specify design parameters $(\alpha^*, 1 - \beta^*, p_0, p_1)$.
2. For $n(> 0)$,

   a. Find the smallest integer a satisfying

   $$B(a|n, p_0) \geq 1 - \alpha^*.$$

   b. Calculate the the power

   $$1 - \beta = 1 - B(a|n, p_1).$$

3. If $1 - \beta \geq 1 - \beta^*$, select n and a as the number of patients required and the critical value, respectively, and stop the procedure. Otherwise, repeat the above step 2 with $n + 1$.

The design identified by this procedure is an optimal single-stage design in the sense that it requires the smallest number of patients among the designs satisfying $(\alpha^*, 1 - \beta^*)$ restriction. Tables 2.1–2.4 list the optimal single-stage designs under various design settings of $(\alpha^*, 1 - \beta^*, p_0, p_1)$.

Example 2.1
Suppose that we want to evaluate an experimental chemotherapy in patients with relapsed or refractory classical Hodgkin's lymphoma (HL). For this patient population, it is known that a standard chemotherapy has $p_0 = 65\%$ response rate. We will be highly interested in the experimental chemotherapy if its response rate is $p_1 = 80\%$ or higher. Given $(\alpha^*, 1 - \beta^*) = (0.1, 0.9)$, the optimal single-stage design is given as $(n, a) = (61, 44)$ from Table 2.4. This design has an exact type I error rate of $\alpha = 0.095$ and a power of $1 - \beta = 0.912$.

Table 2.1 Single-stage designs, and minimax and optimal two-stage designs for $(\alpha^*, 1-\beta^*) = (0.05, 0.8)$

p_0	p_1	Single-Stage Design			Minimax Design				Optimal Design			
		a/n	α	$1-\beta$	$a_1/n_1, a/n$	α	$1-\beta$	EN	$a_1/n_1, a/n$	α	$1-\beta$	EN
0.05	0.15	5/52	0.045	0.812	1/30, 5/52	0.045	0.802	39.8	1/23, 5/56	0.045	0.800	33.6
	0.20	3/27	0.044	0.818	0/13, 3/27	0.044	0.801	19.8	0/10, 3/29	0.044	0.801	17.6
	0.25	2/16	0.043	0.803	0/12, 2/16	0.043	0.801	13.8	0/9, 2/17	0.043	0.812	12.0
0.10	0.25	7/40	0.042	0.818	2/22, 7/40	0.042	0.803	28.8	2/18, 7/43	0.042	0.800	24.7
	0.30	5/25	0.033	0.807	1/15, 5/25	0.033	0.802	19.5	1/10, 5/29	0.033	0.805	15.0
0.15	0.30	11/48	0.048	0.819	3/23, 11/48	0.048	0.804	34.5	3/19, 12/55	0.048	0.801	30.4
	0.35	7/28	0.049	0.818	2/15, 7/28	0.049	0.803	20.1	1/9, 8/34	0.049	0.811	19.0
0.20	0.35	16/56	0.043	0.806	6/31, 15/53	0.043	0.802	40.4	5/22, 19/72	0.043	0.800	35.4
	0.40	11/35	0.034	0.805	4/18, 10/33	0.034	0.801	22.3	3/13, 12/43	0.034	0.800	20.6
0.25	0.40	21/62	0.043	0.803	16/51, 20/60	0.043	0.803	52.0	5/20, 23/71	0.043	0.802	39.5
	0.45	13/36	0.046	0.817	4/17, 13/36	0.046	0.800	25.1	5/17, 14/41	0.046	0.803	22.6
0.30	0.45	26/67	0.047	0.815	16/46, 25/65	0.047	0.803	49.6	9/27, 30/81	0.047	0.802	41.7
	0.50	16/39	0.050	0.832	6/19, 16/39	0.050	0.804	25.7	5/15, 18/46	0.050	0.803	23.6
0.35	0.50	30/68	0.046	0.802	22/55, 29/66	0.046	0.801	57.0	10/27, 33/77	0.046	0.801	43.5
	0.55	19/41	0.048	0.831	8/21, 18/39	0.048	0.801	26.3	5/14, 20/44	0.048	0.800	24.8
0.40	0.55	35/71	0.044	0.802	28/59, 34/70	0.044	0.802	60.1	11/26, 40/84	0.044	0.805	44.9
	0.60	22/42	0.038	0.803	17/34, 20/39	0.038	0.802	34.4	7/16, 23/46	0.038	0.801	24.5
0.45	0.60	38/70	0.047	0.804	19/42, 38/70	0.047	0.800	53.9	12/26, 41/77	0.047	0.804	45.1
	0.65	24/42	0.042	0.818	16/30, 22/39	0.042	0.806	31.2	7/15, 24/43	0.042	0.804	24.7
0.50	0.65	41/69	0.046	0.802	39/66, 40/68	0.046	0.801	66.1	15/28, 48/83	0.046	0.802	43.7
	0.70	23/37	0.049	0.807	12/23, 23/37	0.049	0.801	27.7	8/15, 26/43	0.049	0.804	23.5
0.55	0.70	45/70	0.045	0.820	20/35, 43/67	0.045	0.800	45.8	15/26, 48/76	0.045	0.805	42.0
	0.75	25/37	0.043	0.806	15/24, 24/36	0.043	0.801	26.1	9/15, 28/43	0.043	0.805	22.3
0.60	0.75	43/62	0.049	0.812	18/30, 43/62	0.049	0.802	43.8	17/27, 46/67	0.049	0.800	39.3
	0.80	26/36	0.045	0.832	8/13, 25/35	0.045	0.808	20.8	7/11, 30/43	0.045	0.802	20.5
0.65	0.80	41/55	0.049	0.803	20/31, 41/55	0.049	0.801	41.9	12/18, 49/67	0.049	0.804	35.4
	0.85	24/31	0.046	0.827	19/25, 23/30	0.046	0.807	25.4	10/14, 25/33	0.046	0.804	18.2
0.70	0.85	39/49	0.048	0.809	16/23, 39/49	0.048	0.801	34.4	14/19, 46/59	0.048	0.807	30.3
	0.90	23/28	0.047	0.858	19/23, 21/26	0.047	0.801	23.2	4/6, 22/27	0.047	0.804	14.8
0.75	0.90	38/45	0.045	0.841	17/22, 33/39	0.045	0.802	27.5	10/13, 40/48	0.045	0.809	24.6
	0.95	20/23	0.049	0.895	14/16, 17/20	0.049	0.805	16.3	2/3, 19/22	0.049	0.800	11.0
0.80	0.95	27/30	0.044	0.812	7/9, 26/29	0.044	0.802	17.7	12/14, 30/34	0.044	0.812	18.0
0.85	0.95	54/59	0.047	0.828	35/39, 52/57	0.047	0.811	41.6	11/13, 59/65	0.047	0.800	33.7

Table 2.2 Single-stage designs, and minimax and optimal two-stage designs for $(\alpha^*, 1-\beta^*) = (0.05, 0.85)$

		Single-Stage Design			Minimax Design				Optimal Design				
p_0	p_1	a/n	α	$1-\beta$	$a_1/n_1, a/n$	α	$1-\beta$	EN	$a_1/n_1, a/n$	α	$1-\beta$	EN	
0.05	0.15	6/63	0.037	0.853	1/38, 6/63	0.037	0.850	52.3	1/25, 6/70	0.037	0.855	41.1	
	0.20	4/35	0.029	0.857	0/17, 4/35	0.029	0.850	27.5	1/17, 4/41	0.029	0.851	22.0	
	0.25	3/23	0.026	0.863	0/12, 3/23	0.026	0.854	17.1	0/8, 3/26	0.026	0.850	14.1	
0.10	0.25	8/47	0.041	0.865	2/24, 8/47	0.041	0.853	34.0	2/20, 8/50	0.041	0.853	29.7	
	0.30	5/27	0.047	0.864	2/18, 5/27	0.047	0.851	20.4	1/11, 6/35	0.047	0.851	18.3	
0.15	0.30	13/57	0.039	0.851	7/39, 13/57	0.039	0.852	42.3	5/28, 14/66	0.039	0.851	36.9	
	0.35	8/33	0.049	0.868	3/19, 8/33	0.049	0.850	23.4	3/16, 10/46	0.049	0.851	22.3	
0.20	0.35	18/65	0.049	0.866	6/31, 18/65	0.049	0.850	45.6	6/27, 21/80	0.049	0.853	42.2	
	0.40	12/40	0.043	0.871	3/17, 11/37	0.043	0.850	26.0	4/17, 14/51	0.043	0.854	25.2	
0.25	0.40	24/73	0.049	0.870	9/36, 23/70	0.049	0.851	50.0	8/30, 26/81	0.049	0.852	46.6	
	0.45	15/42	0.042	0.854	6/25, 15/42	0.042	0.850	32.5	5/18, 17/50	0.042	0.850	27.0	
0.30	0.45	29/76	0.049	0.861	10/35, 29/76	0.049	0.850	55.1	9/29, 32/86	0.049	0.853	49.7	
	0.50	18/44	0.044	0.854	14/37, 17/42	0.044	0.851	37.6	7/21, 19/48	0.044	0.850	28.5	
0.35	0.50	35/81	0.050	0.867	30/71, 34/79	0.050	0.850	71.7	13/34, 41/98	0.050	0.851	51.8	
	0.55	21/46	0.050	0.870	19/42, 20/44	0.050	0.852	42.1	6/17, 22/49	0.050	0.851	29.2	
0.40	0.55	41/85	0.049	0.874	25/56, 39/81	0.049	0.851	61.0	14/33, 44/93	0.049	0.850	52.1	
	0.60	23/45	0.048	0.856	11/27, 23/45	0.048	0.851	34.0	8/19, 25/50	0.048	0.851	29.3	
0.45	0.60	44/82	0.046	0.855	41/77, 43/81	0.046	0.851	77.2	17/35, 52/100	0.046	0.853	52.9	
	0.65	26/46	0.043	0.853	20/37, 25/45	0.043	0.851	37.8	9/19, 27/49	0.043	0.852	28.9	
0.50	0.65	47/80	0.046	0.854	43/74, 46/79	0.046	0.850	74.3	18/34, 53/92	0.046	0.851	51.6	
	0.70	27/44	0.048	0.861	11/22, 27/44	0.048	0.851	31.1	9/17, 31/52	0.048	0.855	28.0	
0.55	0.70	49/77	0.050	0.863	21/38, 49/77	0.050	0.852	54.6	18/31, 58/93	0.050	0.854	49.7	
	0.75	28/42	0.045	0.857	25/38, 27/41	0.045	0.852	38.2	8/14, 33/51	0.045	0.850	26.5	
0.60	0.75	51/74	0.044	0.858	21/34, 50/73	0.044	0.851	47.8	16/26, 55/81	0.044	0.851	46.0	
	0.80	28/39	0.045	0.859	24/34, 27/38	0.045	0.852	34.3	10/16, 29/41	0.045	0.854	24.2	
0.65	0.80	48/65	0.049	0.860	21/32, 48/65	0.049	0.850	45.4	20/29, 56/77	0.049	0.851	41.7	
	0.85	27/35	0.042	0.856	10/15, 26/34	0.042	0.851	21.7	8/12, 28/37	0.042	0.851	20.7	
0.70	0.85	45/57	0.049	0.862	15/22, 45/57	0.049	0.850	39.3	17/23, 55/71	0.049	0.851	35.9	
	0.90	23/28	0.047	0.858	9/13, 23/28	0.047	0.852	19.3	8/11, 26/32	0.047	0.854	17.6	
0.75	0.90	42/50	0.045	0.878	37/44, 39/47	0.045	0.851	44.2	14/18, 44/53	0.045	0.857	28.7	
	0.95	20/23	0.049	0.895	9/11, 19/22	0.049	0.856	13.2	8/10, 20/23	0.049	0.857	13.2	
0.80	0.95	33/37	0.045	0.888	20/23, 31/35	0.045	0.861	24.6	10/12, 36/41	0.045	0.856	20.0	
0.85	0.95	62/68	0.047	0.876	48/53, 59/65	0.047	0.853	54.0	20/23, 67/74	0.047	0.852	38.7	

Table 2.3 Single-stage designs, and minimax and optimal two-stage designs for $(\alpha^*, 1 - \beta^*) = (0.05, 0.9)$

p_0	p_1	Single-Stage Design			Minimax Design				Optimal Design				
		a/n	$1-\beta$	α	$a_1/n_1, a/n$	α	$1-\beta$	EN	$a_1/n_1, a/n$	α	$1-\beta$	EN
0.05	0.15	7/77	0.907	0.038	2/46, 7/77	0.038	0.901	58.6	2/37, 7/84	0.038	0.901	50.2
	0.20	4/38	0.901	0.040	1/29, 4/38	0.040	0.900	32.9	1/21, 4/41	0.040	0.902	26.7
	0.25	3/25	0.904	0.034	0/15, 3/25	0.034	0.901	20.4	0/9, 3/30	0.034	0.902	16.8
0.10	0.25	9/55	0.911	0.044	3/31, 9/55	0.044	0.901	40.0	2/21, 10/66	0.044	0.902	36.8
	0.30	6/33	0.906	0.042	2/22, 6/33	0.042	0.902	26.2	2/18, 6/35	0.042	0.902	22.5
0.15	0.30	14/64	0.903	0.049	6/42, 14/64	0.049	0.900	51.8	5/30, 17/82	0.049	0.901	45.1
	0.35	9/38	0.904	0.049	3/23, 9/38	0.049	0.901	29.9	3/19, 10/44	0.049	0.905	26.9
0.20	0.35	21/77	0.905	0.045	8/42, 21/77	0.045	0.900	58.4	8/37, 22/83	0.045	0.901	51.4
	0.40	14/47	0.901	0.037	5/24, 13/45	0.037	0.900	31.2	4/19, 15/54	0.037	0.904	30.4
0.25	0.40	27/83	0.900	0.047	13/57, 27/83	0.047	0.900	72.1	10/37, 31/99	0.047	0.900	56.2
	0.45	17/49	0.905	0.046	6/26, 17/49	0.046	0.900	37.1	6/22, 19/57	0.046	0.900	32.5
0.30	0.45	35/93	0.908	0.045	27/77, 33/88	0.045	0.901	78.5	13/40, 40/110	0.045	0.901	60.8
	0.50	21/53	0.916	0.049	7/24, 21/53	0.049	0.902	36.6	8/24, 24/63	0.049	0.903	34.7
0.35	0.50	41/96	0.908	0.047	16/46, 40/94	0.047	0.900	67.4	16/43, 44/105	0.047	0.900	62.7
	0.55	24/53	0.900	0.045	12/37, 24/53	0.045	0.900	45.9	7/20, 26/59	0.045	0.901	35.6
0.40	0.55	45/94	0.900	0.049	24/62, 45/94	0.049	0.900	78.9	19/45, 49/104	0.049	0.900	64.0
	0.60	28/56	0.917	0.049	12/29, 27/54	0.049	0.901	38.1	11/25, 32/66	0.049	0.902	36.0
0.45	0.60	52/98	0.902	0.044	49/93, 50/95	0.044	0.902	93.1	19/40, 60/116	0.044	0.900	64.0
	0.65	30/54	0.904	0.045	14/31, 30/54	0.045	0.900	40.6	11/23, 33/61	0.045	0.901	34.9
0.50	0.65	54/93	0.901	0.048	28/57, 54/93	0.048	0.900	75.0	22/42, 60/105	0.048	0.901	62.3
	0.70	32/53	0.914	0.049	14/27, 32/53	0.049	0.900	36.1	13/24, 36/61	0.049	0.901	34.0
0.55	0.70	58/92	0.909	0.048	50/81, 56/89	0.048	0.901	81.7	22/38, 68/110	0.048	0.900	59.8
	0.75	33/50	0.902	0.043	20/33, 32/49	0.043	0.902	36.3	10/18, 35/54	0.043	0.901	32.1
0.60	0.75	58/85	0.904	0.047	48/72, 57/84	0.047	0.900	73.2	21/34, 64/95	0.047	0.901	55.6
	0.80	32/45	0.901	0.045	15/26, 32/45	0.045	0.900	35.9	12/19, 37/53	0.045	0.901	29.5
0.65	0.80	55/75	0.900	0.049	34/52, 55/75	0.049	0.900	61.8	21/31, 67/93	0.049	0.902	50.3
	0.85	32/42	0.911	0.043	28/37, 30/40	0.043	0.902	37.2	10/15, 33/44	0.043	0.902	25.2
0.70	0.85	54/69	0.915	0.048	33/44, 53/68	0.048	0.902	48.5	18/25, 61/79	0.048	0.904	43.4
	0.90	30/37	0.929	0.044	13/18, 26/32	0.044	0.901	22.7	11/15, 29/36	0.044	0.905	21.2
0.75	0.90	46/55	0.906	0.045	19/25, 45/54	0.045	0.902	36.0	18/23, 52/63	0.045	0.900	34.3
	0.95	25/29	0.945	0.046	19/22, 22/26	0.046	0.902	22.2	7/9, 24/28	0.046	0.901	14.7
0.80	0.95	39/44	0.933	0.044	31/35, 35/40	0.044	0.900	35.3	16/19, 37/42	0.044	0.903	24.4
0.85	0.95	69/76	0.914	0.050	35/40, 68/75	0.050	0.901	49.2	26/30, 75/83	0.050	0.905	47.0

Table 2.4 Single-stage designs, and minimax and optimal two-stage designs for $(\alpha^*, 1-\beta^*) = (0.1, 0.9)$

		Single-Stage Design			Minimax Design					Optimal Design				
p_0	p_1	a/n	α	$1-\beta$	$a_1/n_1, a/n$	α	$1-\beta$	EN		$a_1/n_1, a/n$	α	$1-\beta$	EN	
0.05	0.15	5/60	0.079	0.903	1/39, 5/60	0.079	0.901	51.3		1/28, 5/66	0.079	0.902	43.6	
	0.20	3/32	0.074	0.907	0/18, 3/32	0.074	0.901	26.4		0/12, 3/37	0.074	0.902	23.5	
	0.25	2/20	0.075	0.909	0/13, 2/20	0.075	0.903	16.4		0/9, 2/24	0.075	0.903	14.5	
0.10	0.25	6/40	0.100	0.904	2/27, 6/40	0.100	0.900	33.7		2/21, 7/50	0.100	0.901	31.2	
	0.30	4/25	0.098	0.910	1/16, 4/25	0.098	0.903	20.4		1/12, 5/35	0.098	0.901	19.8	
0.15	0.30	11/53	0.091	0.909	5/34, 11/53	0.091	0.900	41.7		3/23, 11/55	0.091	0.901	37.7	
	0.35	7/32	0.096	0.918	2/17, 7/32	0.096	0.905	24.2		3/19, 7/33	0.096	0.904	23.4	
0.20	0.35	16/61	0.088	0.905	6/33, 15/58	0.088	0.900	45.5		5/27, 16/63	0.088	0.902	43.6	
	0.40	10/36	0.089	0.910	3/19, 10/36	0.089	0.902	28.3		3/17, 10/37	0.089	0.903	26.0	
0.25	0.40	20/64	0.099	0.905	9/39, 20/64	0.099	0.900	52.1		7/29, 22/72	0.099	0.901	48.1	
	0.45	13/39	0.086	0.905	5/23, 13/39	0.086	0.901	31.5		3/14, 14/44	0.086	0.901	28.4	
0.30	0.45	26/71	0.091	0.904	16/50, 25/69	0.091	0.902	56.0		9/30, 29/82	0.091	0.901	51.4	
	0.50	15/39	0.094	0.900	7/28, 15/39	0.094	0.900	35.0		7/22, 17/46	0.094	0.905	29.9	
0.35	0.50	30/72	0.096	0.903	14/43, 30/72	0.096	0.900	59.3		12/34, 33/81	0.096	0.902	53.2	
	0.55	19/44	0.099	0.922	15/36, 18/42	0.099	0.903	36.9		7/20, 20/47	0.099	0.905	30.8	
0.40	0.55	35/75	0.098	0.909	18/45, 34/73	0.098	0.900	57.2		16/38, 40/88	0.098	0.900	54.5	
	0.60	20/41	0.097	0.903	11/28, 20/41	0.097	0.901	33.8		7/18, 22/46	0.097	0.900	30.2	
0.45	0.60	39/75	0.091	0.902	34/67, 38/74	0.091	0.902	68.0		14/32, 40/78	0.091	0.901	54.2	
	0.65	24/44	0.078	0.901	9/21, 22/41	0.078	0.900	30.8		9/20, 24/45	0.078	0.900	30.2	
0.50	0.65	41/72	0.097	0.904	19/40, 41/72	0.097	0.900	58.0		18/35, 47/84	0.097	0.900	53.0	
	0.70	23/39	0.100	0.906	11/23, 23/39	0.100	0.902	31.0		11/21, 26/45	0.100	0.902	29.0	
0.55	0.70	44/71	0.096	0.909	35/58, 43/70	0.096	0.901	60.1		19/34, 46/75	0.096	0.900	50.1	
	0.75	25/39	0.095	0.914	20/32, 24/38	0.095	0.902	32.9		10/18, 26/41	0.095	0.901	27.0	
0.60	0.75	43/64	0.095	0.901	25/43, 43/64	0.095	0.900	54.4		21/34, 47/71	0.095	0.904	47.1	
	0.80	25/36	0.090	0.911	18/27, 24/35	0.090	0.900	28.5		6/11, 26/38	0.090	0.904	25.4	
0.65	0.80	44/61	0.095	0.912	22/33, 43/60	0.095	0.901	42.6		20/30, 45/63	0.095	0.900	41.8	
	0.85	24/32	0.082	0.904	8/13, 23/31	0.082	0.904	22.0		10/15, 25/34	0.082	0.904	21.7	
0.70	0.85	41/53	0.091	0.909	15/22, 40/52	0.091	0.903	36.8		14/20, 45/59	0.091	0.901	36.2	
	0.90	20/25	0.090	0.902	11/16, 20/25	0.090	0.902	20.0		6/9, 22/28	0.090	0.910	17.8	
0.75	0.90	33/40	0.096	0.900	20/27, 33/40	0.096	0.900	33.1		12/16, 39/48	0.096	0.904	29.0	
	0.95	17/20	0.091	0.925	6/8, 16/19	0.091	0.904	12.0		5/7, 17/20	0.091	0.904	12.8	
0.80	0.95	28/32	0.093	0.926	5/7, 27/31	0.093	0.905	20.8		7/9, 32/37	0.093	0.907	21.2	
0.85	0.95	54/60	0.097	0.921	40/45, 52/58	0.097	0.906	47.3		25/29, 53/59	0.097	0.901	39.5	

2.2 Two-Stage Designs

For ethical reasons, most clinical trials are required to have sequential designs. Yet, for practical reasons, they are usually conducted as multistage experiments instead of being fully sequential. Two-stage designs are commonly used for phase II cancer clinical trials because of simplicity and diminishing returns beyond two stages. In this section, we discuss various two-stage phase II trial design methods.

2.2.1 Gehan's Design

Gehan (1961) proposes a two-stage phase II trial design method. Let p denote the true response rate of the experimental therapy of a phase II trial. At the first stage, n_1 patients are treated with an experimental therapy to test hypotheses $H_0 : p \leq p_0$ vs. $H_1 : p > p_0$ for a specified value p_0. Let X_1 denote the number of responders among the n_1 patients. Given α, such as 0.05 or 0.1, n_1 is chosen as the largest integer satisfying that the probability of observing no responders among n_1 treated patients is no larger than α when $p = p_0$, that is, $P(X > 0|p_0) \leq \alpha$. For example, with $p_0 = 0.2$, we have $n_1 = 14$ if $\alpha = 0.05$ and $n_1 = 11$ if $\alpha = 0.1$.

If no responders are observed among the n_1 patients, then the study is stopped after the first stage, concluding H_0. Otherwise, the study proceeds to the second stage to treat an additional n_2 patients. The stage 2 sample size n_2 is chosen so that the asymptotic standard error for the estimated response rate from $n = (n_1 + n_2)$ patients, $\text{SE} = \sqrt{p(1-p)/n}$, is smaller than a prespecified value. Noting that SE depends on the unknown true response rate p, Gehan proposed using the upper 75% confidence limit of p from stage 1 as an estimate of p in calculating SE. This estimate of p would provide a conservative estimation of SE when the existing cancer drugs had low response rates in the early years of cancer treatment. Using $p = 0.5$ will result in a most conservative estimation of SE and n_2.

2.2.2 Simon's Optimal Design

We consider a two-stage trial that is conducted as follows. During stage 1, n_1 patients are enrolled and treated. If the number of responders X_1 is less than or equal to a_1, the trial is terminated for lack of efficacy, and it is concluded that the treatment does not warrant further investigation. Otherwise, the study is continued to stage 2, during which an additional n_2 patients are enrolled and treated. Let X_2 denote the number of responders from stage 2. If the cumulative number of responders after stage 2, $X = X_1 + X_2$, does not exceed a, it is concluded that the treatment lacks sufficient efficacy. Otherwise, it is concluded that the treatment has sufficient activity, and the treatment will be considered for further investigation in subsequent trials.

A two-stage design is defined by the number of patients to be accrued during stages 1 and 2, n_1 and n_2, and the rejection values a_1 and a $(a_1 < a)$, so we denote any two-stage design by $(a_1/n_1, a/n)$, where $n = n_1 + n_2$ called the *maximum sample size*. The values of $(a_1/n_1, a/n)$ are determined based on some prespecified design parameters $(p_0, p_1, \alpha^*, 1 - \beta^*)$ as in the single-stage design cases described in the previous section.

Noting that, for $k = 1, 2$, X_k are independent $B(n_k, p)$ random variables, the probability of rejecting the treatment (or equivalently failing to reject $H_0 : p \le p_0$) for a two-stage design is expressed as

$$R(p) = P(X_1 \le a_1 \text{ or } X \le a|p)$$
$$= B(a_1|n_1, p) + \sum_{x_1=a_1+1}^{\min(n_1,a)} b(x_1|n_1, p)B(a - x_1|n_2, p)$$

when the true response rate is p. Note that the probability of early termination after stage 1 is given as $\text{PET}(p) \equiv B(a_1|n_1, p)$. The constraints on type I error probability and power are expressed as $R(p_0) \ge 1 - \alpha^*$ and $R(p_1) \le \beta^*$. Given $(p_0, p_1, \alpha^*, 1 - \beta^*)$, there are many two-stage designs $(a_1/n_1, a/n)$ satisfying the constraints.

Simon (1989) proposes two criteria to select a good two-stage design among these designs. The *minimax design* minimizes the maximum sample size, n, among the designs satisfying the $(\alpha^*, 1 - \beta^*)$-constraint. On the other hand, the so-called *optimal design* minimizes the expected sample size EN under the null hypothesis determined by

$$\text{EN} = \text{PET}(p_0) \times n_1 + \{1 - \text{PET}(p_0)\} \times n.$$

Tables 2.1–2.4 present Simon's minimax and optimal two-stage designs under various design settings of $(p_0, p_1, \alpha^*, 1 - \beta^*)$. Note that under each design setting the maximum sample size for the two-stage minimax design is slightly smaller than or equal to the sample size of the single-stage design. Furthermore, if the maximum sample size for the two-stage minimax design equals the sample size of the single-stage design, then the rejection value of the second stage for the two-stage design is the same as the rejection value of the corresponding single-stage design.

2.2.3   Admissible Designs

Simon's minimax and optimal designs have both been widely used, and other designs have largely been ignored in the past for such two-stage phase II cancer clinical trials. However, Simon's designs may result in highly divergent sample size requirements, as shown in the example below. For example, the minimax design may have an excessively large EN as compared to the optimal design, or the optimal design may have an excessively large maximum sample size n as compared to the minimax design. This results from the discrete nature of the binomial distribution.

Example 2.2

For the design parameters $(p_0, p_1, \alpha^*, 1 - \beta^*) = (0.1, 0.3, 0.05, 0.85)$, the minimax design is given by $(a_1/n_1, a/n) = (2/18, 5/27)$ and the optimal design by $(1/11, 6/35)$ from Table 2.2. The maximum sample size n for the minimax design is eight less than that for the optimal design. However, under H_0 the expected sample size $EN = 18.3$ for the optimal design is only slightly smaller than $EN = 20.4$ for the minimax design.

Simon's designs are to some extent mathematical niceties. Also, as indicated above, the minimax and optimal designs can be quite different. Often, practical compromises are possible without changing the statistical operating characteristics appreciably. To avoid these discrepancies in the maximum sample size and the expected sample size under the null hypothesis between the minimax and the optimal designs, Jung, Carey, and Kim (2001) proposed a heuristic graphical method to search for compromise designs, neither minimax nor optimal, but with more desirable and practically appealing features.

Example 2.3 (Example 2.2 revisited)

For the same design parameters $(p_0, p_1, \alpha^*, 1 - \beta^*) = (0.1, 0.3, 0.05, 0.85)$, the design given by $(a_1/n_1, a/n) = (1/13, 5/28)$ requires only one more patient in the maximum sample size n than the minimax design, but its expected sample size EN under H_0 is very comparable to that of the optimal design (18.7 vs. 18.3). Jung, Carey, and Kim (2001) recommend this design as a good compromise between the minimax design and the optimal design.

For a given maximum sample size n, the designs satisfying the $(\alpha^*, 1 - \beta^*)$-constraint can be determined by an exhaustive enumeration. This can be achieved readily by changing $n_1 (= 1, \ldots, n - 1)$, a_1, and a ($0 \le a_1 \le a \wedge n_1$; $a_1 \le a \le a_1 + n - n_1$). From these designs, the one that minimizes EN is determined. This design dominates (in terms of n and EN) all other designs for the given n. So, our search procedure for a good design will go through only these dominating designs within a range of n values. We will call them candidate designs. If n is too small, there may exist no designs satisfying the $(\alpha^*, 1 - \beta^*)$-constraint, and as a result no candidate design either. This process is repeated by increasing n by 1 each time until an arbitrary upper limit, say N, is reached. Typically, N may represent the number of available subjects that can be accrued in a reasonable time period.

A program is developed to plot EN of the candidate designs against n given the design parameters $(p_0, p_1, \alpha^*, 1 - \beta^*)$ and N. The plot starts with Simon's minimax design and ends with $n = N$. From the plot, the design minimizing EN within the range can be easily identified and is marked as "optimal." When N is large enough, this local optimal design is Simon's optimal design. This program, available from the author upon request, is written in Java and is thus platform-independent.

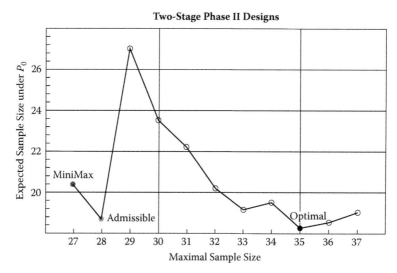

Figure 2.1 Two-stage designs for $(p_0, p_1, \alpha^*, 1 - \beta^*) = (0.1, 0.3, 0.05, 0.85)$ with $N = 37$.

Figure 2.1 shows the plot of EN against n for $(p_0, p_1, \alpha^*, 1 - \beta^*) = (0.1, 0.3, 0.05, 0.85)$ and $N = 37$ discussed in Example 2.2. Simon's minimax design is given by $(a_1/n_1, a/n) = (2/18, 5/27)$ and optimal design by $(1/11, 6/35)$, which is also Simon's optimal design. The program provides the specification of a design $(a_1/n_1, a/n)$ along with EN, PET(p_0), PET(p_1), and the exact type I error rate and power when the circle representing the candidate design, actually (n, EN), is clicked with a pointer. Table 2.5 summarizes the operating characteristics of various designs.

2.2.3.1   A Class of Admissible Designs

In this section, we will use formal statistical criteria to define a class of admissible designs according to which compromise designs between the minimax and the optimal designs as proposed by Jung, Carey, and Kim (2001) can be justified. In order to identify appropriate designs, we need to specify $(p_0, p_1, \alpha^*, 1 - \beta^*)$ and N.

Given $(p_0, p_1, \alpha^*, 1 - \beta^*)$ and N, let $\mathcal{D}$ denote the space of all candidate designs with $n \leq N$ satisfying the $(\alpha^*, 1 - \beta^*)$ constraint. We consider two outcomes, $\omega_1 = n$ and $\omega_2 = \text{EN}$, from each design $d \in \mathcal{D}$. We use notations $n(d)$ and EN(d), in place of n and EN, to relate each design to its outcomes. Define a loss function

$$L(\omega, d) = n(d)I(\omega = \omega_1) + \text{EN}(d)I(\omega = \omega_2)$$

in $\Omega \times \mathcal{D}$, where $\Omega = \{\omega_1, \omega_2\}$ and $I(\cdot)$ is an indicator function. This loss function is justified on the ethical grounds that it is desirable to minimize both the maximum number and the expected number of patients under the null hypothesis in two-stage phase II cancer clinical trials.

Let Q be a probability distribution defined over Ω as $Q(\omega = \omega_1) = q$ and $Q(\omega = \omega_2) = 1 - q$ for $q \in [0, 1]$. For any design $d \in \mathcal{D}$, the expected loss, or risk, is defined as

$$\rho(Q, d) = \int_{\Omega} L(\omega, d) dQ(\omega) = q \times n(d) + (1 - q) \times \text{EN}(d).$$

By considering only the designs with $n \leq N$ with N prespecified, $\rho(Q, d)$ is finite for every $d \in \mathcal{D}$. For a probability distribution Q, the Bayes risk is defined as

$$\rho^*(Q) = \inf_{d \in \mathcal{D}} \rho(Q, d).$$

Any design $d^* \in \mathcal{D}$ whose risk equals the Bayes risk is called a Bayes design against the distribution Q under the specified loss function. Note that the minimax design is a Bayes design against Q with $q = 1$ and Simon's optimal design is a Bayes design against Q with $q = 0$. Since Q is uniquely defined by a constant $q \in [0, 1]$, we may use q and Q interchangeably.

A design d^* is admissible if it is a Bayes design against a distribution Q. Equivalently, a design $d \in \mathcal{D}$ is inadmissible if it is not a Bayes design for any choice of $q \in [0, 1]$, that is, there exists $d_q \in \mathcal{D}$ such that, for some $q \in [0, 1]$,

$$\rho(q, d) > \rho(q, d_q).$$

For $d_1, d_2 \in \mathcal{D}$, it is said that d_1 dominates d_2 if $n(d_1) \leq n(d_2)$ and $\text{EN}(d_1) < \text{EN}(d_2)$, or $n(d_1) < n(d_2)$ and $\text{EN}(d_1) \leq \text{EN}(d_2)$. In this case, d_2 cannot be an admissible design.

This approach can be easily modified to handle any number of stages and different loss functions. Unlike Bayesian multistage designs or designs based on predictive probabilities which have to assign a prior probability to the probability of success, this method assumes that the probability of success is fixed. Instead, we combine some existing optimality criteria, that is, assign prior probabilities to the criteria, and identify admissible designs under the criteria defined by various combinations of the existing criteria.

2.2.3.2 Search for Admissible Designs

Suppose that we want to find a Bayes design against the distribution with a specified q in $[0, 1]$ according to the derivation given in the previous section. There are two ways to identify admissible designs.

The first approach is to consider a straight line $q \times n + (1 - q) \times \text{EN} = \rho$ determined by ρ on the (n, EN)-plane, that is, a line with slope $-q/(1-q)$ and intercept $\rho/(1-q)$. Starting from a small ρ, we move the straight line upward until it touches a design. The first design touched by the line is a Bayes design with Bayes risk ρ^*, where $\rho^*/(1-q)$ is the intercept of the straight line when it touches the Bayes design.

Suppose that we choose $q = 1/2$ for Example 2.2. Then, from Figure 2.1, design $(a_1/n_1, a/n) = (1/13, 5/28)$ is a unique Bayes design. Noting that $n = 28$ and EN $= 18.7$ for this design, we obtain Bayes risk $\rho^* = q \times n(d) + (1-q) \times \text{EN}(d) = 23.3$. Again, Table 2.5 shows the two-stage designs discussed above, that is, Simon's minimax and optimal designs and a compromise design by Jung, Carey, and Kim (2001) for the design parameters $(p_0, p_1, \alpha^*, 1 - \beta^*) = (0.1, 0.3, 0.05, 0.85)$ in Example 2.3. It also summarizes their operating characteristics such as the expected sample size EN under the null hypothesis, exact type I error probability and power, the probability of early termination both under the null and alternative hypotheses, and the distribution Q specified by q against which the design is admissible.

In designing a phase II study, $q \in [0, 1]$ may be chosen depending on the relative importance of n and EN. For example, if the study is on a rare disease so that the accrual is very low, then we may choose a larger q to favor the minimax design. On the other hand, if the accrual is not a problem but we want to stop the study as early as possible when the treatment is inactive, then we may choose a small q to favor the optimal design. Whichever is the case, given $(p_0, p_1, \alpha^*, 1 - \beta^*)$ and N, a design may be regarded as a good one if it is a Bayes design over a wide range of q in $[0, 1]$. In Figure 2.1, the compromise design $(a_1/n_1, a/n) = (1/13, 5/28)$, which is admissible, can be identified by any straight line with slope $-q/(1-q)$ between -1.72 and -0.06, that is, for $q \in [0.057, 0.632]$. Similarly we can show that Simon's minimax and optimal designs are Bayes designs for $q \in [0.632, 1]$ and $q \in [0, 0.057]$, respectively.

The second approach is to consider a convex hull formed by connecting candidate designs between Simon's minimax design and the optimal design. According to DeGroot (1970, pp. 125–127), any designs on the convex hull are admissible. This procedure is implemented in our Java program so that other admissible designs besides Simon's minimax and optimal designs can be automatically identified.

Table 2.5   Two-stage admissible designs for $(p_0, p_1, \alpha^*, 1 - \beta^*) = (0.1, 0.3, 0.05, 0.85)$

$(r_1/n_1, r/n)$	**EN**	α	$1 - \beta$	**PET**(p_0)	**PET**(p_1)	q
$(2/18, 5/27)$	20.4	0.0444	0.851	0.734	0.060	$[0.632, 1]$
$(1/13, 5/28)$	18.7	0.0498	0.858	0.621	0.063	$[0.057, 0.632]$
$(1/11, 6/35)$	18.3	0.0422	0.851	0.697	0.113	$[0, 0.057]$

Note: The first and the third designs are Simon's minimal and optimal designs, respectively.

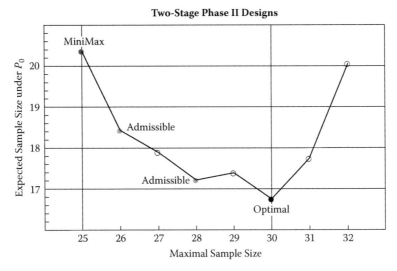

Figure 2.2 Two-stage designs for $(p_0, p_1, \alpha^*, 1-\beta^*) = (0.05, 0.25, 0.05, 0.9)$ with $N = 32$.

In Figure 2.1, the design given by $(a_1/n_1, a/n) = (1/13, 5/28)$ is the only admissible design except for the minimax and the optimal designs. Figure 2.2 shows candidate two-stage designs for $(p_0, p_1, \alpha^*, 1 - \beta^*) = (0.05, 0.25, 0.05, 0.9)$ with $N = 32$. Admissible designs are highlighted at $n = 25$ (minimax design), 26, 28, and 30 (Simon's optimal design). The designs with $n = 26$ and 28 are admissible for $q \in [0.377, 0.660]$ and $q \in [0.187, 0.377]$, respectively. Table 2.6 summarizes admissible two-stage designs identified in Figure 2.2 along with their operating characteristics.

Table 2.6 Two-stage admissible designs for $(p_0, p_1, \alpha, 1 - \beta^*) = (0.05, 0.25, 0.05, 0.9)$

$(r_1/n_1, r/n)$	EN	α	$1 - \beta$	PET(p_0)	PET(p_1)	q
$(0/15, 3/25)$	20.4	0.0336	0.901	0.463	0.013	$[0.660, 1]$
$(0/12, 3/26)$	18.4	0.0365	0.905	0.540	0.032	$[0.377, 0.660]$
$(0/10, 3/28)$	17.2	0.0426	0.906	0.599	0.056	$[0.187, 0.372]$
$(0/9, 3/30)$	16.8	0.0489	0.902	0.630	0.075	$[0, 0.187]$

Note: The first and the last designs are Simon's minimal and optimal designs, respectively.

2.3 Two-Stage Designs with Both Upper and Lower Stopping Values

When the experimental therapy of a phase II trial seems to be efficacious at an interim analysis, there usually is no ethical rule to continue the trial and collect more data to be used to design a future phase III trial. So, most two-stage phase II cancer clinical trials use a lower (or futility) stopping value only as in the previous sections. Sometimes, however, one may want to consider stopping early when the experimental therapy is efficacious too.

A two-stage phase II trial with design $\{(a_1, b_1)/n_1, a/n\}$ proceeds as follows.

Stage 1: Treat n_1 patients, and observe the number of responders X_1.

(a) IF $X_1 \le a_1$, reject the experimental therapy and stop the trial.
(b) IF $X_1 \ge b_1$, accept the experimental therapy and stop the trial.
(c) IF $a_1 < X_1 < b_1$, continue to stage 2.

Stage 2: Treat n_2 patients, and observe the number of responders X_2.

(a) IF $X_1 + X_2 \le a$, reject the experimental therapy.
(b) IF $X_1 > a$, accept the experimental therapy.

For a two-stage design $\{(a_1, b_1)/n_1, a/n\}$, the probability of rejecting the therapy is given as

$$R(p) = B(a_1|n_1, p) + \sum_{x=a_1+1}^{b_1-1} b(x|n_1, p)B(a - x|n_2, p).$$

The constraint on type I error probability and power is expressed as $R(p_0) \ge 1 - \alpha^*$ and $R(p_1) \le \beta^*$.

Given (p_0, p_1), there are many designs satisfying a type I error rate and power constraint $(\alpha^*, 1 - \beta^*)$. Among them, the minimax design minimizes the maximum number of patients $n = n_1 + n_2$. For a response probability p, the expected sample size is given as

$$\text{EN}(p) = \text{PET}(p) \times n_1 + \{1 - \text{PET}(p)\} \times n,$$

where $\text{PET}(p) = B(a_1|n_1, p) + 1 - B(b_1|n_1, p)$ is the probability of early termination after stage 1. Then the optimal design minimizes the average of the expected sample sizes for $p = p_0$ and $p = p_1$ which is given as

$$\text{EN} = \{\text{EN}(p_0) + \text{EN}(p_1)\}/2$$

among the designs satisfying $(\alpha^*, 1 - \beta^*)$.

Tables 2.7–2.10 list minimax and optimal two-stage designs with both upper and lower stopping values under various design settings of $(\alpha^*, 1 - \beta^*, p_0, p_1)$. Here, $\text{EN}_0 = \text{EN}(p_0)$ and $\text{EN}_1 = \text{EN}(p_1)$.

Table 2.7 Two-stage designs with both upper and lower stopping values $(\alpha^*, 1 - \beta^*) = (0.05, 0.8)$

		Minimax Design							Optimal Design						
p_0	p_1	$(a_1, b_1)/n_1, a/n$	α	$1-\beta$	EN_0	EN_1	EN	$(a_1, b_1)/n_1, a/n$	α	$1-\beta$	EN_0	EN_1	EN
0.05	0.15	(1, 5)/32, 5/51	0.046	0.801	40.7	40.1	40.4	(1, 4)/25, 6/60	0.050	0.800	36.3	38.2	37.3
	0.20	(0, 3)/12, 3/27	0.049	0.802	18.6	19.3	19.0	(0, 3)/11, 3/28	0.050	0.806	18.1	20.0	19.1
	0.25	(0, 3)/12, 2/16	0.043	0.801	13.8	13.4	13.6	(0, 3)/9, 2/17	0.047	0.812	11.9	13.2	12.5
0.10	0.25	(4, 7)/33, 7/38	0.048	0.803	33.9	33.9	33.9	(2, 5)/18, 8/47	0.050	0.801	24.9	29.1	27.0
	0.30	(0, 4)/13, 5/24	0.049	0.800	20.8	17.5	19.2	(1, 4)/11, 5/27	0.048	0.812	15.5	18.3	16.9
0.15	0.30	(4, 9)/29, 11/47	0.049	0.801	36.6	36.9	36.8	(4, 8)/24, 12/53	0.049	0.805	31.7	37.2	34.4
	0.35	(3, 7)/18, 7/28	0.048	0.805	20.7	22.7	21.7	(2, 5)/13, 9/35	0.050	0.801	19.0	21.5	20.3
0.20	0.35	(9, 15)/39, 15/53	0.049	0.800	42.3	46.6	44.4	(7, 11)/30, 18/64	0.049	0.802	37.3	43.1	40.2
	0.40	(2, 7)/15, 10/32	0.049	0.800	24.9	24.9	24.9	(3, 7)/14, 11/37	0.047	0.802	20.7	27.1	23.9
0.25	0.40	(7, 16)/38, 20/59	0.050	0.800	53.8	49.3	51.6	(9, 13)/32, 27/79	0.050	0.801	42.6	48.3	45.4
	0.45	(4, 9)/17, 13/36	0.049	0.805	24.9	28.5	26.7	(5, 9)/18, 14/39	0.048	0.801	23.5	27.9	25.7
0.30	0.45	(13, 20)/43, 25/64	0.049	0.800	51.3	53.2	52.3	(10, 15)/30, 30/79	0.049	0.801	42.4	55.0	48.7
	0.50	(8, 14)/27, 15/36	0.049	0.800	30.7	31.3	31.0	(7, 11)/20, 17/42	0.050	0.802	24.6	30.0	27.3
0.35	0.50	(22, 29)/55, 29/66	0.050	0.801	56.9	60.7	58.8	(14, 19)/36, 34/78	0.049	0.801	45.6	54.7	50.1
	0.55	(7, 13)/19, 18/39	0.050	0.801	25.6	33.8	29.7	(8, 12)/20, 21/46	0.050	0.808	25.7	31.8	28.7
0.40	0.55	(16, 24)/41, 34/69	0.050	0.801	54.2	57.4	55.8	(13, 19)/31, 37/76	0.050	0.801	45.7	57.9	51.8
	0.60	(17, 20)/34, 20/39	0.050	0.804	34.3	35.1	34.7	(9, 13)/20, 24/47	0.049	0.807	26.0	32.3	29.2
0.45	0.60	(19, 26)/41, 38/70	0.050	0.802	51.3	57.1	54.2	(15, 21)/32, 41/76	0.049	0.802	46.6	57.7	52.2
	0.65	(16, 22)/30, 22/39	0.050	0.806	31.2	35.8	33.5	(10, 14)/20, 26/46	0.048	0.805	25.9	32.0	29.0
0.50	0.65	(39, 41)/66, 40/68	0.049	0.801	66.0	66.2	66.1	(19, 24)/35, 47/80	0.049	0.802	45.3	56.3	50.8
	0.70	(10, 16)/20, 23/37	0.050	0.802	26.9	32.1	29.5	(11, 15)/20, 26/42	0.049	0.801	25.1	30.3	27.7
0.55	0.70	(26, 34)/48, 42/65	0.050	0.800	56.0	55.9	56.0	(18, 23)/31, 50/78	0.049	0.806	44.1	54.8	49.5
	0.75	(15, 20)/24, 24/36	0.050	0.802	26.0	31.6	28.8	(8, 12)/14, 28/42	0.049	0.805	23.0	31.0	27.0
0.60	0.75	(22, 28)/35, 43/62	0.050	0.800	43.0	51.3	47.1	(19, 24)/30, 47/68	0.050	0.801	40.4	50.8	45.6
	0.80	(10, 15)/17, 24/33	0.049	0.802	24.0	27.4	25.7	(12, 15)/18, 32/44	0.047	0.801	22.6	27.5	25.0
0.65	0.80	(20, 27)/31, 41/55	0.050	0.802	41.8	48.7	45.3	(24, 28)/34, 46/62	0.050	0.801	38.9	45.4	42.1
	0.85	(19, 22)/25, 23/30	0.048	0.807	25.4	26.8	26.1	(10, 14)/14, 29/38	0.048	0.808	18.8	25.9	22.4
0.70	0.85	(22, 27)/30, 39/49	0.049	0.803	35.2	41.6	38.4	(19, 23)/26, 44/55	0.048	0.800	33.8	39.9	36.9
	0.90	(19, 21)/23, 21/26	0.046	0.801	23.1	23.6	23.4	(9, 12)/12, 23/28	0.048	0.815	15.8	21.7	18.8
0.75	0.90	(18, 23)/23, 33/39	0.050	0.801	27.5	36.4	32.0	(17, 20)/21, 41/49	0.050	0.804	25.8	34.5	30.2
	0.95	(14, 16)/16, 17/20	0.049	0.806	16.2	17.5	16.8	(10, 12)/12, 22/25	0.048	0.835	13.6	16.4	15.0
0.80	0.95	(16, 19)/19, 27/30	0.050	0.818	21.4	25.1	23.3	(13, 15)/15, 41/46	0.049	0.804	19.1	26.3	22.7
0.85	0.95	(35, 39)/39, 52/57	0.050	0.811	41.6	52.2	46.9	(24, 27)/27, 60/66	0.049	0.803	34.6	50.4	42.5

Table 2.8 Two-stage designs with both upper and lower stopping values $(\alpha^*, 1-\beta^*) = (0.05, 0.85)$

p_0	p_1	Minimax Design						Optimal Design					
		$(a_1, b_1)/n_1, a/n$	α	$1-\beta$	EN_0	EN_1	EN	$(a_1, b_1)/n_1, a/n$	α	$1-\beta$	EN_0	EN_1	EN
0.05	0.15	(3, 6)/52, 6/60	0.050	0.850	53.7	53.2	53.5	(2, 5)/33, 7/78	0.044	0.852	42.2	47.7	44.9
	0.20	(2, 4)/28, 4/31	0.050	0.850	28.3	28.3	28.3	(0, 3)/14, 4/35	0.047	0.854	24.1	22.5	23.3
	0.25	(1, 3)/16, 3/21	0.046	0.852	16.7	16.7	16.7	(1, 3)/13, 3/27	0.041	0.853	14.6	15.9	15.2
0.10	0.25	(6, 8)/41, 8/44	0.049	0.852	41.2	41.2	41.2	(2, 6)/23, 8/47	0.050	0.856	32.3	33.1	32.7
	0.30	(1, 5)/14, 5/27	0.047	0.851	19.3	21.0	20.1	(2, 5)/16, 6/33	0.041	0.855	19.3	22.0	20.6
0.15	0.30	(4, 11)/37, 12/53	0.050	0.850	47.4	43.7	45.6	(5, 9)/30, 14/62	0.050	0.852	38.4	41.4	39.9
	0.35	(1, 7)/20, 8/32	0.049	0.850	29.6	25.0	27.3	(3, 6)/17, 10/41	0.050	0.850	22.1	24.6	23.4
0.20	0.35	(8, 17)/48, 17/61	0.050	0.850	56.2	54.1	55.1	(9, 13)/37, 21/78	0.050	0.851	43.9	50.5	47.2
	0.40	(3, 9)/17, 11/37	0.049	0.851	26.0	32.1	29.0	(5, 9)/21, 12/41	0.048	0.851	25.3	29.6	27.4
0.25	0.40	(15, 21)/56, 23/69	0.050	0.850	59.8	59.6	59.7	(8, 13)/30, 28/86	0.050	0.852	47.1	57.1	52.1
	0.45	(13, 15)/39, 15/41	0.047	0.851	39.1	39.1	39.1	(6, 10)/21, 17/49	0.048	0.855	27.6	32.6	30.1
0.30	0.45	(24, 28)/69, 29/75	0.050	0.852	69.7	69.8	69.8	(14, 19)/42, 34/89	0.048	0.852	52.8	59.3	56.1
	0.50	(14, 18)/37, 17/42	0.050	0.851	37.5	38.4	37.9	(7, 11)/21, 21/52	0.050	0.850	28.8	33.6	31.2
0.35	0.50	(21, 28)/57, 34/78	0.050	0.850	63.5	64.7	64.1	(14, 20)/38, 38/88	0.050	0.853	53.9	62.6	58.2
	0.55	(19, 21)/42, 20/44	0.050	0.852	42.1	42.2	42.1	(8, 13)/22, 22/48	0.050	0.853	30.7	35.1	32.9
0.40	0.55	(22, 31)/57, 39/80	0.050	0.850	68.7	66.2	67.5	(18, 23)/41, 49/102	0.050	0.852	54.6	64.8	59.7
	0.60	(13, 19)/30, 23/45	0.048	0.851	34.2	37.8	36.0	(10, 14)/23, 30/58	0.049	0.852	31.8	35.7	33.8
0.45	0.60	(22, 31)/50, 43/80	0.049	0.850	64.6	66.1	65.4	(21, 26)/43, 53/99	0.050	0.851	55.6	63.6	59.6
	0.65	(20, 25)/37, 25/45	0.050	0.851	37.8	40.5	39.2	(13, 17)/26, 30/53	0.048	0.851	31.6	35.3	33.5
0.50	0.65	(43, 46)/74, 46/79	0.050	0.851	74.2	74.6	74.4	(20, 26)/38, 52/89	0.048	0.850	53.1	64.6	58.9
	0.70	(11, 17)/22, 27/44	0.049	0.854	31.0	36.3	33.6	(12, 16)/22, 33/54	0.049	0.856	29.5	35.3	32.4
0.55	0.70	(42, 46)/69, 48/75	0.050	0.850	69.6	70.0	69.8	(23, 28)/39, 59/93	0.048	0.852	51.5	61.9	56.7
	0.75	(25, 28)/38, 27/41	0.050	0.852	38.2	38.6	38.4	(13, 17)/22, 32/48	0.050	0.856	28.5	32.6	30.6
0.60	0.75	(22, 30)/38, 49/71	0.049	0.850	55.6	58.5	57.0	(21, 26)/33, 58/85	0.049	0.850	46.4	59.4	52.9
	0.80	(24, 27)/34, 27/38	0.049	0.852	34.2	35.0	34.6	(14, 17)/21, 38/53	0.050	0.854	26.2	30.8	28.5
0.65	0.80	(28, 34)/41, 48/65	0.050	0.854	47.4	54.0	50.7	(23, 27)/33, 61/83	0.049	0.851	43.1	52.6	47.9
	0.85	(15, 19)/21, 26/34	0.050	0.851	23.5	28.1	25.8	(13, 17)/19, 27/35	0.048	0.851	23.5	27.1	25.3
0.70	0.85	(25, 30)/34, 45/57	0.050	0.853	39.9	46.3	43.1	(23, 27)/31, 52/66	0.050	0.860	38.7	45.8	42.3
	0.90	(10, 14)/14, 23/28	0.049	0.852	18.9	24.2	21.5	(12, 15)/16, 28/34	0.047	0.867	20.0	23.5	21.7
0.75	0.90	(37, 39)/44, 39/47	0.047	0.851	44.1	44.4	44.2	(17, 21)/22, 42/50	0.050	0.859	30.6	38.8	34.7
	0.95	(15, 18)/18, 20/23	0.050	0.895	18.6	20.7	19.7	(10, 12)/12, 26/30	0.049	0.862	14.3	18.1	16.2
0.80	0.95	(21, 24)/24, 31/35	0.048	0.856	25.2	30.5	27.9	(15, 18)/18, 34/38	0.047	0.869	23.1	28.9	26.0
0.85	0.95	(48, 51)/53, 59/65	0.050	0.853	53.9	57.5	55.7	(31, 34)/35, 71/78	0.049	0.861	42.9	53.6	48.3

Table 2.9 Two-stage designs with both upper and lower stopping values $(\alpha^*, 1 - \beta^*) = (0.05, 0.9)$

		Minimax Design						Optimal Design					
p_0	p_1	$(a_1, b_1)/n_1, a/n$	α	$1-\beta$	EN_0	EN_1	EN	$(a_1, b_1)/n_1, a/n$	α	$1-\beta$	EN_0	EN_1	EN
0.05	0.15	(5, 7)/66, 7/73	0.049	0.901	66.5	66.4	66.4	(1, 5)/32, 7/78	0.049	0.901	53.1	51.7	52.4
	0.20	(1, 4)/24, 4/38	0.050	0.901	28.3	27.2	27.8	(0, 3)/14, 5/46	0.046	0.901	29.4	26.9	28.2
	0.25	(0, 3)/13, 3/25	0.045	0.903	18.5	16.7	17.6	(0, 3)/11, 3/26	0.042	0.901	17.2	17.2	17.2
0.10	0.25	(6, 9)/47, 9/53	0.049	0.901	47.9	47.6	47.7	(2, 6)/24, 10/60	0.049	0.902	38.7	37.8	38.2
	0.30	(1, 5)/16, 6/33	0.047	0.900	24.0	23.2	23.6	(2, 5)/17, 7/41	0.048	0.901	22.2	24.5	23.3
0.15	0.30	(5, 12)/38, 14/64	0.050	0.901	51.2	51.3	51.2	(5, 9)/31, 19/86	0.049	0.901	46.6	48.8	47.7
	0.35	(4, 9)/26, 9/38	0.049	0.901	30.1	30.6	30.4	(3, 7)/20, 10/42	0.049	0.900	27.3	28.2	27.7
0.20	0.35	(13, 19)/62, 21/76	0.048	0.900	66.5	64.6	65.6	(8, 13)/37, 24/89	0.049	0.901	52.1	57.1	54.6
	0.40	(4, 10)/25, 13/44	0.050	0.901	35.7	32.9	34.3	(5, 9)/23, 16/54	0.045	0.901	31.6	33.4	32.5
0.25	0.40	(15, 22)/57, 27/83	0.050	0.900	65.5	65.9	65.7	(13, 18)/46, 32/100	0.050	0.901	57.8	63.8	60.8
	0.45	(7, 13)/28, 17/49	0.048	0.901	36.2	37.7	36.9	(7, 11)/25, 21/61	0.050	0.904	33.8	36.5	35.2
0.30	0.45	(27, 34)/77, 33/88	0.050	0.901	78.4	80.8	79.6	(16, 22)/49, 37/99	0.050	0.900	62.2	68.3	65.2
	0.50	(9, 17)/34, 20/50	0.050	0.900	43.3	40.8	42.1	(10, 14)/29, 25/63	0.049	0.901	35.8	38.8	37.3
0.35	0.50	(33, 38)/84, 40/93	0.049	0.900	85.3	85.2	85.2	(18, 24)/48, 46/108	0.049	0.900	64.6	71.2	67.9
	0.55	(10, 17)/30, 24/53	0.049	0.901	41.0	41.1	41.1	(12, 16)/30, 30/67	0.049	0.901	37.0	40.5	38.8
0.40	0.55	(20, 31)/53, 45/94	0.050	0.900	76.3	79.0	77.7	(22, 28)/52, 53/110	0.050	0.900	68.4	71.3	69.9
	0.60	(16, 22)/36, 27/54	0.050	0.902	40.1	43.9	42.0	(11, 16)/26, 31/62	0.050	0.905	37.0	41.4	39.2
0.45	0.60	(49, 51)/93, 50/95	0.050	0.902	93.0	93.1	93.1	(23, 29)/48, 60/114	0.049	0.902	65.6	74.4	70.0
	0.65	(15, 21)/32, 30/54	0.049	0.901	39.3	41.3	40.3	(12, 17)/25, 34/62	0.049	0.902	35.7	42.5	39.1
0.50	0.65	(30, 39)/59, 54/93	0.050	0.900	72.2	75.8	74.0	(26, 32)/49, 63/109	0.049	0.902	64.7	72.8	68.7
	0.70	(17, 24)/34, 31/51	0.049	0.900	41.1	41.4	41.3	(11, 16)/22, 36/59	0.049	0.900	36.4	39.3	37.8
0.55	0.70	(50, 55)/81, 56/89	0.050	0.901	81.6	82.8	82.2	(29, 34)/49, 71/113	0.049	0.900	62.1	69.7	65.9
	0.75	(23, 28)/37, 32/49	0.050	0.902	38.7	41.7	40.2	(16, 21)/27, 34/52	0.048	0.900	33.3	38.9	36.1
0.60	0.75	(48, 54)/72, 57/84	0.050	0.900	73.1	76.4	74.8	(26, 31)/41, 72/106	0.050	0.901	57.1	66.1	61.6
	0.80	(14, 20)/24, 32/45	0.050	0.902	34.0	35.1	34.5	(14, 18)/22, 39/55	0.048	0.904	30.7	35.2	33.0
0.65	0.80	(30, 38)/46, 55/75	0.050	0.900	58.3	62.6	60.5	(28, 33)/41, 63/86	0.050	0.901	52.3	58.4	55.4
	0.85	(28, 30)/37, 30/40	0.050	0.902	37.1	37.3	37.2	(15, 18)/21, 43/57	0.049	0.901	27.0	32.0	29.5
0.70	0.85	(29, 36)/41, 51/65	0.050	0.900	50.5	54.9	52.7	(26, 30)/35, 64/82	0.050	0.902	44.7	52.0	48.4
	0.90	(20, 23)/26, 27/33	0.049	0.901	27.0	27.5	27.2	(12, 15)/16, 34/42	0.049	0.905	21.7	26.8	24.3
0.75	0.90	(27, 32)/34, 45/54	0.049	0.901	38.3	46.5	42.4	(21, 25)/27, 51/61	0.048	0.903	36.5	42.9	39.7
	0.95	(19, 21)/22, 22/26	0.049	0.902	22.2	22.8	22.5	(15, 17)/18, 28/32	0.049	0.916	19.3	20.4	19.8
0.80	0.95	(31, 33)/35, 35/40	0.050	0.901	35.2	35.8	35.5	(15, 18)/18, 39/44	0.049	0.904	24.6	32.2	28.4
0.85	0.95	(51, 55)/57, 68/75	0.049	0.903	59.2	65.7	62.4	(38, 41)/43, 90/99	0.049	0.910	52.7	59.9	56.3

Table 2.10 Two-stage designs with both upper and lower stopping values $(\alpha^*, 1-\beta^*) = (0.1, 0.9)$

		Minimax Design						Optimal Design					
p_0	p_1	$(a_1, b_1)/n_1, a/n$	α	$1-\beta$	EN_0	EN_1	EN	$(a_1, b_1)/n_1, a/n$	α	$1-\beta$	EN_0	EN_1	EN
0.05	0.15	(2, 5)/46, 5/58	0.097	0.902	49.9	47.6	48.8	(1, 4)/29, 6/71	0.087	0.900	44.7	41.3	43.0
	0.20	(0, 3)/18, 3/31	0.090	0.901	25.1	21.3	23.2	(0, 3)/16, 3/32	0.087	0.903	24.3	21.2	22.7
	0.25	(0, 3)/13, 2/20	0.074	0.903	16.2	15.2	15.7	(0, 2)/10, 3/26	0.100	0.907	15.0	13.0	14.0
0.10	0.25	(1, 6)/22, 6/40	0.100	0.901	33.6	31.0	32.3	(2, 5)/23, 8/50	0.098	0.901	32.0	29.3	30.7
	0.30	(0, 4)/11, 4/25	0.099	0.903	20.3	18.7	19.5	(0, 3)/9, 5/30	0.099	0.906	20.8	17.9	19.3
0.15	0.30	(3, 8)/28, 11/52	0.099	0.900	41.8	36.4	39.1	(4, 8)/27, 12/59	0.098	0.903	37.9	38.3	38.1
	0.35	(2, 6)/19, 7/31	0.099	0.905	25.1	22.4	23.7	(2, 5)/15, 9/40	0.096	0.904	23.4	22.3	22.8
0.20	0.35	(6, 13)/33, 15/58	0.100	0.901	45.3	48.3	46.8	(7, 11)/34, 18/68	0.098	0.900	44.4	42.8	43.6
	0.40	(5, 9)/27, 10/35	0.099	0.903	30.1	28.3	29.2	(4, 7)/19, 13/47	0.100	0.906	26.3	25.7	26.0
0.25	0.40	(10, 17)/42, 20/64	0.100	0.902	52.3	51.8	52.1	(8, 13)/33, 23/73	0.098	0.901	48.9	47.5	48.2
	0.45	(8, 12)/32, 13/38	0.098	0.900	34.0	32.8	33.4	(4, 8)/17, 15/46	0.097	0.905	28.2	29.0	28.6
0.30	0.45	(17, 23)/52, 25/69	0.100	0.901	56.4	58.0	57.2	(10, 15)/33, 30/83	0.100	0.901	50.8	52.6	51.7
	0.50	(7, 13)/26, 15/39	0.097	0.901	32.7	31.3	32.0	(6, 10)/20, 18/47	0.097	0.901	29.3	29.6	29.4
0.35	0.50	(12, 20)/38, 30/72	0.099	0.901	57.8	56.6	57.2	(12, 17)/34, 37/89	0.098	0.900	53.6	54.4	54.0
	0.55	(8, 14)/26, 18/41	0.098	0.902	34.3	31.4	32.9	(6, 10)/18, 23/52	0.096	0.900	31.3	30.5	30.9
0.40	0.55	(18, 27)/45, 34/73	0.100	0.900	57.1	63.7	60.4	(15, 21)/38, 37/79	0.100	0.900	55.0	54.7	54.8
	0.60	(8, 14)/22, 20/41	0.100	0.900	32.0	32.0	32.0	(9, 13)/22, 24/49	0.098	0.902	30.7	30.7	30.7
0.45	0.60	(18, 27)/45, 38/73	0.100	0.900	63.7	57.1	60.4	(17, 23)/38, 41/79	0.100	0.900	54.7	55.0	54.8
	0.65	(12, 18)/26, 22/41	0.098	0.902	31.4	34.3	32.9	(8, 12)/18, 28/52	0.100	0.904	30.5	31.3	30.9
0.50	0.65	(18, 26)/38, 41/72	0.099	0.901	56.6	57.8	57.2	(17, 22)/34, 51/89	0.100	0.902	54.4	53.6	54.0
	0.70	(13, 19)/26, 23/39	0.099	0.903	31.3	32.7	32.0	(10, 14)/20, 28/47	0.099	0.903	29.6	29.3	29.4
0.55	0.70	(29, 35)/52, 43/69	0.099	0.900	58.0	56.4	57.2	(18, 23)/33, 52/83	0.099	0.900	52.6	50.8	51.7
	0.75	(20, 24)/32, 24/38	0.100	0.902	32.8	34.0	33.4	(9, 13)/17, 30/46	0.095	0.903	29.0	28.2	28.6
0.60	0.75	(25, 32)/42, 43/64	0.098	0.900	51.8	52.3	52.1	(20, 25)/33, 49/73	0.099	0.902	47.5	48.9	48.2
	0.80	(18, 22)/27, 24/35	0.097	0.901	28.3	30.1	29.2	(12, 15)/19, 33/47	0.094	0.900	25.7	26.3	26.0
0.65	0.80	(20, 27)/33, 42/58	0.099	0.900	48.3	45.3	46.8	(23, 27)/34, 49/68	0.100	0.902	42.8	44.4	43.6
	0.85	(13, 17)/19, 23/31	0.095	0.901	22.4	25.1	23.7	(10, 13)/15, 30/40	0.096	0.904	22.3	23.4	22.8
0.70	0.85	(20, 25)/28, 40/52	0.100	0.901	36.4	41.8	39.1	(19, 23)/27, 46/59	0.097	0.902	38.3	37.9	38.1
	0.90	(7, 11)/11, 20/25	0.097	0.901	18.7	20.3	19.5	(6, 9)/9, 24/30	0.094	0.901	17.9	20.8	19.3
0.75	0.90	(16, 21)/22, 33/40	0.099	0.900	31.0	33.6	32.3	(18, 21)/23, 41/50	0.099	0.902	29.3	32.0	30.7
	0.95	(10, 13)/13, 17/20	0.097	0.926	15.2	16.2	15.7	(8, 10)/10, 22/26	0.093	0.900	13.0	15.0	14.0
0.80	0.95	(15, 18)/18, 27/31	0.099	0.910	21.3	25.1	23.2	(13, 16)/16, 28/32	0.097	0.913	21.2	24.3	22.7
0.85	0.95	(41, 44)/46, 52/58	0.098	0.903	47.6	49.9	48.8	(25, 28)/29, 64/71	0.100	0.912	41.3	44.7	43.0

Chang et al. (1987) and Therneau et al. (1990) use the same optimality criterion, but they search for optimal (a_1, b_1, b) with n or (n_1, n_2) fixed, while we search for optimal designs for all possible (n_1, n_2) values.

References

Chang, M.N., Therneau, T.M., Wieand, H.S., and Cha, S.S. (1987). Designs for group sequential phase II clinical trials. *Biometrics*, 43, 865–874.

DeGroot, M.H. (1970). *Optimal Statistical Decisions*. McGraw-Hill, New York.

Gehan, E.A. (1961). The determination of the number of patients required in a follow-up trial of a new chemotherapeutic agent. *Journal of Chronic Diseases*, 13, 346–353.

Jung, S.H., Carey, M., and Kim, K.M. (2001). Graphical search for two-stage designs for phase II clinical trials. *Controlled Clinical Trials*, 22, 367–372.

Simon, R. (1989). Optimal two-stage designs for phase II clinical trials. *Controlled Clinical Trials*, 10, 1–10.

Therneau, T.M., Wieand, H.S., and Chang, M. (1990). Optimal designs for a group sequential trial *Biometrics*, 46, 771–781.

Chapter 3

Inference on the Binomial Probability in Single-Arm Multistage Clinical Trials

Because of ethical and economical reasons, clinical trials are often designed as sequential experiments, as discussed in Chapter 2. A multistage sequential design can be described as follows: At each stage of the trial, a predetermined number of patients are treated. Then the accumulated number of treatment responses is compared to the stopping boundaries. If the accumulated number of responders is smaller than or equal to the lower boundary, the trial is terminated for lack of treatment efficacy. If the accumulated number of responders is larger than or equal to the upper boundary, the trial may be terminated for high treatment efficacy. Obviously, early termination for high efficacy in this setting is not as ethically imperative. Otherwise, an additional fixed number of patients will be treated at the next stage. This will continue until early termination or until the predetermined number of stages. Multistage designs have been described and investigated by Schultz, Nichol, Elfring, and Weed (1973), Herson (1979), Fleming (1982), and Chang, Therneau, Wieand, and Cha (1987), among others.

When a multistage trial is ended, we also want to estimate the true response probability p of the new therapy. The most commonly used estimator is the sample response rate, that is, the maximum likelihood estimator (MLE). However, in multistage designs, we observe only extreme cases by crossing either the lower or upper boundary, and hence the MLE is biased. This is known as the optional sampling effect. The bias of the MLE tends to be larger in studies with lower stopping boundaries only (as in most multistage phase II studies) than in studies with both upper and lower the stopping boundaries. Let M denote the stage at which a trial is terminated, and S denote the cumulative number of responders at stage M. We show that (M, S) is a complete and sufficient statistic for p for the aforementioned multistage designs. Hence, noting that the sample proportion after the first stage is an unbiased estimator, we can obtain the uniformly minimum variance unbiased estimator (UMVUE) by taking the conditional expectation of the first stage sample proportion given $(M, S) = (m, s)$ according to the Rao–Blackwell theorem, where m and s denote specific observations of random variables M and S, respectively.

In multistage designs involving continuous observations, Liu and Hall (1999) proved that the stopping stage and the cumulated sum of observations up to the stopping stage are sufficient but not complete for the unknown mean. Hence, in this case, the conditional expectation of the first stage sample mean given the sufficient statistics is only an efficient estimator, but not necessarily the UMVUE, contrary to Emerson and Fleming (1990). We will discuss a general result developed by Jung and Kim (2004) for multistage designs for phase II clinical trials in cancer drug screening. Specifically, we will derive the UMVUE for the binomial probability following multistage testing.

Jennison and Turnbull (1983) and Duffy and Santner (1987) propose confidence intervals for p based on (M, S). To construct a confidence interval, we need a stochastic ordering among all possible (m, s) values. We show that the ordering by the magnitude of the UMVUE is the same as that used by Jennison and Turnbull (1983).

In analyzing phase II trials, investigators usually report an estimate of p and its confidence interval, and whether the treatment is accepted or not. However, none of these exactly tell us how significant evidence is against $H_0 : p = p_0$ that we observe from the data. We obtain this information by calculating the p-value. Calculation of p-value for the testing associated with a multistage phase II trial requires a linear ordering of the outcomes in the two-dimensional sample space. Emerson and Fleming (1990) and Chang, Gould, and Snapinn (1995) study p-values of sequential testings using continuous observations. Usually, phase II trials have small sample sizes (about 50), so that these continuous variable approaches do not provide a good approximation for these trials with binary outcomes. In this chapter, we also investigate calculation of p-values based on exact binomial sequential distributions. We will consider the ordering by MLE and UMVUE. We also briefly investigate the performance of the p-value based on the likelihood ratio ordering by Emerson and Fleming (1990) as a normal approximation to binary data.

Lastly, we investigate application of the confidence interval and p-value methods to the cases when the realized sample size of a multistage phase II is different from that specified at the design stage.

3.1   Point Estimation

Let K be the number of stages, and n_k and X_k denote the number of patients accrued and the number of responders, respectively, during stage k, $1 \leq k \leq K$. And let $S_k = \sum_{i=1}^{k} X_i$ denote the cumulative number of responders by stage k. In designing a multistage phase II study to test hypotheses on response probability, we usually select lower and upper boundaries a_k and b_k $(a_k < b_k)$ to stop the study after stage k if $S_k \leq a_k$, concluding that the treatment under consideration is not very promising, or if $S_k \geq b_k$, concluding that it is very promising. We set $a_K = b_K - 1$ to make sure that the study terminates before or at stage K. To allow early termination only for lack of clinical efficacy, we choose any number larger than $n_1 + \cdots + n_k$ as b_k. This is justified as there is no compelling reason to terminate the trial early if the treatment appears to have the desired effect and only terminate early if the treatment lacks such an effect. There may be circumstances where the opposite is true.

Let M denote the stopping stage, and let $S = S_M$ denote the total number of responders accumulated up to the stopping stage. The MLE of p is given as $\tilde{p} = p(m, s) = s / \sum_{k=1}^{m} n_k$. As is derived in Appendix 3.A, the probability mass function of the random vector (M, S) is given by

$$f(m, s|p) = c_{m,s} \, p^s (1-p)^{n_1 + \cdots + n_m - s} \tag{3.1}$$

with support $\mathcal{S} = \cup_{m=1}^{K} \mathcal{S}_m$, where

$$\mathcal{S}_m = \{(m, s) : a_{m-1} + 1 \leq s \leq a_m \quad \text{or} \quad b_m \leq s \leq n_m + b_{m-1} - 1\}$$

and $a_0 = -1$ and $b_0 = 1$. Here $c_{1,s} = \binom{n_1}{s}$ and, for $m \geq 2$,

$$c_{m,s} = \sum_{x_1} \cdots \sum_{x_m} \binom{n_1}{x_1} \cdots \binom{n_m}{x_m}$$

with the summations over the set

$$\mathcal{R}(m, s) = \{(x_1, \ldots, x_m) : x_1 + \cdots + x_m = s,$$
$$a_k + 1 \leq x_1 + \cdots + x_k \leq b_k - 1 \text{ for } k = 1, \ldots, m-1\}.$$

Note that the dimension of $\mathcal{R}(m, s)$ is $m - 1$.

In Appendix 3.A, we also prove that (M, S) is a complete and sufficient statistic. Since $\tilde{p}_1 = X_1/n_1$ is an unbiased estimator of p, the UMVUE of p is obtained as $\hat{p} = \mathrm{E}\{\tilde{p}_1|(m, s)\}$ by the Rao–Blackwell theorem. For observation (m, s), the UMVUE is given by

$$\hat{p} = \frac{\sum \cdots \sum_{\mathcal{R}(m,s)} x_1 \binom{n_1}{x_1} \cdots \binom{n_m}{x_m}}{n_1 c_{m,s}} = \frac{\sum \cdots \sum_{\mathcal{R}(m,s)} \binom{n_1 - 1}{x_1 - 1} \binom{n_2}{x_2} \cdots \binom{n_m}{x_m}}{\sum \cdots \sum_{\mathcal{R}(m,s)} \binom{n_1}{x_1} \cdots \binom{n_m}{x_m}}, \tag{3.2}$$

where we define $\binom{n}{x} = 0$ if $x < 0$. See Appendix 3.B for the detailed derivation. Note that calculation of the UMVUE requires specification of the stopping boundaries for stages up to $m - 1$, that is, (a_k, b_k) for $1 \leq k \leq m - 1$, as well as the summary statistic value (m, s). At stage m, we may accrue slightly more (or possibly fewer) patients than n_m, especially in multicenter trials; see Green and Dahlberg (1992) and Herndon (1998). In this case, we do not have to delete the extra patients (or temporarily reopen the study to accrue more patients) for the UMVUE calculation. Since UMVUE does not require specification of the stopping boundaries at stage m, we can use all patients accrued in the estimation.

Girshick, Mosteller, and Savage (1946) and Lehmann (1983) prove that the number of successes X and the number of failures Y at the termination of a study are jointly complete and sufficient statistics for p and derive the UMVUE for a family of sequential binomial trials. Noting that the family includes the multistage phase II study design and (M, S) and (X, Y) are one-to-one, the two UMVUE's are identical.

It is easy but tedious to show that the ordering of the sample space for (M, S) by the magnitude of the UMVUE is the same as that by Jennison and Turnbull (1983). See also Armitage (1958) and Tsiatis, Rosner, and Mehta (1984). In other words, we have

$$
\begin{aligned}
\hat{p}(1, 0) &< \hat{p}(1, 1) < \cdots < \hat{p}(1, a_1) \\
&< \hat{p}(2, a_1 + 1) < \cdots < \hat{p}(2, a_2) \\
&\quad\vdots \\
&< \hat{p}(K, a_{K-1} + 1) < \cdots < \hat{p}(K, a_K) \\
&< \hat{p}(K, b_K) < \cdots < \hat{p}(K, b_{K-1} - 1 + n_K) \\
&< \hat{p}(K - 1, b_{K-1}) < \cdots < \hat{p}(K - 1, b_{K-2} - 1 + n_{K-1}) \\
&\quad\vdots \\
&< \hat{p}(1, b_1) < \cdots < \hat{p}(1, n_1)
\end{aligned}
\tag{3.3}
$$

where $\hat{p}(m, s)$ is the UMVUE for $(M, S) = (m, s)$. The stochastic ordering for the distribution of the UMVUE is proved in Appendix 3.C in the case of two-stage designs, as discussed in the next section.

3.1.1   Two-Stage Designs

Very often in cancer clinical trials, the number of stages is chosen to be 2. Let p_0 denote the maximum unacceptable probability of response and p_1 denote the minimum acceptable probability of response $(p_0 < p_1)$.

For two-stage designs, the UMVUE given in formula (3.2) simplifies to

$$
\hat{p} =
\begin{cases}
\dfrac{s}{n_1} & m = 1 \\[2ex]
\dfrac{\sum_{x_1 = (a_1 + 1) \vee (s - n_2)}^{s \wedge (b_1 - 1)} \binom{n_1 - 1}{x_1 - 1}\binom{n_2}{s - x_1}}{\sum_{x_1 = (a_1 + 1) \vee (s - n_2)}^{s \wedge (b_1 - 1)} \binom{n_1}{x_1}\binom{n_2}{s - x_1}} & m = 2
\end{cases},
\tag{3.4}
$$

where $a \wedge b = \min(a, b)$ and $a \vee b = \max(a, b)$. Note that $\hat{p} = \tilde{p}$ when $m = 1$. In a two-stage design with lower and upper boundaries a_1 and b_1 for stage 1, the MLE can be written specifically as

$$
\tilde{p} = \frac{X_1}{n_1} I(X_1 \leq a_1 \text{ or } X_1 \geq b_1) + \frac{X_1 + X_2}{n_1 + n_2} I(a_1 < X_1 < b_1) = \frac{s}{\sum_{k=1}^{m} n_k}.
$$

From formula (3.1), the probability mass function of (M, S) in a two-stage design with lower stopping boundaries only is given as

$$f(m, s|p) = \begin{cases} p^s(1-p)^{n_1-s} \binom{n_1}{s} & m = 1, \quad 0 \le s \le a_1 \\ p^s(1-p)^{n_1+n_2-s} \sum_{x_1=a_1+1}^{n_1 \wedge s} \binom{n_1}{x_1}\binom{n_2}{s-x_1} & m = 2, \quad a_1+1 \le s \cdot \\ & \hspace{3.5em} \le n_1 + n_2 \end{cases} \quad (3.5)$$

As an example, we consider $p_0 = 0.2$ as the maximum unacceptable probability of response and $p_1 = 0.4$ as the minimum acceptable probability of response. In this setting, we may consider a two-stage design with lower stopping boundaries only. In the first stage, we treat $n_1 = 13$ patients, of which if we observe $a_1 = 3$ or fewer responders, we conclude that the true response probability is at most p_0 and stop the trial, and otherwise go on to the second stage. In the second stage, we treat an additional $n_2 = 30$ patients. Out of the total of $n(= n_1 + n_2) = 43$ patients treated, if we observe $a(= a_2) = 12$ or fewer responders, we also conclude that the true response probability is at most p_0, and otherwise we conclude that the true response probability is at least p_1 and we consider further investigation of the therapy. From Table 2.1 in Chapter 2, this is Simon's optimal design for $(p_0, p_1, \alpha^*, 1 - \beta^*) = (0.2, 0.4, 0.05, 0.8)$.

Table 3.1 gives the UMVUE and the MLE for observations from a two-stage design with $n_1 = 13$ and $n_2 = 30$ and lower boundaries $a_1 = 3$ and $a_2 = 12$ as given above. This design is optimal according to Simon (1989) for $p_0 = 0.2$ and $p_1 = 0.4$ with $\alpha^* = 0.05$ and $\beta^* = 0.2$. When $m = 1$, two estimates are exactly the same as noted earlier. When $m = 2$, the MLE is much smaller than UMVUE for small s values. We also calculated the probability mass function $f(m, s|p)$ of (M, S) for the true response probabilities $p = 0.1 : 0.5(0.1)$ according to formula (3.5).

The probability mass functions for the UMVUE and for the MLE following termination of this two-stage design based on $f(m, s|p)$ are plotted in Figure 3.1. Note that for the observations for which the UMVUE and the MLE are very different, the probability mass function has very small values. The difference is largest at $(m, s) = (2, a_1 + 1)$, where $\tilde{p} = (a_1 + 1)/(n_1 + n_2)$ while $\hat{p} = (a_1 + 1)/n_1$ from formula (3.2). For $(2, s)$ with large s, the UMVUE and the MLE are very similar. Overall, the UMVUE and the MLE tend to be close to each other as $p \to 0.5$. Most significantly, the distributions of the UMVUE are stochastically increasing in p, whereas those for the MLE are not.

3.1.2 Numerical Studies

To understand the extent of the bias of the MLE following two-stage phase II clinical trials and the relative efficiency of the UMVUE as compared to the MLE defined as the ratio of the mean squared error (MSE) of the MLE to the variance of the UMVUE, we conducted numerical studies based on two-stage designs with lower stopping boundaries only as they are the most commonly used designs.

Table 3.1   UMVUE, MLE, and probability mass for true p at each observation in a two-stage design with $n_1 = 13$ and $n_2 = 30$ and lower boundaries $a_1 = 3$ and $a_2 = 12$ to test $H_0 : p_0 = 0.2$ versus $H_1 : p_1 = 0.4$ with $\alpha = 0.05$ and $\beta = 0.2$

				$f(m, s|p)$ for p				
m	s	UMVUE	MLE	0.1	0.2	0.3	0.4	0.5
1	0	0.000	0.000	0.254	0.055	0.010	0.001	0.000
1	1	0.077	0.077	0.367	0.179	0.054	0.011	0.002
1	2	0.154	0.154	0.245	0.268	0.139	0.045	0.010
1	3	0.231	0.231	0.100	0.246	0.218	0.111	0.035
2	4	0.308	0.093	0.001	0.000	0.000	0.000	0.000
2	5	0.312	0.116	0.004	0.002	0.000	0.000	0.000
2	6	0.317	0.140	0.007	0.006	0.001	0.000	0.000
2	7	0.322	0.163	0.008	0.015	0.002	0.000	0.000
2	8	0.328	0.186	0.006	0.027	0.006	0.000	0.000
2	9	0.335	0.209	0.004	0.038	0.015	0.001	0.000
2	10	0.343	0.233	0.002	0.043	0.030	0.003	0.000
2	11	0.351	0.256	0.001	0.041	0.049	0.008	0.000
2	12	0.360	0.279	0.000	0.033	0.068	0.018	0.001
2	13	0.371	0.302	0.000	0.023	0.081	0.033	0.003
2	14	0.382	0.326	0.000	0.014	0.084	0.054	0.006
2	15	0.395	0.349	0.000	0.007	0.076	0.076	0.013
2	16	0.409	0.372	0.000	0.003	0.062	0.096	0.025
2	17	0.424	0.395	0.000	0.001	0.044	0.107	0.042
2	18	0.440	0.419	0.000	0.001	0.029	0.108	0.063
2	19	0.458	0.442	0.000	0.000	0.017	0.098	0.085
2	20	0.477	0.465	0.000	0.000	0.009	0.080	0.105
2	21	0.496	0.488	0.000	0.000	0.004	0.059	0.116
2	22	0.517	0.512	0.000	0.000	0.002	0.040	0.118
2	23	0.538	0.535	0.000	0.000	0.001	0.025	0.108
2	24	0.560	0.558	0.000	0.000	0.000	0.014	0.091
2	25	0.582	0.581	0.000	0.000	0.000	0.007	0.069
2	26	0.605	0.605	0.000	0.000	0.000	0.003	0.048
2	27	0.628	0.628	0.000	0.000	0.000	0.001	0.030
2	28	0.651	0.651	0.000	0.000	0.000	0.001	0.017
2	29	0.674	0.674	0.000	0.000	0.000	0.000	0.009
2	30	0.698	0.698	0.000	0.000	0.000	0.000	0.004
2	31	0.721	0.721	0.000	0.000	0.000	0.000	0.002
2	32	0.744	0.744	0.000	0.000	0.000	0.000	0.001
2	33	0.767	0.767	0.000	0.000	0.000	0.000	0.000
2	34	0.791	0.791	0.000	0.000	0.000	0.000	0.000
2	35	0.814	0.814	0.000	0.000	0.000	0.000	0.000
2	36	0.837	0.837	0.000	0.000	0.000	0.000	0.000
2	37	0.861	0.861	0.000	0.000	0.000	0.000	0.000
2	38	0.884	0.884	0.000	0.000	0.000	0.000	0.000
2	39	0.907	0.907	0.000	0.000	0.000	0.000	0.000
2	40	0.930	0.930	0.000	0.000	0.000	0.000	0.000
2	41	0.954	0.954	0.000	0.000	0.000	0.000	0.000
2	42	0.977	0.977	0.000	0.000	0.000	0.000	0.000
2	43	1.000	1.000	0.000	0.000	0.000	0.000	0.000

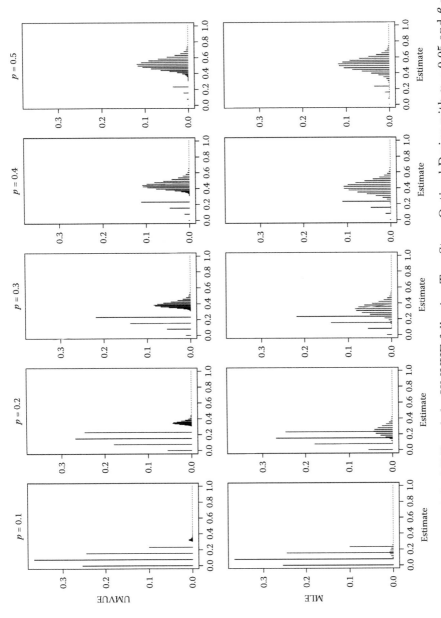

Figure 3.1 Distribution of the MLE and the UMVUE following Two-Stage Optimal Design with $\alpha = 0.05$ and $\beta = 0.2$ for $p_0 = 0.2$ and $p_1 = 0.4$.

Based on the probability mass function, we can evaluate the bias of the MLE explicitly by

$$\text{bias}(\tilde{p}|p) = \sum_{(m,s)\in\mathcal{S}} \tilde{p}(m,s) f(m,s|p) - p.$$

However, noting that X_1 and X_2 are independent binomial random variables, we can determine the bias explicitly as

$$\text{bias}(\tilde{p}|p) = -\frac{n_2}{n_1(n_1+n_2)} \sum_{x_1=a_1+1}^{b_1-1} (x_1 - n_1 p)\binom{n_1}{x_1} p^{x_1}(1-p)^{n_1-x_1}. \qquad (3.6)$$

The MSE of the MLE can be determined directly using the probability mass function of the sufficient statistics (M, S) according to formula (3.1) as follows:

$$\text{MSE}\{\tilde{p}(m,s)\} = \sum_{(m,s)\in\mathcal{S}} \{\tilde{p}(m,s) - p\}^2 f(m,s|p).$$

The variance of the UMVUE is obtained by replacing $\tilde{p}$ with $\hat{p}$ in this expression.

For various two-stage optimal and minimax designs according to Simon (1989), we evaluate the bias of the MLE according to formula (3.6). We also evaluate the MSE of the MLE and the variance of UMVUE for these designs. Two sets of numerical studies have been performed; the first set (a) with fixed type I and II error probabilities but with varying p_0 and p_1 and the second set (b) with fixed p_0 and p_1 but with varying type I and II error probabilities.

In the first set of numerical studies (a), we consider Simon's optimal and minimax designs $(a_1/n_1, a_2/(n_1 + n_2))$ with $\alpha = 0.05$ and $\beta = 0.1$ for the following binomial probabilities:

a.I $p_0 = 0.1$ and $p_1 = 0.3$: optimal $= (2/18, 6/35)$, minimax $= (2/22, 6/33)$

a.II $p_0 = 0.2$ and $p_1 = 0.4$: optimal $= (4/19, 15/54)$, minimax $= (5/24, 13/45)$

a.III $p_0 = 0.3$ and $p_1 = 0.5$: optimal $= (8/24, 24/63)$, minimax $= (7/24, 21/53)$

These numerical studies are conducted to evaluate the bias of the MLE and the relative efficiency of the UMVUE as compared to the MLE for different values of the true binomial probability.

In the second set of numerical studies (b), we consider Simon's optimal and minimax designs to test $p_0 = 0.2$ versus $p_1 = 0.4$ with the following type I and II error probabilities:

b.I $\alpha = 0.1$ and $\beta = 0.1$: optimal $= (3/17, 10/37)$, minimax $= (3/19, 10/36)$

b.II $\alpha = 0.05$ and $\beta = 0.2$: optimal $= (3/13, 12/43)$, minimax $= (4/18, 10/33)$

b.III $\alpha = 0.05$ and $\beta = 0.1$: optimal $= (4/19, 15/54)$, minimax $= (5/24, 13/45)$

These numerical studies are conducted to evaluate the bias of the MLE and the relative efficiency of the UMVUE as compared to the MLE for different values of the type I and II error probabilities.

Figures 3.2a and 3.2b display bias of the MLE for designs a.I, a.II, and a.III and for designs b.I, b.II, and b.III, respectively, for a range of true p values, including p_0 and p_1. The bias of the MLE is bigger at p values around the middle of p_0 and p_1, but somewhat closer to p_0 rather than at the extreme values. Overall, the bias of the MLE tends to be bigger with optimal designs than with minimax designs.

Figures 3.3a and 3.3b display the relative efficiency of the UMVUE as compared to the MLE, that is, the ratio of the MSE of the MLE to the variance of the UMVUE, for designs a.I, a.II, and a.III and for designs b.I, b.II, and b.III, respectively, for a range of true p values, including p_0 and p_1. For all designs, the MLE has smaller MSE for smaller p values than UMVUE, but larger MSE for larger p values. There appears to be some efficiency loss with

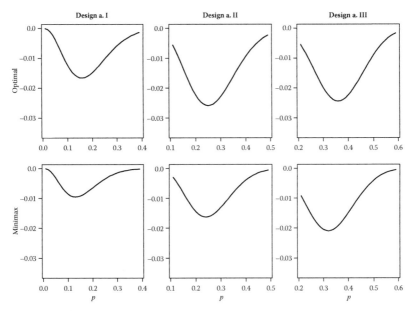

Figure 3.2(a) Bias of the MLE for Two-Stage Optimal and Minimax Designs with $\alpha = 0.05$ and $\beta = 0.1$: I ($p_0 = 0.1$ and $p_1 = 0.3$), II ($p_0 = 0.2$ and $p_1 = 0.4$), III ($p_0 = 0.3$ and $p_1 = 0.5$).

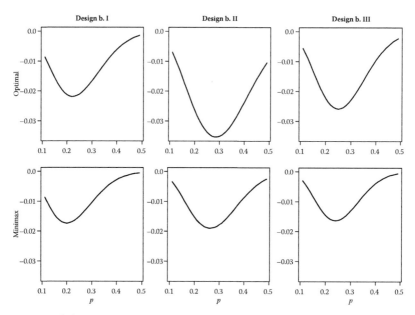

Figure 3.2(b) Bias of the MLE for Two-Stage Optimal and Minimax Designs for $p_0 = 0.2$ and $p_1 = 0.4$: I ($\alpha = 0.1$ and $\beta = 0.1$), II ($\alpha = 0.5$ and $\beta = 0.2$), III ($\alpha = 0.05$ and $\beta = 0.1$).

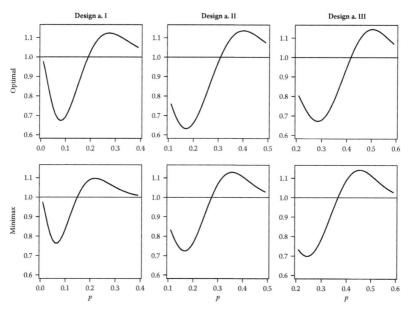

Figure 3.3(a) Relative Efficiency of the UMVUE for Two-Stage Optimal and Minimax Designs with $\alpha = 0.05$ and $\beta = 0.1$: I ($p_0 = 0.1$ and $p_1 = 0.3$), II ($p_0 = 0.2$ and $p_1 = 0.4$), III ($p_0 = 0.3$ and $p_1 = 0.5$).

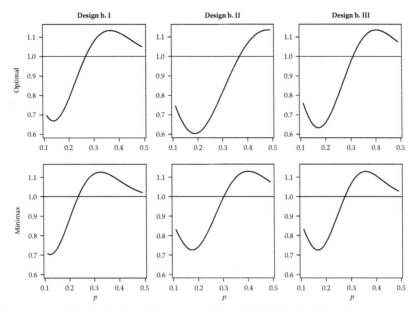

Figure 3.3(b) Relative Efficiency of the UMVUE for Two-Stage Optimal and Minimax Designs for $p_0 = 0.2$ and $p_1 = 0.4$: I ($\alpha = 0.1$ and $\beta = 0.1$), II ($\alpha = 0.5$ and $\beta = 0.2$), III ($\alpha = 0.05$ and $\beta = 0.1$).

the UMVUE as compared to the MLE, particularly for optimal designs, a reasonable price for unbiasedness.

With a moderate n_1 (with $n_1 p \geq 5$ as a rule of thumb), the binomial mass function is approximately symmetric about $n_1 p$, so that the right-hand side of formula (3.6) becomes very small for p such that $n_1 p \approx (a_1 + b_1)/2$. Similarly, the bias tends to be negative (positive) in studies with lower (upper) boundaries only. Also, the MLE will be more biased in studies with one-sided stopping boundaries than in those with lower and upper boundaries. Chang, Wieand, and Chang (1989) provide a study of bias of the MLE in studies with lower and upper boundaries proposed by Chang, Therneau, Wieand, and Cha (1987).

3.2 Confidence Intervals

The confidence intervals determined according to Clopper and Pearson (1934) and the stochastic ordering based on the magnitude of the UMVUE are the same as those by Jennison and Turnbull (1983) by considering tail probabilities. With the UMVUE $\hat{p}(m, s)$, an exact $100(1 - \alpha)\%$ equal tail confidence interval (p_L, p_U) for p is given by

$$\Pr(\hat{p}(M, S) \geq \hat{p}(m, s)|p = p_L) = \alpha/2$$

and

$$\Pr(\hat{p}(M, S) \le \hat{p}(m, s)|p = p_U) = \alpha/2.$$

Confidence limits p_L and p_U can be obtained by a linear search procedure, such as the bisection method, solving the equations.

For example, suppose that we observed $(m, s) = (2, 7)$ from a two-stage study with lower boundaries only, $(n_1, n_2, a_1, a_2) = (13, 30, 3, 12)$. In this case, we have $b_1 = 14$, $(a_1 + 1) \vee (s - n_2) = (3+1) \vee (7-30) = 4$, and $s \wedge (b_1 - 1) = 7 \wedge (14 - 1) = 7$. From (3.2) or (3.4) in the following section, the UMVUE is

$$\hat{p}(2, 7) = \frac{\sum_{x_1=4}^{7} \binom{13-1}{x_1-1}\binom{30}{7-x_1}}{\sum_{x_1=4}^{7} \binom{13}{x_1}\binom{30}{7-x_1}} = 0.322.$$

Using (3.1), we have

$$\Pr(\hat{p}(M, S) \ge .322|p = .103) = .025,$$

$$\Pr(\hat{p}(M, S) \le .322|p = .538) = .025,$$

so that a 95% confidence interval on p is given as $(.103, .538)$, which is the same as the one according to Jennison and Turnbull (1983). In contrast, a naive 95% confidence interval by Clopper and Pearson (1934) ignoring the group sequential aspect of the study is given as $(.068, .307)$. Note that the latter is narrower than the former by ignoring the group sequential aspect of the study. Furthermore, the former is slightly shifted to the right from the latter to reflect the fact that the study has been continued to stage 2 after observing more responders than $a_1 = 3$ in stage 1.

3.3   P-Values

If one ignores the multistage design aspect of the study, S may be regarded as a binomial random variable from $N_m = n_1 + \cdots + n_m$ independent Bernoulli trials. This leads to a naive p-value

$$v = \Pr(S \ge s|p_0) = \sum_{i=s}^{N_m} \binom{N_m}{i} p_0^i (1 - p_0)^{N_m - i}$$

for observed values $(M, S) = (m, s)$. However, the naive p-value does not have the property that a proper p-value should have that is, the distribution of the naive p-value $V = v(M, S)$ under H_0 does not have the property $\Pr(V \le v|H_0) = v$ for the observable p-values, $v \in [0, 1]$. This occurs because the assumed binomial distribution for S is incorrect under the two-stage design.

The true null distribution of $V = v(M, S)$ is calculated using the probability mass function $f(m, s|p_0)$ of (M, S). From (3.1), the probability mass function of the random vector (M, S) is given by

$$f(m, s|p) = c_{m,s} \, p^s (1 - p)^{N_m - s}$$

with support $S = \cup_{m=1}^{K} S_m$, where

$$S_m = \{(m, s) : a_{m-1} + 1 \le s \le a_m \text{ or } b_m \le s \le n_m + b_{m-1} - 1\}$$

and $a_0 = -1$ and $b_0 = 1$. Here $c_{1,s} = \binom{n_1}{s}$ and, for $m \ge 2$,

$$c_{m,s} = \sum_{x_1} \cdots \sum_{x_m} \binom{n_1}{x_1} \cdots \binom{n_m}{x_m}$$

with the summations over the set

$$\mathcal{R}(m, s) = \{(x_1, \ldots, x_m) : x_1 + \cdots + x_m$$
$$= s, a_k + 1 \le x_1 + \cdots + x_k \le b_k - 1 \quad \text{for } k = 1, \ldots, m - 1\}.$$

We define $\binom{n}{x} = 0$ if $x < 0$ or $x > n$.

Let $\hat{\theta}(M, S)$ denote an estimator of p. Then, a p-value may be defined as the probability of obtaining more extreme estimates toward H_1 than the observed one when H_0 is true. Hence, for testing $H_0 : p = p_0$ against $H_1 : p > p_0$, the p-value for an estimate $\hat{\theta}(m, s)$ will be given as

$$\Pr(\hat{\theta}(M, S) \ge \hat{\theta}(m, s)|p_0) = \sum_{\{(i,j):\hat{\theta}(i,j) \ge \hat{\theta}(m,s)\}} f(i, j|p_0).$$

We consider two estimators, MLE $\tilde{p}(M, S)$ and UMVUE $\hat{p}(M, S)$, in this section.

By minimizing $f(m, s|p)$ with respect to p, we obtain the well-known MLE as

$$\tilde{p}(m, s) = \frac{s}{N_m}.$$

Note that the naive p-value is also based on the ordering of MLE, but without using the correct probability density function $f(m, s|p_0)$ for the outcomes.

As shown in Appendix 3.C, the UMVUE has a natural stochastic ordering of

$$\hat{p}(1, 0) < \hat{p}(1, 1) < \cdots < \hat{p}(1, a_1)$$
$$< \hat{p}(2, a_1 + 1) < \cdots < \hat{p}(2, a_2)$$

$$\vdots$$

$$< \hat{p}(K, a_{K-1} + 1) < \cdots < \hat{p}(K, a_K)$$
$$< \hat{p}(K, b_K) < \cdots < \hat{p}(K, b_{K-1} - 1 + n_K)$$
$$< \hat{p}(K - 1, b_{K-1}) < \cdots < \hat{p}(K - 1, b_{K-2} - 1 + n_{K-1})$$

$$\vdots$$

$$< \hat{p}(1, b_1) < \cdots < \hat{p}(1, n_1).$$

The probability mass function $f(m, s|p)$ depends on the stopping boundaries only up to stage $m-1$, that is, $\{(a_k, b_k), 1 \leq k \leq m-1\}$. This property combined with the monotonicity of the above stochastic ordering implies that, given $(M, S) = (m, s)$, the p-value based on UMVUE can be calculated if p_0 and the stopping boundaries up to stage $m-1$ are given since

$$\text{p-value} = \begin{cases} \sum_{\{(i,j):\hat{p}(i,j) \geq \hat{p}(m,s)\}} f(i, j|p_0) & \text{if } s \geq b_m \\ 1 - \sum_{\{(i,j):\hat{p}(i,j) < \hat{p}(m,s)\}} f(i, j|p_0) & \text{if } s \leq a_m \end{cases}$$

In contrast, calculation of the p-value based on the MLE requires one to know all stopping boundaries since there may be observations (i, j) with smaller or larger MLE values than $\tilde{p}(m, s)$ in the later stages. Cook (2002) discusses similar issues for the cases with a continuous variable.

Whatever estimator is used, the p-values depend on the stochastic ordering, but not on the estimates. So, two estimators will result in exactly the same p-values if they have the same stochastic ordering. Chang, Wieand, and Chang (1989) correct the bias of the MLE using Whitehead's (1986) approach. The bias-corrected estimator has exactly the same ordering as the MLE (see Appendix 3.D for the proof for two-stage designs), so that the two estimators result in the same p-values. Further, both MLE and UMVUE increase in s for each m. Hence, the two estimators will have the same ordering as long as their ordering matches at the boundaries, that is, for all $k = 1, \ldots, K-1$, $\tilde{p}(k, a_k) < \tilde{p}(k+1, a_k+1)$ and $\tilde{p}(k, b_k) > \tilde{p}(k+1, n_{k+1}+b_k-1)$.

3.3.1   P-Values under Two-Stage Designs

From Section 3.1.1, for a two-stage study, the probability mass function is given as

$$f(m, s|p) = \begin{cases} p^s(1-p)^{n_1-s} \binom{n_1}{s} & m = 1, 0 \leq s \leq a_1 \\ & \text{or } b_1 \leq s \leq n_1 \\ p^s(1-p)^{n_1+n_2-s} \sum_{x_1=a_1+1}^{b_1-1} \binom{n_1}{x_1}\binom{n_2}{s-x_1} & m = 2, a_1+1 \leq s \\ & \leq b_1+n_2-1 \end{cases}$$

and the UMVUE of p given as to

$$\hat{p}(m, s) = \begin{cases} \dfrac{s}{n_1} & m = 1 \\ \dfrac{\sum_{x_1=(a_1+1)\vee(s-n_2)}^{s\wedge(b_1-1)} \binom{n_1-1}{x_1-1}\binom{n_2}{s-x_1}}{\sum_{x_1=(a_1+1)\vee(s-n_2)}^{s\wedge(b_1-1)} \binom{n_1}{x_1}\binom{n_2}{s-x_1}} & m = 2 \end{cases}$$

where $a \wedge b = \min(a, b)$ and $a \vee b = \max(a, b)$. Note that $\hat{p} = \tilde{p}$ when $m = 1$.

Example 3.1 (Minimax design)
For $H_0 : p_0 = .4$ versus $H_1 : p_1 = .6$, the two-stage design $(n_1, n_2, a_1, b_1, a_2) = (34, 5, 17, 35, 20)$ is the minimax design according to Simon (1989) among those with $\alpha \leq 0.05$, $1-\beta \geq 0.8$ and a lower early stopping boundary only.

Table 3.2 MLE and UMVUE, and p-values using these estimators for a two-stage design with $(n_1, n_2, a_1, b_1, a_2) = (34, 5, 17, 35, 20)$ and $p_0 = .4$

m	s	$f(m,s\|p_0)$	Estimate		p-value		
			UMVUE	MLE	UMVUE	MLE	Naive
1	0	0.0000	0.0000	0.0000	1.0000	1.0000	1.0000
1	1	0.0000	0.0294	0.0294	1.0000	1.0000	1.0000
1	2	0.0000	0.0588	0.0588	1.0000	1.0000	1.0000
1	3	0.0001	0.0882	0.0882	1.0000	1.0000	1.0000
1	4	0.0003	0.1176	0.1176	0.9999	0.9999	0.9999
1	5	0.0010	0.1471	0.1471	0.9997	0.9997	0.9997
1	6	0.0034	0.1765	0.1765	0.9986	0.9986	0.9986
1	7	0.0090	0.2059	0.2059	0.9952	0.9952	0.9952
1	8	0.0203	0.2353	0.2353	0.9862	0.9862	0.9862
1	9	0.0391	0.2647	0.2647	0.9659	0.9659	0.9659
1	10	0.0652	0.2941	0.2941	0.9268	0.9268	0.9268
1	11	0.0948	0.3235	0.3235	0.8617	0.8617	0.8617
1	12	0.1211	0.3529	0.3529	0.7669	0.7669	0.7669
1	13	0.1366	0.3824	0.3824	0.6458	0.6458	0.6458
1	14	0.1366	0.4118	0.4118	0.5092	0.5092	0.5092
1	15	0.1214	0.4412	0.4412	0.3726	0.3726	0.3726
1	16	0.0961	0.4706	0.4706	**0.2512**	**0.2478**	0.2512
1	17	0.0679	0.5000	0.5000	**0.1550**	**0.1388**	0.1550
2	18	0.0033	0.5294	0.4615	**0.0872**	**0.2512**	0.2653
2	19	0.0129	0.5337	0.4872	**0.0838**	**0.1517**	0.1713
2	20	0.0219	0.5403	0.5128	0.0709	0.0709	0.1021
2	21	0.0217	0.5508	0.5385	0.0490	0.0490	0.0559
2	22	0.0145	0.5672	0.5641	0.0273	0.0273	0.0280
2	23	0.0075	0.5897	0.5897	0.0128	0.0128	0.0128
2	24	0.0033	0.6154	0.6154	0.0053	0.0053	0.0053
2	25	0.0013	0.6410	0.6410	0.0020	0.0020	0.0020
2	26	0.0005	0.6667	0.6667	0.0007	0.0007	0.0007
2	27	0.0002	0.6923	0.6923	0.0002	0.0002	0.0002
2	28	0.0000	0.7179	0.7179	0.0001	0.0001	0.0001
2	29	0.0000	0.7436	0.7436	0.0000	0.0000	0.0000
2	30	0.0000	0.7692	0.7692	0.0000	0.0000	0.0000
2	31	0.0000	0.7949	0.7949	0.0000	0.0000	0.0000
2	32	0.0000	0.8205	0.8205	0.0000	0.0000	0.0000
2	33	0.0000	0.8462	0.8462	0.0000	0.0000	0.0000
2	34	0.0000	0.8718	0.8718	0.0000	0.0000	0.0000
2	35	0.0000	0.8974	0.8974	0.0000	0.0000	0.0000
2	36	0.0000	0.9231	0.9231	0.0000	0.0000	0.0000
2	37	0.0000	0.9487	0.9487	0.0000	0.0000	0.0000
2	38	0.0000	0.9744	0.9744	0.0000	0.0000	0.0000
2	39	0.0000	1.0000	1.0000	0.0000	0.0000	0.0000

Table 3.2 displays the p-values for MLE and UMVUE, the naive p-values, and the probability mass function at $p_0 = 0.4$ for each sample point in the descending order for UMVUE. For example, for $(m, s) = (2, 19)$, we have

$$\tilde{p} = s/(n_1 + n_2) = 19/(34 + 5) = 0.4872$$

and

$$\hat{p} = \frac{\sum_{x_1=(17+1)\vee(19-5)}^{19\wedge(35-1)} \binom{34-1}{x_1-1}\binom{5}{19-x_1}}{\sum_{x_1=(17+1)\vee(19-5)}^{19\wedge(35-1)} \binom{34}{x_1}\binom{5}{19-x_1}} = \frac{\binom{33}{17}\binom{5}{1} + \binom{33}{18}\binom{5}{0}}{\binom{34}{18}\binom{5}{1} + \binom{34}{19}\binom{5}{0}} = 0.5337.$$

Also, when $(m, s) = (2, 19)$ is observed, we calculate the p-value based on MLE as

$$
\begin{aligned}
\Pr(\tilde{p}(M, S) \geq .4872 | p_0) &= f(1, 17 | p_0) + \sum_{j=19}^{39} f(2, j | p_0) \\
&= .0679 + (.0129 + .0219 + .0217 + .0145 + .0075 \\
&\quad + .0033 + .0013 + .0005 + .0002 + .0000 + \cdots \\
&\quad + .0000) \\
&= .1517
\end{aligned}
$$

and that based on UMVUE as

$$
\begin{aligned}
\Pr(\hat{p}(M, S) \geq .5337 | p_0) &= \sum_{j=19}^{39} f(2, j | p_0) \\
&= .0129 + .0219 + .0217 + .0145 + .0075 + .0033 \\
&\quad + .0013 + .0005 + .0002 + .0000 + \cdots + .0000 \\
&= .0838
\end{aligned}
$$

In Table 3.2, the p-values that differ for MLE and UMVUE are boldfaced. The p-values by the two estimators are different around the stopping boundary, especially around $(m, s) = (a_1 + 1, 2)$. The naive p-values exactly match with those based on UMVUE in stage 1, but in stage 2 they are closer to those by MLE than to those by UMVUE.

Example 3.2 (With both lower and upper stopping boundaries)
Under the same setting as in Example 3.1, $(p_0, p_1, \alpha, 1 - \beta) = (.4, .6, .05, .8)$, $(n_1, n_2, a_1, b_1, a_2) = (20, 27, 9, 13, 24)$ minimizes $(\text{EN}_0 + \text{EN}_1)/2$ among the two stages with both lower and upper early stopping boundaries, where EN_k $(k = 0, 1)$ is the expected sample size when $p = p_k$; see Chang et al. (1987). Table 3.3 displays the p-values for the observations listed in descending order for UMVUE. The p-values by the two estimators are different around the upper and lower stopping boundaries. The stopping boundaries may be

Table 3.3 MLE and UMVUE, and p-values using these estimators for a two-stage design with $(n_1, n_2, a_1, b_1, a_2) = (20, 27, 9, 13, 24)$ and $p_0 = .4$

m	s	$f(m,s\|p_0)$	Estimate		p-value		
			UMVUE	**MLE**	**UMVUE**	**MLE**	**Naive**
1	0	0.0000	0.0000	0.0000	1.0000	1.0000	1.0000
1	1	0.0005	0.0500	0.0500	1.0000	1.0000	1.0000
1	2	0.0031	0.1000	0.1000	0.9995	0.9995	0.9995
1	3	0.0123	0.1500	0.1500	0.9964	0.9964	0.9964
1	4	0.0350	0.2000	0.2000	0.9840	0.9840	0.9840
1	5	0.0746	0.2500	0.2500	0.9490	0.9490	0.9490
1	6	0.1244	0.3000	0.3000	**0.8744**	**0.8738**	0.8744
1	7	0.1659	0.3500	0.3500	**0.7500**	**0.7438**	0.7500
1	8	0.1797	0.4000	0.4000	**0.5841**	**0.5543**	0.5841
1	9	0.1597	0.4500	0.4500	**0.4044**	**0.2891**	0.4044
2	10	0.0000	0.5000	0.2128	**0.2447**	**0.9490**	0.9980
2	11	0.0000	0.5016	0.2340	**0.2447**	**0.9490**	0.9947
2	12	0.0000	0.5034	0.2553	**0.2447**	**0.8744**	0.9871
2	13	0.0001	0.5055	0.2766	**0.2446**	**0.8744**	0.9721
2	14	0.0005	0.5077	0.2979	**0.2445**	**0.8743**	0.9450
2	15	0.0016	0.5101	0.3191	**0.2440**	**0.7494**	0.9012
2	16	0.0040	0.5128	0.3404	**0.2425**	**0.7478**	0.8370
2	17	0.0085	0.5156	0.3617	**0.2385**	**0.5779**	0.7514
2	18	0.0151	0.5188	0.3830	**0.2300**	**0.5694**	0.6472
2	19	0.0228	0.5221	0.4043	**0.2149**	**0.3746**	0.5316
2	20	0.0295	0.5256	0.4255	**0.1921**	**0.3518**	0.4139
2	21	0.0331	0.5294	0.4468	**0.1625**	**0.3222**	0.3040
2	22	0.0323	0.5334	0.4681	0.1294	0.1294	0.2098
2	23	0.0276	0.5375	0.4894	0.0970	0.0970	0.1356
2	24	0.0206	0.5418	0.5106	0.0695	0.0695	0.0819
2	25	0.0135	0.5462	0.5319	0.0489	0.0489	0.0460
2	26	0.0078	0.5508	0.5532	0.0354	0.0354	0.0241
2	27	0.0039	0.5553	0.5745	0.0276	0.0276	0.0117
2	28	0.0017	0.5599	0.5957	0.0237	0.0237	0.0052
2	29	0.0007	0.5644	0.6170	0.0220	0.0220	0.0022
2	30	0.0002	0.5689	0.6383	0.0213	0.0213	0.0008
2	31	0.0001	0.5733	0.6596	**0.0211**	**0.0065**	0.0003
2	32	0.0000	0.5775	0.6809	**0.0210**	**0.0065**	0.0001
2	33	0.0000	0.5815	0.7021	**0.0210**	**0.0016**	0.0000
2	34	0.0000	0.5853	0.7234	**0.0210**	**0.0016**	0.0000
2	35	0.0000	0.5888	0.7447	**0.0210**	**0.0016**	0.0000
2	36	0.0000	0.5920	0.7660	**0.0210**	**0.0003**	0.0000
2	37	0.0000	0.5950	0.7872	**0.0210**	**0.0003**	0.0000
2	38	0.0000	0.5976	0.8085	**0.0210**	**0.0000**	0.0000
2	39	0.0000	0.6000	0.8298	**0.0210**	**0.0000**	0.0000
1	13	0.0146	0.6500	0.6500	**0.0210**	**0.0211**	0.0210
1	14	0.0049	0.7000	0.7000	0.0065	0.0065	0.0065
1	15	0.0013	0.7500	0.7500	0.0016	0.0016	0.0016
1	16	0.0003	0.8000	0.8000	0.0003	0.0003	0.0003
1	17	0.0000	0.8500	0.8500	0.0000	0.0000	0.0000
1	18	0.0000	0.9000	0.9000	0.0000	0.0000	0.0000
1	19	0.0000	0.9500	0.9500	0.0000	0.0000	0.0000
1	20	0.0000	1.0000	1.0000	0.0000	0.0000	0.0000

interpreted as follows: using $\hat{p}(M, S)$ as the test statistic, we reject H_0 if $\hat{p}(m, s) \geq 0.5462 = \hat{p}(2, b_2)$, where $b_2 = a_2 + 1 = 25$. Since the p-value for the critical value $\hat{p}(2, 25)$ is 0.0489, the exact type I error for the two-stage design is 0.0489, which satisfies the restriction of $\alpha \leq 0.05$. We can make a similar statement with respect to the MLE. However, with the MLE, the outcome $(m, s) = (1, 9)$, on which the study will be stopped due to a low response rate after stage 1, has a smaller p-value than those between $(m, s) = (2, 10)$ and $(2, 21)$, which only occurs when the study proceeds to stage 2 after observing a promising response rate from stage 1. In this sense, the UMVUE ordering may be considered to be more in accordance with the multistage design for phase II trials than the MLE ordering. As in the designs with a lower stopping boundary only, the naive p-values exactly match those based on UMVUE in stage 1, but they are closer to those by MLE in stage 2 than those by UMVUE.

Chang and O'Brien (1985) propose to use the likelihood-ratio

$$\frac{f(m, s|\tilde{p})}{f(m, s|p_0)} = \left(\frac{\tilde{p}}{p_0}\right)^s \left(\frac{1 - \tilde{p}}{1 - p_0}\right)^{N_m - s}$$

to measure how far the MLE $\tilde{p} = \hat{p}(m, s)$ is from p_0. The ordering of the sample space based on the likelihood-ratio is two-sided in nature, so that it can be used to derive confidence intervals (Chang and O'Brien, 1987). As discussed previously, phase II trials ordinarily have one-sided hypotheses, so that this ordering is not appropriate to derive p-values for phase II trials.

Assuming the normal approximation of the binomial random variables, the likelihood ratio ordering can be expressed as follows: (m, s) is more extreme from $H_0 : p = p_0$ toward $H_1 : p > p_0$ than (m', s') if and only if

$$\sqrt{N_m}|\tilde{p}(m, s) - p_0| > \sqrt{N_{m'}}|\tilde{p}(m', s') - p_0|.$$

Emerson and Fleming (1990) drop the absolute value signs and refer to the linear ordering

$$\sqrt{N_m}\{\tilde{p}(m, s) - p_0\} > \sqrt{N_{m'}}\{\tilde{p}(m', s') - p_0\} \tag{3.7}$$

as the likelihood ratio ordering. The latter has been used in the literature under the name of the likelihood ratio ordering, including Chang, Gould, and Snapinn (1995) and Cook (2002). The two orderings are different because $p_m(m, s) - p_0$ can take negative values for some outcomes. Furthermore, if $\tilde{p}(m, s) = \tilde{p}(m', s') < p_0$ and $m < m'$, then (m, s) is more in favor of $H_1 : p > p_0$ by (3.7). The p-value for (m, s) based on (3.7) is obtained by

$$v_r(m, s) = \sum_{(i,j) \in \mathcal{S}} I\{\sqrt{N_i}(\tilde{p}(i, j) - p_0) > \sqrt{N_m}(\tilde{p}(m, s) - p_0)\} f(i, j|p_0)$$

where $I(\cdot)$ is the indicator function. As an example, we consider the design $(n_1, n_2, a_1, b_1, a_2) = (30, 30, 9, 31)$ with $p_0 = 0.3$. Under the design, both $(m, s) = (1, 9)$ and $(2, 18)$ have the same MLE of 0.3, but the p-value $v_r(1, 9) = 0.4602$ is smaller than $v_r(2, 18) = 0.5037$. This is against the concept of a group sequential testing with lower stopping boundaries only in the sense that, between the two outcomes with the same MLE, the outcome which accepts H_0 and stops after stage 1 is more supportive for H_1 than the other which proceeds to stage 2.

It is obvious from (3.3) that UMVUE gives p-values satisfying the following properties: (a) the p-values in the acceptance region of H_0 are larger than those in the rejection region, and (b) the p-values for the critical value matches with the type I error probability of the sequential testing. These properties may not be satisfied by p-values defined by other orderings.

3.4 When Realized Sample Size Is Different from That Specified in Design

At the design stage of a trial, we determine the required number of patients (sample size) and a critical value for a specified type I error rate corresponding to the sample size. When the study is over, however, the resulting sample size is often different from the planned one due to ineligibilities and dropouts. In this case, the prespecified critical value may not be appropriate anymore. One of the common approaches to this problem is to assume that the realized sample size is the planned one and recalculate the critical value corresponding to the realized sample size and the prespecified type I error rate.

More specifically in a multistage phase II trial, the prespecified critical values at the terminal stage is not applicable if the realized sample size is different from the one determined at the design stage. In this case, we can use the confidence interval or p-value approaches to test $H_0 : p = p_0$ against $H_1 : p > p_0$ based on the prespecified type I error rate α. This is possible because the UMVUE-based calculation of confidence interval and p-value discussed in this chapter does not require specification of the critical values at the terminal stage.

For example, Simon's optimal two-stage design for $(p_0, p_1, \alpha^*, 1 - \beta^*) = (0.4, 0.6, 0.1, 0.9)$ is $(a_1/n_1, a/n) = (7/18, 22/46)$. Suppose that the study is completed with 23 responders from cumulative 48 eligible patients after the second stage. Note that the statistical tests for phase II trials are one-sided. Hence, we have to compare the lower confidence limit of $100(1 - 2\alpha)\%$ two-sided confidence interval with p_0 if we want to use a confidence interval method for testing. Using the resulting data $(M, S) = (2, 23)$ and the realized design $(a_1/n_1, n) = (7/18, 48)$, the 80% confidence interval is obtained as $(0.387, 0.599)$. Since the lower limit 0.387 of the confidence interval is smaller than $p_0 = 0.4$, we cannot reject $H_0 : p_0 = 0.4$ at $\alpha = 0.1$ level. Similarly, the p-value for $(M, S) = (2, 23)$ with respect to the realized design

$(a_1/n_1, n) = (7/18, 48)$ is given as p-value= 0.1360. Since the p-value is larger than $\alpha = 0.1$, we fail to reject H_0, too. For a significant outcome of the study, we need at least $S = 25$ responders out of the realized $n = 48$ after the second stage, for which case we have a 80% confidence interval of $(0.423, 0.628)$ and p-value $= 0.0896$.

APPENDIX 3.A: Completeness and Sufficiency of (M, S)

We consider a K-stage phase II trial design. The probability mass of a sample path with $x_1, \ldots, x_m$ successes $(a_k + 1 \leq x_1 + \cdots + x_k \leq b_k - 1$ for $k = 1, \ldots, m - 1$, and $x_1 + \cdots + x_m \leq a_m$ or $\geq b_m)$ is given as

$$p^{x_1 + \cdots + x_m}(1 - p)^{(n_1 + \cdots + n_m) - (x_1 + \cdots + x_m)}.$$

The sufficiency of (M, S) follows from the factorization theorem. In order to prove completeness, we first derive the probability mass function $f(m, s|p)$ of random vector (M, S). For $m = 1, \ldots, K$ and $s = a_{m-1} + 1, \ldots, a_m, b_m, \ldots, n_m + b_{m-1} - 1$,

$$
\begin{aligned}
f(m, s|p) &= \Pr(M = m, S = s|p) \\
&= \Pr(S_m = s, a_k + 1 \leq S_k \leq b_k - 1, \ k = 1, \ldots, m - 1|p) \\
&= \sum_{x_1} \cdots \sum_{x_m} \Pr(X_1 = x_1, \ldots, X_m = x_m|p),
\end{aligned}
$$

where the summations are subject to

$$\mathcal{R}(m, s) = \{(x_1, \ldots, x_m) : x_1 + \cdots + x_m = s, a_k + 1 \leq s_k \leq b_k - 1, \ k = 1, \ldots, m - 1\}.$$

Hence, we have

$$
\begin{aligned}
f(m, s|p) &= \sum \cdots \sum_{\mathcal{R}(m,s)} \binom{n_1}{x_1} p^{x_1}(1 - p)^{n_1 - x_1} \cdots \binom{n_m}{x_m} p^{x_m}(1 - p)^{n_m - x_m} \\
&= p^s(1 - p)^{n_1 + \cdots + n_m - s} \sum \cdots \sum_{\mathcal{R}(m,s)} \binom{n_1}{x_1} \cdots \binom{n_m}{x_m}.
\end{aligned}
$$

Let $c_{m,s} = \sum \cdots \sum_{\mathcal{R}(m,s)} \binom{n_1}{x_1} \cdots \binom{n_m}{x_m}$. Then the probability mass function of (M, S) is given as

$$f(m, s|p) = c_{m,s} p^s(1 - p)^{n_1 + \cdots + n_m - s} \tag{3.A.1}$$

with support $\mathcal{S} = \cup_{m=1}^{K} \mathcal{S}_m$ where

$$\mathcal{S}_m = \{(m, s) : a_{m-1} + 1 \leq s \leq a_m \text{ or } b_m \leq s \leq n_m + b_{m-1} - 1\}.$$

Now we prove the completeness of (M, S). From (3.A.1), $h(p) = E_p\{g(M, S)\}$ is obtained as

$$\sum_{m=1}^{K} \sum_{s=a_{m-1}+1}^{a_m} g(m, s) f(m, s|p) + \sum_{m=1}^{K} \sum_{s=b_m}^{n_m+b_{m-1}-1} g(m, s) f(m, s|p)$$

$$= \sum_{m=1}^{K} \left\{ \sum_{s=a_{m-1}+1}^{a_m} g(m, s) c_{m,s} p^s (1-p)^{n_1 + \cdots + n_m - s} \right.$$

$$\left. + \sum_{s=b_m}^{n_m+b_{m-1}-1} g(m, s) c_{m,s} p^s (1-p)^{n_1 + \cdots + n_m - s} \right\}. \qquad (A.2)$$

We need to show that $h(p) = 0$ for all $p \in [0, 1]$ ensures $g(m, s) \equiv 0$ for all (m, s) in the support of (M, S). If $p = 0$, then, from (A.2), we have $g(1, 0) = 0$. If $1 - p = 0$, then, also from (A.2), we have $g(1, n_1) = 0$. Now, for $p \in (0, 1)$, let $P_k(p) = h(p)/p^k$ and $Q_l(p) = h(p)/(1-p)^l$. Each term, say, term i, in (A.2) has the factor $p^{k_i}(1-p)^{l_i}$ for some nonnegative integers k_i and l_i. Since all terms have different factors, that is, $(k_i, l_i) \neq (k_j, l_j)$ if $i \neq j$, any subset of the terms in (A.2) has a unique minimum either among the k_i's or the l_i's. If k_i's have a unique minimum k, then, since $P_k(p) = 0$ for all $p \in (0, 1)$, letting $p \to 0$ shows $g(m, s) = 0$, where $g(m, s)$ is the coefficient of the term with p^k factor. On the other hand, if l_i's have a unique minimum l, then, since $Q_l(p) = 0$ for all $p \in (0, 1)$, letting $p \to 1$ shows $g(m, s) = 0$, where $g(m, s)$ is the coefficient of the term with $(1-p)^l$ factor. Whichever coefficient is 0, we remove that term from $h(p)$ before next step. Starting from $k = 1$ and $l = 1$, we continue this procedure until all terms in (A.2) are removed, concluding that $g(m, s) \equiv 0$ for all (m, s) in the support of (M, S).

APPENDIX 3.B: UMVUE of p

Since (M, S) is complete and sufficient by Appendix 3.A, and $\tilde{p}_1 = X_1/n_1$ is unbiased, by the Rao–Blackwell theorem, the UMVUE of p is given as $\hat{p} = E\{X_1|(m, s)\}/n_1$. If $M = 1$, we have $\hat{p} = \tilde{p}_1$. On the other hand, if $2 \leq M \leq K$, the conditional probability mass function of X_1 given $(M, S) = (m, s)$ in $\mathcal{S}$ is, for $a_1 + 1 \leq x_1 \leq b_1 - 1$,

$$\frac{\Pr(X_1 = x_1, M = m, S = s|p)}{\Pr(M = m, S = s|p)}$$

$$= \frac{\Pr(X_1 = x_1, S_m = s, a_k < S_k < b_k \text{ for } k = 2, \ldots, m-1|p)}{f(m, s|p)}$$

$$= \frac{\sum_{x_2} \cdots \sum_{x_m} \binom{n_1}{x_1} p^{x_1}(1-p)^{n_1-x_1} \cdots \binom{n_m}{x_m} p^{x_m}(1-p)^{n_m-x_m}}{f(m, s|p)}$$

where the summations in the numerator are over the set

$$\mathcal{R}(m, s|x_1) = \{(x_2, \ldots, x_m) : x_2 + \cdots + x_m = s - x_1, a_k + 1 \le s_k \le b_k - 1,$$
$$k = 2, \ldots, m - 1\}.$$

Hence, the conditional probability mass function is simplified to

$$\frac{\binom{n_1}{x_1} \sum \cdots \sum_{\mathcal{R}(m,s|x_1)} \binom{n_2}{x_2} \cdots \binom{n_m}{x_m}}{\sum \cdots \sum_{\mathcal{R}(m,s)} \binom{n_1}{x_1} \cdots \binom{n_m}{x_m}}.$$

Therefore,

$$\hat{p} = \frac{E\{X_1|(m,s)\}}{n_1} = \frac{\sum_{x_1} x_1 \binom{n_1}{x_1} \sum \cdots \sum_{\mathcal{R}(m,s|x_1)} \binom{n_2}{x_2} \cdots \binom{n_m}{x_m}}{n_1 \sum \cdots \sum_{\mathcal{R}(m,s)} \binom{n_1}{x_1} \cdots \binom{n_m}{x_m}}.$$

Since $\sum_{x_1} \sum \cdots \sum_{\mathcal{R}(m,s|x_1)} = \sum \cdots \sum_{\mathcal{R}(m,s)}$,

$$\hat{p} = \frac{\sum \cdots \sum \binom{n_1-1}{x_1-1} \binom{n_2}{x_2} \cdots \binom{n_m}{x_m}}{\sum \cdots \sum \binom{n_1}{x_1} \cdots \binom{n_m}{x_m}}$$

with the summations over $\mathcal{R}(m, s)$ in the numerator and in the denominator.

APPENDIX 3.C: Stochastic Ordering among $\hat{p}(m, s)$

We consider a two-stage design with lower stopping boundaries only (that is, $b_1 = n_1 + 1$) and assume that $s \le n_1$. The proof under other situations can be conducted similarly. We want to prove $\hat{p}(1, 0) < \hat{p}(1, 1) < \cdots < \hat{p}(1, a_1) < \hat{p}(2, a_1 + 1) < \cdots < \hat{p}(2, n_1 + n_2)$.

It is trivial that $\hat{p}(1, s) < \hat{p}(1, s + 1)$ for $0 \le s \le a_1 - 1$. Also, since $\hat{p}(2, a_1 + 1) = (a_1 + 1)/n_1$, $\hat{p}(1, a_1) = a_1/n_1 < \hat{p}(2, a_1 + 1)$. Now, we complete the proof by showing that $\hat{p}(2, s) < \hat{p}(2, s + 1)$ for $a_1 + 1 \le s \le n_1 + n_2 - 1$. Since

$$\hat{p}(2, s + 1) - \hat{p}(2, s) = \frac{\sum_{x_1=a_1+1}^{s+1} x_1 \binom{n_1}{x_1} \binom{n_2}{s+1-x_1}}{n_1 \sum_{x_1=a_1+1}^{s+1} \binom{n_1}{x_1} \binom{n_2}{s+1-x_1}} - \frac{\sum_{x_1=a_1+1}^{s} x_1 \binom{n_1}{x_1} \binom{n_2}{s-x_1}}{n_1 \sum_{x_1=a_1+1}^{s} \binom{n_1}{x_1} \binom{n_2}{s-x_1}},$$

after reduction of the fractions to the common denominator, the numerator of $n_1\{\hat{p}(2, s + 1) - \hat{p}(2, s)\}$ is given as

$$\left\{ \sum_{x_1=a_1+1}^{s} x_1 \binom{n_1}{x_1} \binom{n_2}{s+1-x_1} + (s+1) \binom{n_1}{s+1} \right\} \sum_{x_1=a_1+1}^{s} \binom{n_1}{x_1} \binom{n_2}{s-x_1}$$

$$- \sum_{x_1=a_1+1}^{s} x_1 \binom{n_1}{x_1} \binom{n_2}{s-x_1} \left\{ \sum_{x_1=a_1+1}^{s} \binom{n_1}{x_1} \binom{n_2}{s+1-x_1} + \binom{n_1}{s+1} \right\}.$$

Noting that $\binom{n_2}{s+1-x_1} = (n_2-s+x_1)/(s+1-x_1)\binom{n_2}{s-x_1}$, the numerator is expressed as

$$\sum_{x_1=a_1+1}^{s} \frac{x_1(n_2-s+x_1)}{s+1-x_1}\binom{n_1}{x_1}\binom{n_2}{s-x_1} \sum_{x_1=a_1+1}^{s}\binom{n_1}{x_1}\binom{n_2}{s-x_1}$$

$$+ (s+1)\binom{n_1}{s+1} \sum_{x_1=a_1+1}^{s}\binom{n_1}{x_1}\binom{n_2}{s-x_1}$$

$$- \sum_{x_1=a_1+1}^{s} x_1\binom{n_1}{x_1}\binom{n_2}{s-x_1} \sum_{x_1=a_1+1}^{s}\frac{n_2-s+x_1}{s+1-x_1}\binom{n_1}{x_1}\binom{n_2}{s-x_1}$$

$$- \binom{n_1}{s+1} \sum_{x_1=a_1+1}^{s} x_1\binom{n_1}{x_1}\binom{n_2}{s-x_1}.$$

The difference between the first and the third terms can be expressed as

$$\left\{ \sum_{x_1=a_1+1}^{s}\binom{n_1}{x_1}\binom{n_2}{s-x_1}\right\}^2 \text{cov}\left(X_1, \frac{n_2-s+X_1}{s+1-X_1}\right)$$

where the covariance is taken with respect to X_1 with mass function

$$h(x_1) = \frac{\binom{n_1}{x_1}\binom{n_2}{s-x_1}}{\sum_{x=a_1+1}^{s}\binom{n_1}{x}\binom{n_2}{s-x}}$$

for $a_1 + 1 \le x_1 \le s$. Since $(n_2 - s + X_1)/(s + 1 - X_1)$ increases in X_1, the covariance is positive. On the other hand, for the second and fourth terms,

$$(s+1) \sum_{x_1=a_1+1}^{s}\binom{n_1}{x_1}\binom{n_2}{s-x_1} > \sum_{x_1=a_1+1}^{s} x_1\binom{n_1}{x_1}\binom{n_2}{s-x_1}.$$

Hence, the numerator (as well as the denominator) of $n_1\{\hat{p}(2, s+1) - \hat{p}(2, s)\}$ is positive.

APPENDIX 3.D: Bias-Corrected Estimator Has Same Stochastic Ordering as MLE

We consider a two-stage design with design parameters $(n_1, n_2, a_1, b_1, a_2)$. Let $n = n_1 + n_2$. By Whitehead (1986), the bias-corrected estimator is obtained by solving

$$\tilde{p} = p + B(p) \tag{3.A.2}$$

with respect to p, where $B(p)$ is the bias of $\tilde{p}$ when the true response probability is p, that is,

$$B(p) = -\frac{n_2}{n_1 n} \sum_{x_1=a_1+1}^{b_1-1} (x_1 - n_1 p) \binom{n_1}{x_1} p^{x_1} (1-p)^{n_1-x_1};$$

see Jung and Kim (2004). From (3.A.2), it suffices to show that $p + B(p)$ is a strictly increasing function in $p \in (0, 1)$. The derivative of $p + B(p)$ with respect to p is

$$1 - \frac{n_2}{n_1 n p(1-p)} \sum_{x_1=a_1+1}^{b_1-1} \{(x_1 - n_1 p)^2 - n_1 p(1-p)\} \binom{n_1}{x_1} p^{x_1} (1-p)^{n_1-x_1}.$$

We have $a_1 + 1 \leq b_1 - 1$ for a two-stage design, so that the derivative for $p \in (0, 1)$ is larger than

$$1 - \frac{n_2}{n_1 n p(1-p)} \sum_{x_1=a_1+1}^{b_1-1} (x_1 - n_1 p)^2 \binom{n_1}{x_1} p^{x_1} (1-p)^{n_1-x_1}. \qquad (3.A.3)$$

Since

$$\sum_{x_1=a_1+1}^{b_1-1} (x_1 - n_1 p)^2 \binom{n_1}{x_1} p^{x_1} (1-p)^{n_1-x_1} < \sum_{x_1=0}^{n_1} (x_1 - n_1 p)^2 \binom{n_1}{x_1} p^{x_1} (1-p)^{n_1-x_1}$$

$$= n_1 p(1-p),$$

(3.A.3) is larger than $1 - n_2/n$, which is positive for a two-stage design. This completes the proof.

References

Armitage, P. (1958). Numerical studies in the sequential estimation of a binomial parameter. *Biometrika*, 45, 1–15.

Chang, M.N., Gould, A.L., and Snapinn, S.M. (1995). P-values for group sequential testing. *Biometrika*, 82, 650–654.

Chang, M.N. and O'Brien, PC. (1985). Confidence intervals following group sequential trials. *Controlled Clinical Trials*, 7, 18–26.

Chang, M.N., Therneau, T.M., Wieand, H.S., and Cha, S.S. (1987). Designs for group sequential phase II clinical trials. *Biometrics*, 43, 865–874.

Chang, M.N., Wieand, H.S., and Chang, V.T. (1989). The bias of the sample proportion following a group sequential phase II clinical trials. *Statistics in Medicine*, 8, 563–570.

Clopper, C.J. and Pearson, E.S. (1934). The use of confidence or fiducial limits illustrated in the case of the binomial. *Biometrika*, 26, 404–413.

Cook, T.D. (2002). *P*-value adjustment in sequential clinical trials. *Biometrics*, 58, 1005–1011.

Duffy, D.E. and Santner, T.J. (1987). Confidence intervals for a binomial parameter based on multistage tests. *Biometrics*, 43, 81–93.

Emerson, S.S. and Fleming, T.R. (1990). Parameter estimation following group sequential hypothesis testing. *Biometrika*, 77, 875–892.

Fleming, T.R. (1982). One sample multiple testing procedure for phase II clinical trials. *Biometrics*, 38, 143–151.

Girshick, M.A., Mosteller, F., and Savage, L.J. (1946). Unbiased estimates for certain binomial sampling problems with application. *Annals of Mathematical Statistics*, 17, 13–23.

Green, S.J. and Dahlberg, S. (1992). Planned versus attained design in phase II clinical trials. *Statistics in Medicine*, 11, 853–862.

Herndon, J. (1998). A design alternative for two-stage, phase II, multicenter cancer clinical trials. *Controlled Clinical Trials*, 19, 440–450.

Herson, J. (1979). Predictive probability early termination plans for phase II clinical trials. *Biometrics*, 35, 775–783.

Jennison, C. and Turnbull, B.W. (1983). Confidence intervals for a binomial parameter following a multistage test with application to MIL-STD 105D and medical trials. *Technometrics*, 25, 49–58.

Jung, S.H. and Kim, K.M. (2004). On the estimation of the binomial probability in multistage clinical trials. *Statistics in Medicine*, 23, 881–896.

Lehmann, E.L. (1983). *Theory of Point Estimation*. Wiley, New York.

Liu, A. and Hall, W.J. (1999). Unbiased estimation following a group sequential test. *Biometrika*, 86, 71–78.

Schultz, J.R., Nichol, F.R., Elfring, G.L., and Weed, S.D. (1973). Multistage procedures for drug screening. *Biometrics*, 29, 293–300.

Simon, R. (1989). Optimal two-stage designs for phase II clinical trials. *Controlled Clinical Trials*, 10, 1–10.

Tsiatis, A.A., Rosner, G.L., and Mehta, C.R. (1984). Exact confidence intervals following a group sequential test. *Biometrics*, 40, 797–803.

Whitehead, J. (1986). On the bias of maximum likelihood estimation following a sequential test. *Biometrika*, 73, 573–581.

Chapter 4

Single-Arm Phase II Clinical Trials with Time-to-Event Endpoints

The most popular primary endpoint in phase II cancer clinical trials is tumor response, resulting in a binary variable. Often, however, a time-to-event endpoint, such as time-to-disease progression or overall survival (meaning time to death by any cause) starting from registration, may be chosen as the primary endpoint of a phase II trial when a typical tumor response endpoint is not applicable or is not clinically relevant. For example, in studies involving blood cancers or in the case of surgical studies with adjuvant chemotherapies, where the tumor is completely resected, so that tumor response is not a meaningful endpoint. Also, cytostatic therapies are to prevent the growth of tumor rather than to shrink it, so that tumor response cannot be a good endpoint for phase II trials on experimental cytotoxic therapies. In these cases, a popular clinical outcome of interest may be the time to a specific event, such as disease progression or death. Because of loss to follow-up or termination of study, event times are subject to right censoring. Based on the standard terminology, we use time-to-event and survival time together regardless of the type of event, in this book.

Let $T_1, \ldots, T_n$, denoting the survival times for n patients who are treated by the experimental therapy of a single-arm phase II clinical trial, be independent and identically distributed random variables with a survival function $S(t) = P(T_i \geq t)$. Because of censoring, we observe $\{(X_i, \delta_i), i = 1, \ldots, n\}$ instead of survival times, where X_i denotes the minimum of survival time T_i and censoring time C_i, and $\delta_i = I(T_i \leq C_i)$ denotes the event indicator taking 1 if an event is observed and 0 otherwise. We assume that the survival and censoring times are independent. In this chapter, we discuss some design and analysis methods for single-arm phase II trials with a survival outcome as the primary endpoint.

4.1 A Test Based on Median Survival Time

Let θ denote the true median survival time for the study population. Then for the cumulative hazard function $\Lambda(t) = -\log S(t)$, we have $\Lambda(\theta) = \log 2$. By Nelson (1969), a consistent estimator of $\Lambda(t)$ is given as

$\hat{\Lambda}(t) = \int_0^t Y^{-1}(t) dN(t)$, where $Y(t) = \sum_{i=1}^n Y_i(t)$, $N(t) = \sum_{i=1}^n N_i(t)$, $Y_i(t) = I(X_i \geq t)$, and $N_i(t) = \delta_i I(X_i \leq t)$. Hence, a consistent estimator of θ is obtained by solving $\hat{\Lambda}(\theta) = \log 2$, or $\hat{S}(\theta) = 1/2$, where $\hat{S}(t)$ denotes the Kaplan–Meier (1958) estimator of $S(t)$.

For large n, $\sqrt{n}\{\hat{\Lambda}(\theta) - \log 2\}$ is approximately distributed as $N(0, \sigma^2)$, where

$$\sigma^2 = \int_0^\theta \frac{1}{S(t)G(t)} d\Lambda(t)$$

and $G(t) = P(C \geq t)$ is the survivor function of the censoring variable C. In deriving the asymptotic distribution of the test statistics on survival data in this chapter, we use the following asymptotic results from Fleming and Harrington (1991):

Theorem 4.1

Let $L_n(t)$ be a predictable process (i.e., a function generated by left-continuous functions) uniformly convergent to a square integrable function $\ell(t)$. Then, as $n \to \infty$, we have following results:

(a) *$n^{-1} \int_0^\infty L_n(t) dN(t)$ almost surely converges to $\int_0^\infty \ell(t) y(t) d\Lambda(t)$, where $y(t) = G(t)S(t)$ is the limit of $n^{-1}Y(t)$.*

(b) *$n^{-1/2} \int_0^\infty L_n(t) dM(t)$ converges to $N(0, v)$, where $dM(t) = dN(t) - Y(t) d\Lambda(t)$ and $v = \int_0^\infty \ell^2(t) y(t) d\Lambda(t)$, which can be consistently estimated by $\hat{v} = n^{-1} \int_0^\infty L_n^2(t) Y(t) d\hat{\Lambda}(t) = n^{-1} \int_0^\infty L_n^2(t) dN(t)$.*

4.1.1   Statistical Testing

For a chosen historical control with a median survival time θ_0, we want to test if the experimental therapy has a larger median survival time than θ_0. So, the associated statistical hypotheses are given as $H_0 : \theta = \theta_0$ and $H_1 : \theta > \theta_0$. Let $S_h(t)$ and $\Lambda_h(t)$ denote the survivor function and the cumulative hazard function, respectively, of the survival distribution under H_h ($h = 0, 1$). A cumulative hazard function is a monotonically increasing function, so that, if H_1 is true, $\Lambda(\theta_0) \to \Lambda_1(\theta_0) < \Lambda_1(\theta_1) = \log 2$, where θ_1 denotes the median survival time under H_1. Hence, we reject H_0 if

$$\frac{\sqrt{n}\{\hat{\Lambda}(\theta_0) - \log 2\}}{\hat{\sigma}} < -z_{1-\alpha},$$

where $z_{1-\alpha}$ is the $100(1-\alpha)$ percentile of the standard normal distribution and

$$\hat{\sigma}^2 = n \int_0^{\theta_0} \frac{dN(t)}{Y^2(t)}$$

is a consistent estimator of σ^2 under H_0 by Theorem 4.1(b), or refer to, for example, Fleming and Harrington (1991).

The test statistic is calculated by using

$$\hat{\Lambda}(\theta_0) = \sum_{i=1}^{n} \frac{\delta_i I(X_i \le \theta_0)}{\sum_{j=1}^{n} I(X_j \ge X_i)}$$

and

$$\hat{\sigma}^2 = n \sum_{i=1}^{n} \frac{\delta_i I(X_i \le \theta_0)}{\{\sum_{j=1}^{n} I(X_j \ge X_i)\}^2}.$$

Note that, for this testing, the maximum follow-up period of the study should be longer than θ_0. But a follow-up time longer than θ_0 does not have any impact on the testing result either. In this sense, we may consider following each subject for a period of θ_0 only, that is, $C_i = \theta_0$, if we are interested in the median survival time only.

This is a nonparametric test since the test statistic and its null distribution do not require any parametric model assumption. However, at the design stage, we have to assume a parametric survival model for sample size calculation as described in the following section.

4.1.2   Sample Size Calculation

The asymptotic distribution of median survival estimators has been widely investigated in the literature, including Brookmeyer and Crowley (1982) and Gardiner et al. (1986). Based on these results, a sample size formula for the median survival test can be summarized as follows. Let us suppose that we want to calculate a sample size n required for power $1 - \beta$ with respect to a specific alternative hypothesis $H_1 : \theta = \theta_1 (> \theta_0)$. It is easy to show that, under H_1, both the limit of $\hat{\sigma}^2$ and the variance of $\sqrt{n}\{\hat{\Lambda}(\theta_0) - \log 2\}$ are identically given as

$$\sigma^2 = \int_0^{\theta_0} \frac{d\Lambda_1(t)}{S_1(t)G(t)}.$$

Then, we have

$$1 - \beta = P\left(\frac{\sqrt{n}\{\hat{\Lambda}(\theta_0) - \log 2\}}{\hat{\sigma}} < -z_{1-\alpha} \middle| H_1 \right)$$

$$\approx P\left(\frac{\sqrt{n}\{\hat{\Lambda}(\theta_1) - \log 2\}}{\sigma} + \frac{\sqrt{n}\{\hat{\Lambda}(\theta_0) - \hat{\Lambda}(\theta_1)\}}{\sigma} < -z_{1-\alpha} \middle| H_1 \right).$$

Let $\Delta = \Lambda_1(\theta_0) - \Lambda_1(\theta_1) = \Lambda_1(\theta_0) - \log 2$. Under H_1, $\sqrt{n}\{\hat{\Lambda}(\theta_0) - \hat{\Lambda}(\theta_1)\}$ is approximated by $\sqrt{n}\Delta$, and

$$\frac{\sqrt{n}\{\hat{\Lambda}(\theta_1) - \log 2\}}{\sigma}$$

is asymptotically $N(0, 1)$. Hence, by solving the above equation, we obtain

$$n = \frac{\sigma^2 (z_{1-\alpha} + z_{1-\beta})^2}{\Delta^2}. \tag{4.1}$$

Formula (4.1) can be used to estimate a sample size based on any specified censoring and survival distributions. In the next section, we consider sample size calculation under some practical distributional assumptions.

4.1.2.1 Under Uniform Accrual and Exponential Survival Models

For a sample size calculation, we have to specify a survival distribution that is simple but well approximates the true distribution. Furthermore, we also have to specify the censoring distribution based on the expected accrual period and missing pattern. For a practical sample size, we may make following assumptions:

(A) Exponential survival distribution: $S(t) = \exp(-\lambda t)$ and $\Lambda(t) = \lambda t$ for a specified hazard rate λ. Given a median survival time θ, we have $\lambda = \theta^{-1} \log 2$.

(B) Uniform censoring distribution: Suppose that patients are expected to be recruited at a constant rate during accrual period a and will be followed for an additional period b after completion of the total accrual. Then, the censoring distribution is $U(b, a + b)$ with survivor function

$$G(t) = \begin{cases} 1 & \text{if } t \le b \\ -t/a + (a+b)/a & \text{if } b < t \le a + b. \\ 0 & \text{if } t > a + b \end{cases}$$

We assume no loss to follow-up due to dropout here.

The variance σ^2 can be calculated only when $G(\theta_0) > 0$. Thus, the follow-up period b should be chosen so that $a + b \ge \theta_0$. Under (A) and (B), we have

$$\sigma^2 = e^{\lambda_1 \theta_0} - 1$$

if $\theta_0 \le b$. On the other hand, if $b \le \theta_0 \le a + b$, then

$$\sigma^2 = e^{\lambda_1 b} - 1 + \lambda_1 \int_b^{\theta_0} \frac{e^{\lambda_1 t}}{(a+b)/a - t/b} dt. \tag{4.2}$$

The integration in the right-hand side can be calculated using a numerical method.

Note that if the additional follow-up period b is longer than θ_0, then the variance in (4.2), and consequently the sample size in (4.1), does not depend on the accrual period a. So, we can conduct the final data analysis when every patient is followed for θ_0 or experiences an event. If θ_0 is not too long, a reasonable choice for the additional follow-up period may be $b = \theta_0$. In this case, we have $\sigma^2 = e^{\lambda_1 \theta_0} - 1$. If $b < \theta_0$, however, the accrual period a should be so large that we need $a + b \geq \theta_0$. In this case, we may want to calculate the expected number of events at the time of data analysis: $D = n \times d$, where d is the probability for a patient to experience an event during the study, that is,

$$d = 1 - P(T > C|H_1) = 1 + \int_0^\infty S_1(t)dG(t) = 1 - \frac{\exp(-b\lambda_1)}{a\lambda_1}\{1 - \exp(-a\lambda_1)\},$$

where $\lambda_1 = \theta_1^{-1} \log 2$.

The assumptions (A) and (B) can be easily extended to a nonexponential survival model and a nonuniform censoring distribution. Typically, in well-designed and well-conducted clinical trials collecting survival times, we do not observe many cases of loss to follow-up during the study, so that most censored cases are administrative. In this sense, we assume no loss to follow-up by (B). If one expects a large proportion of dropouts, it can be easily reflected in the sample size calculation. Let E denote the time to loss to follow-up from entry with a specific distribution, such as an exponential distribution, and $\tilde{C}$ denote the time to administrative censoring whose distribution is determined by accrual and follow-up periods; then the censoring variable for each patient is given as $C = \min(E, \tilde{C})$ with a survivor function $G(t) = P(E > t)P(\tilde{C} > t)$ since the loss to follow-up of a patient is usually independent of the administrative censoring. Suppose that $\tilde{C} \tilde{U}(b, a + b)$ as in (B) and E follows an exponential distribution with hazard rate λ_E. Then we have

$$G(t) = \begin{cases} \exp(-\lambda_E t) & \text{if } t \leq b \\ (1 + b/a - t/b)\exp(-\lambda_E t) & \text{if } b < t \leq a + b \, . \\ 0 & \text{if } t > a + b \end{cases}$$

Example 4.1
Suppose that the median progression-free survival (PFS) for a standard therapy is known to be $\theta_0 = 1$ year. We will be interested in the experimental therapy if its median PFS is $\theta_1 = 1.5$ years or longer. Under the exponential PFS model, we have corresponding hazard rates $\lambda_0 = 0.693$ and $\lambda_1 = 0.462$. Assuming no loss to follow-up and $b = 1(= \theta_0)$ year of follow-up for each patient, we need $n = 73$ patients for $1 - \beta = 90\%$ power by the median survival test with one-sided $\alpha = 10\%$. A simulation study is conducted to investigate the small sample performance of the testing and sample size calculation method. The test statistic was applied to each of $B = 10{,}000$ simulation samples with $n = 73$ that were generated under the design settings. The empirical type I error rate and power were 11.8% and 86%, respectively. The sample size for the median survival test seems to be slightly underpowered.

4.1.2.2   When Accrual Rate Is Given

Recall that, if the follow-up period of each patient is longer than θ_0 (that is, $b > \theta_0$), the required sample size does not depend on the the accrual period a (or accrual rate). However, if the additional follow-up period b is not so long that $b < \theta_0$ ($\leq a + b$), then the variance in (4.2), and consequently the sample size in (4.1), depends on the accrual period a. In this case, the above sample size formula is required to specify an accrual period a. When designing a clinical trial, however, we usually can estimate an expected accrual rate r, rather than an accrual period a, based on the number of patients accrued from the member sites recently. In this case, assumption (B) should be replaced by

(B′) Patients are accrued following a Poisson distribution with rate r, and are followed for a period b after the completion of accrual.

With $(r, \lambda_0, \lambda_1, \alpha, 1 - \beta, b)$ specified, $\sigma = \sigma(a)$ is a function of a as given in (4.2). Hence, under (A) and (B), (4.1) is expressed as

$$n = \frac{\sigma^2(a)(z_{1-\alpha} + z_{1-\beta})^2}{\Delta^2}. \tag{4.3}$$

On the other hand, under the Poisson accrual distribution (B′), we have

$$n = a \times r. \tag{4.4}$$

Now, we have two equations (4.3) and (4.4) with two unknowns n and a. Let a^* denote the solution to the equation that is obtained by equating the right-hand sides of (4.3) and (4.4), that is,

$$a \times r = \frac{\sigma^2(a)(z_{1-\alpha} + z_{1-\beta})^2}{\Delta^2}.$$

Finally, given an accrual rate r (instead of an accrual period a), we obtain the required sample size by $n = a^* \times r$. This equation is solved by a numerical method such as the bisection method. Note that, at each replication, the accrual period a should be large enough that the total study period is no smaller than θ_0, that is, $a + b \geq \theta_0$, and σ^2 is calculable. If θ_0 is so large that the solution a^* to the equation is too large, then the median survival method is not appropriate for a phase II trial.

4.2   Maximum Likelihood Method for Exponential Distribution

Since the family of exponential distributions is indexed by only one parameter (hazard rate) and the distributions of most real survival data are closely approximated by exponential distributions, these distributions have been widely used for parametric analysis of survival data or as a hypothetical model in the sample size calculation of nonparametric analysis method. In this section, we discuss design and analysis methods of phase II trials based on exponential maximum likelihood estimator (MLE). This approach can be easily extended to other survival distribution models, such as Weibull distribution.

Suppose that the survival times of n subjects $T_1, \ldots, T_n$ are IID random variables with hazard rate λ whose survival and probability density functions are given as $f(t) = \lambda \exp(-\lambda t)$ and $S(t) = \exp(-\lambda t)$ for $t \geq 0$, respectively. With the observed survival data $\{(X_i, \delta_i), i = 1, \ldots, n\}$, the log-likelihood function is given by

$$l(\lambda) = \log \prod_{i=1}^{n} \left\{ f(X_i)^{\delta_i} S(X_i)^{1-\delta_i} \right\} = \log(\lambda) \sum_{i=1}^{n} \delta_i - \lambda \sum_{i=1}^{n} X_i.$$

From this likelihood function, the MLE of λ is obtained as

$$\hat{\lambda} = \frac{D}{X},$$

where $D = \sum_{i=1}^{n} \delta_i$ denotes the total number of events and $X = \sum_{i=1}^{n} X_i$ denotes the total observed survival time. By the standard procedure on MLE, $\hat{\lambda}$ is asymptotically normal with mean λ and variance λ^2/D.

By Miller (1981), the normality approximation is improved by taking a log-transformation of the MLE. That is, by applying the delta method to this result, we can show that $\log \hat{\lambda}$ is approximately normal with mean $\log \lambda$ and variance $1/D$. Alternatively, Sprott (1973) proposes another transformation $\hat{\lambda}^{1/3}$ to improve the normality. We consider the log-transformed estimator in this section.

4.2.1 Statistical Testing

Suppose that the survival distribution of a chosen historical control is known to have a hazard rate of λ_0. We want to test $H_0 : \lambda = \lambda_0$ versus $H_1 : \lambda < \lambda_0$. By Miller (1981), $\sqrt{D}(\log \hat{\lambda} - \log \lambda_0)$ is approximately $N(0, 1)$ under H_0. So, we reject H_0 in favor of H_1 if $\sqrt{D}(\log \hat{\lambda} - \log \lambda_0) < -z_{1-\alpha}$.

4.2.2 Sample Size Calculation

Let $\lambda_1 (< \lambda_0)$ denote a hazard rate which is a clinically meaningful improvement from λ_0 for the experimental therapy. We want to estimate the required sample size for a specified power under $H_1 : \lambda = \lambda_1$. Given a number of events D, the power function is given as

$$1 - \beta = P\{\sqrt{D}(\log \hat{\lambda} - \log \lambda_0) < -z_{1-\alpha} | H_1\}$$
$$= P\{\sqrt{D}(\log \hat{\lambda} - \log \lambda_1) < \sqrt{D} \log \Delta - z_{1-\alpha} | H_1\},$$

where $\Delta = \lambda_0/\lambda_1$ denotes the hazard ratio. Since $\sqrt{D}(\log\hat{\lambda} - \log\lambda_1)$ is approximately $N(0, 1)$ under H_1, the required number of events for power $1 - \beta$ is obtained by

$$D = \frac{(z_{1-\alpha} + z_{1-\beta})^2}{(\log\Delta)^2}. \tag{4.5}$$

Let $d = P(T \le C|\lambda_1)$ denote the probability that a patient has an event during the study. Since $D = n \times d$, from (4.5), the required sample size is obtained as

$$n = \frac{(z_{1-\alpha} + z_{1-\beta})^2}{d(\log\Delta)^2}. \tag{4.6}$$

For a specified survivor function of a specified censoring distribution $G(t) = P(C \ge t)$, we calculate

$$d = 1 - \mathrm{P}(T > C|H_1) = E\{1 - \exp(-\lambda_1 C)\} = 1 + \int_0^\infty e^{-\lambda_1 t} dG(t).$$

4.2.2.1   Under a Uniform Accrual Model

Suppose that patients are accrued at a constant rate during accrual period a and followed for an additional period b. Then, the censoring distribution is $U(b, a + b)$ with

$$G(t) = \begin{cases} 1 & \text{if } t \le b \\ -t/a + (a+b)/a & \text{if } b < t \le a+b \\ 0 & \text{if } t > a+b \end{cases}$$

In this case, we have

$$d = 1 - \frac{e^{-\lambda_1 b}}{\lambda_1 a}(1 - e^{-\lambda_1 a}). \tag{4.7}$$

4.2.2.2   When Accrual Rate Is Known

Suppose that the accrual rate r is known instead of accrual period a. In this case, the accrual period a is an unknown output variable at a sample size calculation. From (4.7), $d = d(a) = 1 - e^{-\lambda b}(1 - e^{-\lambda a})/(\lambda a)$ is a function of the accrual period a. By replacing $n = a \times r$ in (4.6), we obtain the required accrual period a^* by solving

$$a \times r \times d(a) = \frac{(z_{1-\alpha} + z_{1-\beta})^2}{(\log\Delta)^2} \tag{4.8}$$

with respect to a. We solve the equation using a numerical method such as the bisection method. Finally, the required sample size is calculated by $n = a^* \times r$.

Example 4.2

Suppose that the median progression-free survival for a standard therapy is known to be 1 year. We will be interested in the experimental therapy if its median PFS is 1.5 years or longer. Under the exponential PFS model, we have $\lambda_0 = 0.693$ and $\lambda_1 = 0.462$ ($\Delta = 1.5$). For one-sided $\alpha = 10\%$ test $1-\beta = 90\%$ power ($z_{1-\alpha} = 1.282 = z_{1-\beta} = 1.282$), the required number of events at the analysis from (4.5) is given as

$$D = \frac{(1.282 + 1.282)^2}{(\log 1.5)^2} = 40.$$

This trial is expected to accrue about 5 patients per month (or $r = 60$ patients per year) based on the recent accrual rate of patients at the study institution. Assuming $b = 1$ year of additional follow-up after completion of patient accrual, we have from (4.7)

$$d(a) = 1 - \frac{e^{-1.5}}{1.5a}(1 - e^{-1.5a}).$$

By plugging this in (4.8), we solve

$$60a\left\{1 - \frac{e^{-1.5}}{1.5a}(1 - e^{-1.5a})\right\} = 40$$

to obtain $a^* = 1.272$ years or $n = 1.272 \times 60 = 77$ patients. The total study will take about 28 months for 16 months of patient accrual and 12 months of additional follow-up period. A simulation study is conducted to investigate the small sample performance of the testing and sample size calculation methods. The test statistic was applied to each of $B = 10,000$ simulation samples with $n = 77$ that were generated under the design settings. The empirical type I error rate and power were 9% and 92.3%, respectively, which are close to their nominal levels.

4.3 One-Sample Log-Rank Test

The median survival test in the previous section and the test on t-year survival in Section 4.5 use the survival estimate at only one time point, so that they may lose statistical efficiency by not fully using the entire information from survival data. While the exponential MLE test uses the whole information on the data, its performance strongly depends on the validity of the parametric model assumption for given a data set. In order to tackle these issues, we propose to use the one-sample log-rank test that was investigated by, for example, Berry (1983) and Finkelstein et al. (2003).

4.3.1 Statistical Testing

Let $\Lambda_0(t)$ denote the cumulative hazard function of a historical control that is chosen for a new single-arm phase II trial. If the historical control data come from a previous study, $\Lambda_0(t)$ may be the Nelson–Aalen estimate (Nelson 1969; Aalen 1978) from the data. Let $\Lambda(t)$ denote the cumulative hazard function of an experimental therapy that will be observed from the new phase II trial. We want to test $H_0 : \Lambda(t) = \Lambda_0(t)$ against $H_1 : \Lambda(t) < \Lambda_0(t)$ for $t > 0$.

Under H_0 for large n,

$$W = n^{-1/2} \sum_{i=1}^{n} \int_0^\infty \{dN_i(t) - Y_i(t)d\Lambda_0(t)\}$$

is approximately normal with mean 0 and its variance can be consistently estimated by

$$\hat{\sigma}^2 = n^{-1} \sum_{i=1}^{n} \int_0^\infty Y_i(t)d\Lambda_0(t).$$

Hence, we reject H_0 with one-sided type I error rate α if $Z = W/\hat{\sigma} < -z_{1-\alpha}$ (Finkelstein et al. 2003).

Note that the standardized test statistic, $W/\hat{\sigma}$ is expressed as

$$Z = \frac{O - E}{\sqrt{E}},$$

where $O = \sum_{i=1}^{n} \int_0^\infty dN_i(t) = \sum_{i=1}^{n} \delta_i$ denotes the observed number of events. On the other hand, under H_0, $n^{-1} \sum_{i=1}^{n} Y_i(t) \to S_0(t)G(t)$ uniformly, so that $E = \sum_{i=1}^{n} \int_0^\infty Y_i(t)d\Lambda_0(t) = \sum_{i=1}^{n} \Lambda_0(X_i)$ is asymptotically identical to $-n \int_0^\infty G(t)dS_0(t)$, which is the expected number of events under H_0. If the historical control has an exponential survival distribution, we have $\tilde{E} = \lambda_0 \sum_{i=1}^{n} X_i$. Hence, the exponential MLE test with no transformation in the previous section is similarly expressed as

$$\frac{O - \tilde{E}}{\tilde{E}/\sqrt{O}}.$$

Note that D and $\lambda_0 X$ in the previous section are denoted as O and $\tilde{E}$ in this section, respectively.

4.3.2 Sample Size Calculation

We calculate the required sample size n for a specified power under a specific alternative hypothesis $H_1 : \Lambda(t) = \Lambda_1(t)(< \Lambda_0(t))$. Under H_1, $n^{-1} \sum_{i=1}^{n} Y_i(t)$ uniformly converges to $G(t)S_1(t)$, so that $\hat{\sigma}^2$ converges to

$$\sigma_0^2 = \int_0^\infty G(t)S_1(t)d\Lambda_0(t). \qquad (4.9)$$

On the other hand, we have

$$W = \frac{1}{\sqrt{n}} \sum_{i=1}^{n} \int_0^{\infty} \{dN_i(t) - Y_i(t)d\Lambda_1(t)\} + \frac{1}{\sqrt{n}} \sum_{i=1}^{n} \int_0^{\infty} Y_i(t)d\{\Lambda_1(t) - \Lambda_0(t)\},$$

so that, under H_1, W is approximately normal with mean

$$\sqrt{n}\omega \equiv \sqrt{n} \int_0^{\infty} G(t)S_1(t)d\{\Lambda_1(t) - \Lambda_0(t)\}$$

and variance $\text{var}(W) = \text{var}(n^{-1/2} \sum_{i=1}^{n} \epsilon_i)$, where

$$\epsilon_i = \int_0^{\infty} \{dN_i(t) - Y_i(t)d\Lambda_1(t)\} + \int_0^{\infty} Y_i(t)d\{\Lambda_1(t) - \Lambda_0(t)\}$$

$$= \int_0^{\infty} \{dN_i(t) - Y_i(t)d\Lambda_1(t)\} + \{\Lambda_1(X_i) - \Lambda_0(X_i)\}.$$

In order to simplify the calculation of $\text{var}(W)$ under H_1, we assume that $\Lambda_1(t)$ and $\Lambda_0(t)$ are close. Under this assumption, the second term of ϵ_i is ignorable and $\text{var}(W)$ under H_1 is approximated by

$$\sigma_1^2 = \int_0^{\infty} G(t)S_1(t)d\Lambda_1(t) = -\int_0^{\infty} G(t)dS_1(t) \tag{4.10}$$

by Theorem 4.1, note that σ_1^2 equals the probability that a patient has an event during the study period when H_1 is true, and $\omega = \sigma_1^2 - \sigma_0^2$.

Hence, we have the power function

$$1 - \beta = P(W/\hat{\sigma} < -z_{1-\alpha}|H_1) = P\left(\frac{W - \sqrt{n}\omega}{\sigma_1} \times \frac{\sigma_1}{\sigma_0} < -\frac{\sqrt{n}\omega}{\sigma_0} - z_{1-\alpha}|H_1\right).$$

By solving this equation and replacing $\omega = \sigma_1^2 - \sigma_0^2$, we obtain the required sample size

$$n = \frac{(\sigma_0 z_{1-\alpha} + \sigma_1 z_{1-\beta})^2}{(\sigma_0^2 - \sigma_1^2)^2}. \tag{4.11}$$

Although the one-sample log-rank test is nonparametric, its sample size calculation requires specification of survival and censoring distributions. We now derive sample size formulas under some practical design settings.

4.3.2.1   Under Proportional Hazards Model Assumption

Under a proportional hazards model assumption, $\Lambda_0(t) = \Delta\Lambda_1(t)$, and from (4.9) and (4.10), we have $\sigma_0^2 = \Delta\sigma_1^2$. Also, since σ_1^2 equals the probability that a patient has an event during the study period, from (4.11), the required number of events $D = n\sigma_1^2$ is expressed as

$$D = \frac{(\sqrt{\Delta}z_{1-\alpha} + z_{1-\beta})^2}{(\Delta - 1)^2}. \tag{4.12}$$

Note that a calculation of the required number of events does not require specification of any parametric models for the survival and censoring distributions. However, calculation of a sample size $n = D/\sigma_1^2$ requires specification of these distributions to calculate σ_1^2.

4.3.2.2   Under Uniform Accrual and Exponential Survival Models

For a practical sample size calculation, we assume that the survival distribution of the experimental therapy is exponential with hazard rate λ_0 under H_0 and λ_1 under H_1. The survival functions are given as $S_0(t) = \exp(-\lambda_0 t)$ and $S_1(t) = \exp(-\lambda_1 t)$, respectively. Under exponential models for survival distributions, we have a proportional hazards model, $\Delta = \lambda_0/\lambda_1$.

Assuming that patients are accrued at a constant rate during period a and followed for an additional period of b, the censoring distribution is given as $U(b, a + b)$ with a survivor function $G(t) = P(C \geq t) = 1$ if $t \leq b$; $= (a + b)/a - t/a$ if $b \leq t \leq a + b$; $= 0$ otherwise.

Under a proportional hazards model, by using (4.12), a sample size estimation requires to calculate only σ_1^2 based on the distributional assumptions:

$$\sigma_1^2 = \lambda_1 \int_0^b e^{-\lambda_1 t}\,dt + \frac{\lambda_1(a+b)}{a} \int_b^{a+b} e^{-\lambda_1 t}\,dt - \frac{\lambda_1}{a} \int_b^{a+b} t e^{-\lambda_1 t}\,dt$$

$$= 1 - e^{-\lambda_1 b} + \left(1 + \frac{b}{a}\right)\left(e^{-\lambda_1 b} - e^{-\lambda_1(a+b)}\right) - \frac{1}{a}\{be^{-\lambda_1 b} - (a+b)e^{-\lambda_1(a+b)}\}$$

$$- \frac{1}{a\lambda_1}\left(e^{-\lambda_1 b} - e^{-\lambda_1(a+b)}\right) = 1 - \frac{e^{-\lambda_1 b}}{a\lambda_1}\left(1 - e^{-\lambda_1 a}\right). \tag{4.13}$$

Hence, by combining $n = D/\sigma_1^2$, (4.12) and (4.13), we obtain

$$n = \frac{(\sqrt{\Delta}z_{1-\alpha} + z_{1-\beta})^2}{\sigma_1^2(\Delta - 1)^2}. \tag{4.14}$$

4.3.2.3   When Accrual Rate Is Given

Now, we consider a sample size calculation when the accrual rate r is given instead of the accrual period a. From (4.13), $\sigma_1^2 = \sigma_1^2(a)$ is a function of the unknown variable a. By replacing n with $a \times r$ in (4.14), we obtain an equation a,

$$a \times r \times \sigma_1^2(a) = \left(\frac{\sqrt{\Delta}z_{1-\alpha} + z_{1-\beta}}{\Delta - 1}\right)^2$$

or simply

$$a \times r \times \sigma_1^2(a) = D \tag{4.15}$$

from $n\sigma_1^2 = D$. In order to use (4.15), we should calculate D using (4.12) first. We solve one of these equations using a numerical method such as the bisection method. Let a^* denote the solution to one of these equations. Then the required sample size is obtained as $n = a^* \times r$.

Example 4.3

Suppose that the PFS for a standard therapy has the exponential distribution with a median of $\theta_0 = 1$ year. We will be interested in the experimental therapy if its median PFS is $\theta_1 = 1.5$ years or longer ($\lambda_0 = 0.693$ and $\lambda_1 = 0.462$). So, we have $\Delta = \lambda_0/\lambda_1 = \theta_1/\theta_0 = 1.5$. We want to design a study to detect this improvement in PFS by the experimental therapy with $1 - \beta = 90\%$ power using the one-sample log-rank test with one-sided $\alpha = 10\%$ ($z_{1-\alpha} = 1.282 = z_{1-\beta} = 1.282$). From (4.12), the required number of events is obtained as

$$D = \frac{(1.282\sqrt{1.5} + 1.282)^2}{(1.5 - 1)^2} = 32.5.$$

Further, suppose that this trial is expected to accrue about 5 patients per month (or $r = 60$ per year) based on the recent accrual rate of patients at the study institution. Assuming $b = 1$ year of additional follow-up after completion of patient accrual, equation (4.15), combined with equation (4.13), is expressed as

$$60a \left\{ 1 - \frac{e^{-0.462}}{0.462a}(1 - e^{-0.462a}) \right\} = 32.5.$$

By solving this equation with respect to a, we obtain an accrual period of $a^* = 1.077$ years (or 13 months), and a required sample size of $n = a^* \times r = 1.077 \times 60 = 65$. The expected total study period is $a^* + b = 25$ months. From $B = 10,000$ simulations with $n = 65$, we observed an empirical type I error of 9.3% and power of 87.7%.

4.4   Two-Stage Trials Using One-Sample Log-Rank Test

The previous sections in this chapter consider single-stage designs. In this section, we investigate design and analysis methods for two-stage phase II trials using the one-sample log-rank test that was discussed in the previous section. The other survival testing methods can be similarly extended to two-stage designs. We consider an interim analysis only for futility testing as in most traditional phase II trials, but one with efficacy only or with both futility and efficacy can be similarly derived.

4.4.1   Two-Stage One-Sample Log-Rank Test

Suppose that n_l patients are treated by the experimental therapy during stage $l(= 1, 2)$. Let $n = n_1 + n_2$ denote the maximal sample size. We conduct an interim analysis at time τ, which may be determined in terms of number of events or by calendar time. In order to avoid treating too many patients when the experimental therapy is shown to be inefficacious, we assume that τ is smaller than the planned accrual period a.

For subject $i(= 1, \ldots, n)$, let T_i denote the survival time with survival distribution $S_h(t)$ and cumulative hazard function $\Lambda_h(t)$ under H_h $(h = 0, 1)$, and e_i denote the entering time $(0 \le e_i \le a)$. Let C_i denote the censoring time at the end of stage 2 with survivor function $G(t) = P(C_i \ge t)$ that is defined by the accrual trend and additional follow-up period. The censoring time at the interim analysis is denoted as $C_{1i} = \max\{\min(\tau - e_i, C_i), 0\}$. If patient i enters the study during stage 1 (that is, $e_i < \tau$), then the censoring variable at the interim analysis has a survivor function $G_1(t) = P\{\min(\tau - e_i, C_i) \ge t\}$.

The observed survival data are expressed as (X_{1i}, δ_{1i}) at the interim analysis and (X_i, δ_i) at the final analysis, where $X_{1i} = \min(T_i, C_{1i})$, $\delta_{1i} = I(T_i \le C_{1i})$, $X_i = \min(T_i, C_i)$, and $\delta_i = I(T_i \le C_i)$. We define at-risk processes $Y_{1i}(t) = I(X_{1i} \ge t)$ and $Y_i(t) = I(X_i \ge t)$, and event processes $N_{1i}(t) = \delta_{1i} I(X_{1i} \le t)$ and $N_i(t) = \delta_i I(X_i \le t)$.

Test statistics at the interim and final analyses are expressed as

$$W_1 = n_1^{-1/2} \sum_{i=1}^{n} \int_0^{\infty} \{dN_{1i}(t) - Y_{1i}(t)d\Lambda_0(t)\}$$

and

$$W = n^{-1/2} \sum_{i=1}^{n} \int_0^{\infty} \{dN_i(t) - Y_i(t)d\Lambda_0(t)\},$$

respectively. For large n_1 and n, the distribution of (W_1, W) under H_0 is approximately bivariate normal with means 0, and variances and covariance that can be approximated by

$$\hat{\sigma}_1^2 = n_1^{-1} \sum_{i=1}^{n} \int_0^{\infty} Y_{1i}(t)d\Lambda_0(t),$$

$$\hat{\sigma}^2 = n^{-1} \sum_{i=1}^{n} \int_0^{\infty} Y_i(t)d\Lambda_0(t),$$

and $\mathrm{cov}(W_1, W) = \hat{\sigma}_1^2$, respectively; see, for example, Tsiatis (1982).

Note that n_1 denotes the number of patients who have entered the study before the interim analysis time τ, that is, $n_1 = \sum_{i=1}^{n} I(e_i \le \tau)$. In the interim analysis, the patients who have not entered the study yet (that is, $e_i > \tau$) have their survival times censored at time 0 (that is, $X_{1i} = 0$ and $\delta_{1i} = 0$), so that they make no contributions to W_1 and $\hat{\sigma}_1^2$. A two-stage trial using the one-sample log-rank test is conducted as follows:

- *Design stage*: Specify $\Lambda_0(t)$ and α, together with an interim analysis time and an early stopping value c_1.
- *Stage 1*: If $W_1/\hat{\sigma}_1 \geq c_1$, then reject the experimental therapy and stop the trial. Otherwise, proceed to Stage 2.
- *Stage 2*: If $W/\hat{\sigma} < c$, then accept the experimental therapy. Here, the critical value c satisfies

$$\alpha = P\left(\frac{W_1}{\hat{\sigma}_1} \leq c_1, \frac{W}{\hat{\sigma}} \leq c \Big| H_0\right). \tag{4.16}$$

Noting that conditioning on $W = w$, W_1 is approximately normal with mean $\hat{\rho}w$ and variance $1 - \hat{\rho}$, we approximate equation (4.16) by

$$\alpha = \int_{-\infty}^{c} \phi(w)\Phi\left(\frac{c_1 - \hat{\rho}w}{\sqrt{1 - \hat{\rho}^2}}\right) dw,$$

where $\hat{\rho} = \hat{\sigma}_1/\hat{\sigma}$, and $\phi(\cdot)$ and $\Phi(\cdot)$ are the probability density and cumulative distribution functions of the $N(0, 1)$ distribution, respectively.

4.4.2   Sample Size Calculation

At first we derive a power function given τ and c_1 together with the accrual period a, follow-up period b, $\Lambda_h(t)$ for $h = 0, 1$, and $(\alpha, 1 - \beta)$. The interim analysis time τ may be determined in terms of calendar time or number of events observed, but at the design stage, we should specify it as a calendar time. If we want to specify it in terms of the number of events at the design stage, we can convert it to a calendar time based on the expected accrual rate and the specified survival distribution. We often choose $c_1 = 0$; that is, we stop the trial early if the experimental therapy does no better than the historical control. But we can choose any value for c_1, depending on how aggressively we want to screen out the experimental therapy at the interim analysis.

The power function is given as

$$1 - \beta = P\left(\frac{W_1}{\hat{\sigma}_1} \leq c_1, \frac{W}{\hat{\sigma}} \leq c \Big| H_1\right).$$

Before deriving a power function, we have to calculate c for a specified type I error rate α, that is,

$$\alpha = P\left(\frac{W_1}{\hat{\sigma}_1} \leq c_1, \frac{W}{\hat{\sigma}} \leq c \Big| H_0\right).$$

So, for a power calculation, we need to derive the limits of $\hat{\sigma}_1^2$ and $\hat{\sigma}^2$ under H_0 and H_1, and $\omega_1 = E(W_1)$, $\omega = E(W)$, var(W_1) and var(W) under H_1.

Under H_0, we have $E(W_1) = E(W) = 0$, and $\hat{\sigma}_1^2$ and $\hat{\sigma}^2$ converge to

$$v_1 = -\int_0^\infty G_1(t)dS_0(t)$$

and

$$v = -\int_0^\infty G(t)dS_0(t),$$

respectively. Note that var$(W_1) = v_1$ and var$(W) = v$ under H_0. By independent increment of the one-sample log-rank statistic, corr(W_1, W) is given as $\rho_0 = \sqrt{v_1/v}$.

Under H_1, we have $E(W_1) = \sqrt{n_1}\omega_1$ and $E(W) = \sqrt{n}\omega$, where

$$\omega_1 = \int_0^\infty G_1(t)S_1(t)d\{\Lambda_1(t) - \Lambda_0(t)\}$$

and

$$\omega = \int_0^\infty G(t)S_1(t)d\{\Lambda_1(t) - \Lambda_0(t)\}.$$

Further, $\hat{\sigma}_1^2$ and $\hat{\sigma}^2$ converge to

$$\sigma_{01}^2 = -\int_0^\infty G_1(t)S_1(t)d\Lambda_0(t)$$

and

$$\sigma_0^2 = -\int_0^\infty G(t)S_1(t)d\Lambda_0(t),$$

respectively. The variances of W_1 and W are given as

$$\sigma_{11}^2 = -\int_0^\infty G_1(t)dS_1(t)$$

and

$$\sigma_1^2 = -\int_0^\infty G(t)dS_1(t),$$

respectively, under H_1. By independent increment of the one-sample log-rank statistic, corr(W_1, W) is given as $\rho_1 = \sigma_{11}/\sigma_1$. Note that $\omega_1 = \sigma_{11}^2 - \sigma_{01}^2$ and $\omega = \sigma_1^2 - \sigma_0^2$, and σ_{11}^2 is the probability that a patient who is accrued during stage 1 experiences an event before the interim analysis time, and σ_1^2 is the probability that a patient in the study experiences an event before the final analysis time. Hence, the expected numbers of events are calculated as $D_1 = n_1\sigma_{11}^2$ and $D = n\sigma_1^2$ at the two analysis times, respectively.

If (X, Y) is a bivariate normal random vector with means μ_x and μ_y, variances σ_x^2 and σ_y^2, and correlation coefficient ρ, then it is well known that the conditional distribution of X given $Y = y$ is normal with mean $\mu_x + (\rho\sigma_x/\sigma_y)(y - \mu_y)$ and variance $\sigma_x^2(1 - \rho^2)$. This result simplifies the calculation of type I error probability and power below.

If the interim analysis time τ and the stopping value c_1 are reasonably chosen, the power of a two-stage design is not much lower than that of the corresponding single-stage design. So, when searching for the required accrual period (or sample size) of a two-stage design, we may start from the accrual period for the single-stage design. Assuming an accrual pattern with a uniform rate, the design procedure of two-stage designs can be summarized as follows:

- Given $(\alpha, 1-\beta, r, b, \Lambda_0(t), \Lambda_1(t))$, calculate the sample size n and accrual period a_0 required for a single-stage design.

- Determine an interim analysis time τ during the accrual period a_0 of the chosen single-stage design (that is, $\tau < a_0$) and the stopping value c_1 at the interim analysis.

- The accrual period required for a two-stage design is obtained around a_0 as follows:

At $a = a_0$ (note that $n_1 = r\tau$ and $n = ra_0$),

    (a) Obtain c by solving, the equation

$$\alpha = \int_{-\infty}^{c} \phi(z)\Phi\left(\frac{c_1 - \rho_0 z}{\sqrt{1 - \rho_0^2}}\right) dz.$$

    (b) Given (n_1, n, c_1, c, α), calculate

$$\text{power} = \int_{-\infty}^{\bar{c}} \phi(z)\Phi\left(\frac{\bar{c}_1 - \rho_1 z}{\sqrt{1 - \rho_1^2}}\right) dz$$

    where

$$\bar{c}_1 = \frac{\sigma_{01}}{\sigma_{11}}\left(c_1 - \frac{\omega_1\sqrt{n_1}}{\sigma_{01}}\right) \quad \text{and} \quad \bar{c} = \frac{\sigma_0}{\sigma_1}\left(c - \frac{\omega\sqrt{n}}{\sigma_0}\right).$$

- If the power is smaller than $1 - \beta$, increase a slightly, and repeat the above procedure until the power is close enough to $1-\beta$. We may want to change the interim analysis time τ when repeating the above procedure with a different accrual period a.

4.4.2.1   Under Uniform Accrual and Exponential Survival Models

Suppose that the survival distribution is exponential with a hazard rate λ_0 under H_0 and λ_1 under H_1. If patients are accrued at a constant rate during period a and followed for an additional period of b, and the interim analysis takes place before completion of patient accrual (that is, $\tau < a$), then the censoring distribution at the interim analysis is $U(0, \tau)$ and that at final analysis is $U(b, a + b)$, for which the survivor functions are given as

$$G_1(t) = \begin{cases} 1 & \text{if } t \leq 0 \\ 1 - t/\tau & \text{if } 0 < t \leq \tau \\ 0 & \text{if } t > \tau \end{cases}$$

and

$$G(t) = \begin{cases} 1 & \text{if } t \leq b \\ -t/a + (a + b)/a & \text{if } b < t \leq a + b, \\ 0 & \text{if } t > a + b \end{cases}$$

respectively. Note that we assume administrative censoring only. If loss to follow-up is expected, then we may incorporate it in the calculation if its distribution can be modeled as in Section 4.1, or we may increase the final sample size by the expected proportion of loss to follow-up.

Under these assumptions, it is easy to show that

$$v_1 = 1 - (1 - e^{-\lambda_0 \tau})/(\tau \lambda_0),$$

$$v = 1 - (1 - e^{-\lambda_0 a})e^{-\lambda_0 b}/(a\lambda_0),$$

$$\sigma_{11}^2 = 1 - (1 - e^{-\lambda_1 \tau})/(\tau \lambda_1),$$

$$\sigma_1^2 = 1 - (1 - e^{-\lambda_1 a})e^{-\lambda_1 b}/(a\lambda_1),$$

$\sigma_{01}^2 = \Delta \sigma_{11}^2$, and $\sigma_0^2 = \Delta \sigma_1^2$, where $\Delta = \lambda_0/\lambda_1$, $\rho_0 = \sqrt{v_1/v}$, $\rho_1 = \sigma_{11}/\sigma_1$, $\bar{c}_1 = c_1 \sqrt{\Delta} - \sigma_{11}(1 - \Delta)\sqrt{n_1}$, and $\bar{c} = c\sqrt{\Delta} - \sigma_1(1 - \Delta)\sqrt{n}$.

Example 4.4

Suppose that the PFS for a standard therapy (historical control) has the exponential distribution with a median of 1 year ($\lambda_0 = 0.693$). We will be interested in the experimental therapy if its median PFS is 1.5 years ($\lambda_1 = 0.462$) or longer. This trial is expected to accrue about 5 patients per month (or $r = 60$ per year) based on the recent accrual rate of patients at the study institution. Assuming $b = 1$ year of additional follow-up after completion of patient accrual, a single-stage design for the one-sample log-rank test with one-sided $\alpha = 5\%$ requires an accrual period of $a = 1.36$ years or a sample size of $n = 82$ for $1 - \beta = 90\%$ power. If we conduct an interim futility testing with $c_1 = 0$ at $\tau = 1$ year, then the power of the two-stage design with one-sided $\alpha = 5\%$ decreases to 88% with $n = 82$. So, by increasing the accrual period and sample size by about 5% for $a = 1.43$ years and $n = 86$, a two-stage design with $\tau = 1$ and $c_1 = 0$ has about 90% power. By the latter design, under H_1, we will have about $D_1 = 12$ events at $\tau = 1$ year and $D = 47$ at the final analysis. From $B = 10,000$ simulations on the design setting of the latter two-stage design ($n = 86$), we observed an empirical type I error of 4.6% and power of 87%.

4.5   Binomial Testing on t-Year Survival Probability

Suppose that t is a clinically relevant landmark time point for a specific disease, and a standard therapy is known to have a survival probability of p_0 at t. Let $S(t)$ denote the survival probability at time t for the experimental therapy of a study. We want to test $H_0 : S(t) = p_0$ against $H_1 : S(t) = p_1(> p_0)$. Considering the small sample sizes of regular single-arm phase II trials, Owzar and Jung (2008) proposed using the exact binomial test on the total number of patients whose event times are at least t, that is, $X = \sum_{i=1}^{n} I(T_i \geq t)$. Through extensive simulations, they claim that the methods on median survival time and the exponential MLE do not perform well for phase II trials with small sample sizes, and the exponential MLE method is sensitive to the validity of a specified survival distribution. The methods discussed in Chapters 2 and 3 can be used for the design and statistical analysis for the binomial testing method.

Example 4.5

Suppose that the median progression-free survival for a standard therapy is known to be 1 year. We will be interested in the experimental therapy if its median PFS is 1.5 years or longer. In this case, a reasonable choice for the landmark time point is $t = 1$ year. Under the exponential PFS model, we have $p_0 = 0.5$ and $p_1 = 0.63$. By the method in Chapter 2, a single-stage design requires $n = 98$ patients for $(\alpha, 1 - \beta) = (0.1, 0.9)$. The sample size for the binomial test will depend on the chosen t. With $t = 1.5$ years, we have $p_0 = 0.35$ and $p_1 = 0.5$ under the exponential PFS model, and we need $n = 77$ under the same design setting. With $t = 1.5$, the required sample size is decreased, but we may have more missing observations (censoring before t) due to the extended follow-up time.

For exact testing, the binomial testing will exclude the patients whose event times are censored before t from analysis. If we want to use them, we may use an asymptotic testing based on the Kaplan–Meier (1958) estimator at time t, but this is not an exact test.

References

Aalen, O.O. (1978). Nonparametric inference for a family of counting processes. *Annals of Statistics*, 6, 701–726.

Berry, G. (1983). The analysis of mortality by the subject-years methods. *Biometrics*, 39, 173–184.

Brookmeyer, R. and Crowley, J. (1982). A confidence interval for the median survival time. *Biometrics*, 38, 29–41.

Finkelstein, D.M., Muzikansky, A., and Schoenfeld, D.A. (2003). Comparing survival of a sample to that of a standard population. *Journal of the National Cancer Institute*, 95, 1434–1439.

Fleming, T.R. and Harrington, D.P. (1991). *Counting Processes and Survival Analysis*, Wiley, New York.

Gardiner, J., Susarla, V., and Van Ryzin, J. (1985). On the estimation of the median survival time under random censorship. In: *Adaptive Statistical Procedures and Related Topics*, IMS Lecture Notes, 8, 350–364.

Kaplan, E.L. and Meier, P. (1958). Nonparametric estimation from incomplete observations. *Journal of the American Statistical Association*, 53, 457–481.

Miller, R.G. (1981). *Survival Analysis*, John Wiley & Sons, New York.

Nelson, W. (1969). Hazard plotting for incomplete failure data. *Journal of Quality Technology*, 1, 27–52.

Owzar, K. and Jung, S.H. (2008). Designing phase II trials in cancer with time-to-event endpoints (with discussion). *Clinical Trials*, 5, 209–221.

Sprott, D.A. (1973). Normal likelihoods and their relation to large sample theory of estimation. *Biometrika* 60, 457–465.

Tsiatis, A.A. (1982). Repeated significance testing for a general class of statistics used in censored survival analysis. *Journal of American Statistical Society*, 77, 855–861.

Chapter 5

Single-Arm Phase II Trials with Heterogeneous Patient Populations: Binary and Survival Outcomes

The patient population for a phase II trial often consists of multiple subgroups, called subpopulations, with different prognosis although the study therapy is expected to be similarly beneficial for all subgroups. In this case, the final decision on the study treatment should be adjusted for the heterogeneity of the patient population.

Suppose that we want to evaluate the tumor response of CD30 antibody, SGN-30, combined with GVD (Gemcitabine, Vinorelbine, Pegylated Liposomal Doxorubicin) chemotherapy in patients with relapsed or refractory classical Hodgkin lymphoma (HL) through a phase II trial. In a previous study, GVD only (a historical control) has led to responses in 65% of patients with relapsed or refractory HL patients who never had a transplant and 75% in the transplant group. About 50% of patients in the previous study never had a transplant. Combining the data from the two subpopulations, the response rate (RR) for the whole patient population is estimated as 70%(= 0.5 × 0.65 + 0.5 × 0.75).

A standard design to account for the heterogeneity of the patient population is a single-arm trial based on a specified prevalence for each subpopulation for testing hypotheses

$$H_0 : p \leq 70\% \qquad \text{against} \qquad H_a : p > 70\%,$$

where p denotes the true RR of the combination therapy in the patient population combining the two subgroups, one for those with prior transplants and the other for those without one. Suppose that we consider an increase in RR by 15% or larger to be clinically significant for each subpopulation. So, we will not be interested in the combination therapy if the true RR, p, is lower than $p_0 = 70\%$ and will be strongly interested if the true RR is higher than $p_a = 85\%$. Then, Simon's (1989) two-stage optimal design for testing

$$H_0 : p_0 = 70\% \qquad \text{against} \qquad H_a : p_a = 85\%$$

with type I error no larger than $\alpha^* = 0.1$ and power no smaller than $1 - \beta^* = 0.9$ is described as follows.

Stage 1 Accrue $n_1 = 20$ patients. If $\bar{a}_1 = 14$ or fewer patients respond, then we stop the trial, concluding that the combination therapy is inefficacious. Otherwise, the trial proceeds to stage 2.

Stage 2 Accrue an additional $n_2 = 39$ patients. If more than $\bar{a} = 45$ patients out of the total $n = 59$ ($= n_1 + n_2$) respond, then the combination therapy will be accepted for further investigation.

Using the fact that the number of responders from the two stages are independent binomial random variables with an RR of p_0 under H_0 and p_a under H_a, we obtain the exact type I error rate and power of the two-stage design as 0.0980 and 0.9029, respectively.

In developing such a standard design, an accurate specification of the prevalence of each subpopulation is critical. If the prevalence is erroneously specified, the type I error of the statistical testing cannot be accurately controlled. Even though the prevalence is accurately specified, the observed proportion of patients from each subpopulation may be quite different from the true one when a study is over. This can easily happen in the standard phase II trials because of their small sample sizes. If a new study accrues a larger number of high-risk (low-risk) patients than expected, then the trial will have a higher false negativity (positivity). This kind of bias will be increase as the difference in RR increases between strata.

Stratified analysis is a popular statistical method to handle the heterogeneity of a study population. When the clinical outcome is binary as in the above example, London and Chang (2005) propose to resolve this issue by choosing rejection values based on a stratified analysis method. They adopt early stopping boundaries for both low- and high-efficacy cases based on a type I error rate and power spending function approach. Sposto and Gaynon (2009) propose a two-stage design with a lower stopping value only based on large sample approximations that may not hold well for phase II trials with small sample sizes.

Noting that there usually exists no compelling reason to stop a phase II trial due to high efficacy, Jung, Chang, and Kang (2011) propose two-stage designs with early stopping based on futility testing only. In this chapter, we investigate their method for binary clinical outcomes. We also discuss stratified one-sample log-rank test for the studies with a survival endpoint.

5.1   Binary Outcome Case

Suppose that we want to design a phase II trial on a new therapy with respect to a patient population with two subpopulations of patients, called the high-risk subpopulation and the low-risk subpopulation. Cases with more than two subpopulations will be discussed later. For subpopulation $j(= 1, 2)$, let p_j denote the RR of the therapy and γ_j denote the prevalence ($\gamma_1 + \gamma_2 = 1$). The RR for the combined population is given as $p = \gamma_1 p_1 + \gamma_2 p_2$. Based on some historical control data, we will not be interested in the new therapy if its RR for subpopulation j is p_{0j} or lower, and will be highly interested in it if its RR is $p_{aj}(= p_{0j} + \Delta_j$ for $\Delta_j > 0$) or higher. Let $p_0 = \gamma_1 p_{01} + \gamma_2 p_{02}$ and $p_a = \gamma_1 p_{a1} + \gamma_2 p_{a2}$.

We want to investigate the performance of unstratified and stratified designs in terms type I error rate and power control.

5.1.1   Single-Stage Designs

At first we consider single-stage designs with a binary study endpoint.

5.1.1.1   Unstratified Testing

A standard single-stage design to test hypotheses $H_0 : p \leq p_0$ versus $H_a : p > p_0$ is to accrue a certain number of patients, say, n, and to reject the therapy (that is, to fail rejecting H_0), if the observed number of responders is smaller than or equal to a chosen rejection value $\bar{a}$. Given a prespecified type I error rate α^*, power $1 - \beta^*$, and clinically significant difference $\Delta_j = p_{aj} - p_{0j}$ for subpopulation $j(=1, 2)$, we choose the smallest n together with an integer $\bar{a}$ satisfying

$$\alpha = P(X > \bar{a} | p = p_0) \leq \alpha^*$$

and

$$1 - \beta = P(X > \bar{a} | p = p_a) \geq 1 - \beta^*, \qquad (5.1)$$

where X denotes the number of responders among n patients. Given $\bar{a}$, we usually calculate the exact type I error α and power $1 - \beta$ by regarding X as a binomial random variable with n independent trials and probability of success $p = \gamma_1 p_1 + \gamma_2 p_2$, that is, $\alpha = B(\bar{a} + 1 | n, p_0)$ and $1 - \beta = B(\bar{a} + 1 | n, p_a)$, where $B(x | n, p) = \sum_{i=x}^{n} b(x | n, p)$ and

$$b(x | n, p) = \binom{n}{x} p^x (1 - p)^{n-x} \qquad \text{for } x = 0, 1, \ldots, n.$$

We call $(n, \bar{a})$ a standard or unstratified design.

Let $b(n, p)$ denote the binomial distribution with n independent trials and probability of success p. Let M_j be a random variable denoting the number of patients from subpopulation j among n patients. Assuming that the population consists of infinitely many patients, we have $M_1 \sim b(n, \gamma_1)$ and $M_2 = n - M_1$. Conditioning on $M_1 = m_1$, the number of responders X_j among m_j patients from subpopulation j follows $b(m_j, p_{0j})$ under H_0. Hence, it is easy to show that the above type I error for a standard design can be calculated also as

$$\alpha = \mathrm{E}^{M_1}\mathrm{P}(X_1 + X_2 > \bar{a}|p_{01}, p_{02}, M_1)$$

$$= \sum_{m_1=0}^{n}\sum_{x_1=0}^{m_1}\sum_{x_2=0}^{n-m_1} I(x_1 + x_2 > \bar{a})b(x_1|m_1, p_{01})b(x_2|n - m_1, p_{02})b(m_1|n, \gamma_1).$$

Power (5.1) can be calculated similarly.

5.1.1.2　Stratified Testing

For a stratified single-stage design, we propose to choose a value a satisfying the α^*-condition given the observed m_1 value while fixing $n(= m_1 + m_2)$ at the sample size of a standard design. Given $M_1 = m_1$ ($m_2 = n - m_1$), the conditional type I error for a rejection value a is calculated as

$$\alpha(m_1) = \mathrm{P}(X_1 + X_2 > a|p_{01}, p_{02}, m_1)$$

$$= \sum_{x_1=0}^{m_1}\sum_{x_2=0}^{n-m_1} I(x_1 + x_2 > a)b(x_1|m_1, p_{01})b(x_2|n - m_1, p_{02}).$$

Given m_1, we want to choose the maximal $a = a(m_1)$ such that $\alpha(m_1) \leq \alpha^*$. For the chosen rejection value $a = a(m_1)$, the conditional power is calculated as

$$1 - \beta(m_1) = \mathrm{P}(X_1 + X_2 > a|p_{a1}, p_{a2}, m_1)$$

$$= \sum_{x_1=0}^{m_1}\sum_{x_2=0}^{n-m_1} I(x_1 + x_2 > a)b(x_1|m_1, p_{a1})b(x_2|n - m_1, p_{a2}). \quad (5.2)$$

In summary, a stratified single-stage design for a population with two subpopulations is chosen as follows:

Step 1. Specify γ_1, $(p_{01}, p_{02}, p_{a1}, p_{a2})$, and $(\alpha^*, 1 - \beta^*)$.

Step 2. Choose a reasonable n as follows:
　(a) Calculate $p_0 = \gamma_1 p_{01} + \gamma_2 p_{02}$ and $p_a = \gamma_1 p_{a1} + \gamma_2 p_{a2}$.
　(b) Choose a standard single-stage design $(n, \bar{a})$ for testing

$$H_0 : p = p_0 \text{ vs. } H_a : p = p_a$$

under the $(\alpha^*, 1 - \beta^*)$-condition. We choose this n (or a little larger number) as the sample size of the stratified design.

Step 3. For $m_1 \in [0, n]$, choose the maximum $a = a(m_1)$ satisfying $\alpha(m_1) \leq \alpha^*$.

Step 4. Given (n, m_1, a), calculate the conditional power $1 - \beta(m_1)$ by (5.2).

The study protocol using a stratified design may provide a table of $\{a(m_1), \alpha(m_1), 1 - \beta(m_1)\}$ for $0 \le m_1 \le n$. When the study is over, we observe m_1 and $x(= x_1 + x_2)$, and reject the study therapy if $x \le a(m_1)$.

Noting that $M_1 \sim b(n, \gamma_1)$, we can calculate the marginal type I error rate and power of the stratified design by

$$\alpha = \mathrm{E}\{\alpha(M_1)\} = \sum_{m_1=0}^{n} \alpha(m_1) b(m_1 | n, \gamma_1)$$

and

$$1 - \beta = \mathrm{E}\{1 - \beta(M_1)\} = \sum_{m_1=0}^{n} \{1 - \beta(m_1)\} b(m_1 | n, \gamma_1),$$

respectively. Since, for each $m_1 \in [0, \dots, n]$, we choose $a = a(m_1)$ so that its conditional type I error does not exceed α^*, the marginal type I error will not exceed α^*.

Example 5.1

Let's consider the example study discussed at the beginning of this chapter using $\Delta_1 = \Delta_2 = 0.15$. Under $\gamma_1 = \gamma_2 = 0.5$ and response rates $(p_{01}, p_{02}) = (0.65, 0.75)$, the hypotheses in terms of the population RR are expressed as $H_0 : p_0 = 0.7$ and $H_a : p_1 = 0.85$. For $(\alpha^*, 1 - \beta^*) = (0.1, 0.9)$, the standard (unstratified) design with the minimal sample size is $(n, \bar{a}) = (53, 41)$, which has $\alpha = 0.0906$ and $1 - \beta = 0.9093$. The type I error and power are valid only when the true prevalence is $\gamma_1 = \gamma_2 = 0.5$.

Suppose that the study observed $(x_1, x_2) = (28, 13)$ and $m_1 = 36$. Note that the observed prevalence for the high-risk subpopulation, $\hat{\gamma}_1 = 36/53 = 0.68$, is much larger than the expected $\gamma_1 = 0.5$. By the unstratified design, $x = 41$ equals the rejection value $\bar{a} = 41$, so that the therapy will be rejected. However, noting that $m_1 = 36$ is much larger than expected, the stratified design lowers the rejection value to $a = 40$, so that, with observation $x = 41$, the therapy will be accepted for further investigation. Similarly, the unstratified Simon's design may falsely accept the therapy if $\hat{\gamma}_1$ is much lower than the specified prevalence $\gamma_1 = 0.5$.

Table 5.1 lists the conditional type I error rate and power of the standard unstratified design for each $m_1 \in [0, n]$. Note that if m_1 is much larger than $n\gamma_1$, that is, too many subpopulation 1 (high risk) patients are accrued, then the standard rejection value $\bar{a} = 41$ is so conservative that the conditional type I error and power become smaller than the specified $\alpha^* = 0.1$ and $1 - \beta^* = 0.9$, respectively. On the other hand, if m_1 is too small compared to $n\gamma_1$, that is, too many subpopulation 2 (low-risk) patients are accrued, then the standard rejection value $\bar{a} = 41$ is so anticonservative that the conditional type I error becomes larger than the specified $\alpha^* = 0.1$ level. Figure 5.1(a) displays the conditional type I error rate and power of the standard (unstratified) design.

Table 5.1 Conditional type I error and power of single-stage standard (unstratified) and stratified designs with $n = 53$ for $(p_{01}, p_{02}, \Delta) = (0.65, 0.75, 0.15)$ and $(\alpha^*, 1 - \beta^*) = (0.1, 0.9)$. The standard design has a fixed critical value $\bar{a} = 41$

	Unstratified		Stratified				Unstratified		Stratified		
m_1	α	$1 - \beta$	a	α	$1 - \beta$	m_1	α	$1 - \beta$	a	α	$1 - \beta$
0	0.2961	0.9947	44	0.0606	0.9215	27	0.0869	0.9081	41	0.0869	0.9081
1	0.2852	0.9939	44	0.0569	0.9142	28	0.0823	0.9011	41	0.0823	0.9011
2	0.2746	0.9930	44	0.0535	0.9065	29	0.0780	0.8938	41	0.0780	0.8938
3	0.2641	0.9919	43	0.0972	0.9517	30	0.0738	0.8862	41	0.0738	0.8862
4	0.2540	0.9908	43	0.0920	0.9467	31	0.0699	0.8782	41	0.0699	0.8782
5	0.2440	0.9896	43	0.0870	0.9414	32	0.0661	0.8699	41	0.0661	0.8699
6	0.2343	0.9882	43	0.0822	0.9357	33	0.0625	0.8612	41	0.0625	0.8612
7	0.2249	0.9866	43	0.0776	0.9296	34	0.0590	0.8523	41	0.0590	0.8523
8	0.2157	0.9849	43	0.0733	0.9232	35	0.0557	0.8430	41	0.0557	0.8430
9	0.2067	0.9830	43	0.0691	0.9163	36	0.0526	0.8334	40	0.0961	0.9049
10	0.1980	0.9810	43	0.0651	0.9091	37	0.0496	0.8236	40	0.0913	0.8981
11	0.1895	0.9787	43	0.0614	0.9015	38	0.0468	0.8134	40	0.0867	0.8909
12	0.1813	0.9763	43	0.0578	0.8935	39	0.0441	0.8029	40	0.0822	0.8835
13	0.1734	0.9736	43	0.0544	0.8851	40	0.0415	0.7922	40	0.0780	0.8757
14	0.1656	0.9707	42	0.0969	0.9368	41	0.0391	0.7812	40	0.0739	0.8677
15	0.1582	0.9676	42	0.0919	0.9311	42	0.0367	0.7699	40	0.0701	0.8593
16	0.1510	0.9642	42	0.0870	0.9250	43	0.0346	0.7584	40	0.0664	0.8506
17	0.1440	0.9606	42	0.0823	0.9186	44	0.0325	0.7467	40	0.0628	0.8417
18	0.1373	0.9566	42	0.0779	0.9119	45	0.0305	0.7347	40	0.0594	0.8325
19	0.1308	0.9525	42	0.0736	0.9048	46	0.0287	0.7225	40	0.0562	0.8230
20	0.1245	0.9480	42	0.0696	0.8973	47	0.0269	0.7102	39	0.0955	0.8886
21	0.1185	0.9432	42	0.0657	0.8895	48	0.0252	0.6977	39	0.0908	0.8813
22	0.1127	0.9382	42	0.0620	0.8813	49	0.0237	0.6850	39	0.0864	0.8738
23	0.1071	0.9328	42	0.0585	0.8727	50	0.0222	0.6722	39	0.0820	0.8659
24	0.1017	0.9271	42	0.0551	0.8638	51	0.0208	0.6592	39	0.0779	0.8578
25	0.0966	0.9211	41	0.0966	0.9211	52	0.0195	0.6462	39	0.0739	0.8495
26	0.0916	0.9148	41	0.0916	0.9148	53	0.0182	0.6330	39	0.0701	0.8408

We observe that the conditional type I error of the standard design widely varies between 0.0182 for $m_1 = 53$ and 0.2961 for $m_1 = 0$. Its conditional power also widely varies around $1 - \beta^* = 0.9$.

The second part of Table 5.1 reports the conditional rejection value $a(m_1)$ and its $\{\alpha(m_1), 1 - \beta(m_1)\}$ for each $m_1 \in [0, n]$. The conditional rejection value $a(m_1)$ decreases from 44 to 39 as m_1 increases. Note that $\bar{a} = a(m_1) = 41$ for m_1 values around $n\gamma_1 = 26.5$. Figure 5.1(a) displays the conditional type I error rate and power of the stratified design. While the conditional type I error of the stratified design $\alpha(m_1)$ is closely controlled below α^*, the conditional power is also well controlled around $1 - \beta^* = 0.9$. If we want $1 - \beta$ to be larger than $1 - \beta^*$ for all $m_1 \in [0, n]$, we have to choose a slightly larger n than 53.

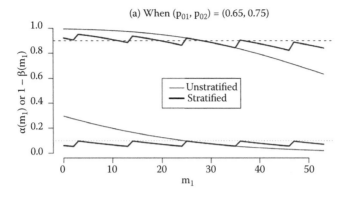

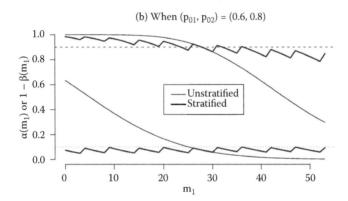

Figure 5.1 Conditional type I error and power of standard (unstratified) and stratified designs with $n = 53$ for $(\alpha^*, 1 - \beta^*, \Delta) = (0.1, 0.9, 0.15)$. The standard design has a fixed critical value $\bar{a} = 41$. The upper lines are conditional powers and the lower lines are conditional type I error.

If the difference of the response probabilities between two subpopulations $|p_{01} - p_{02}|$ is larger, then the range of the rejection values for the stratified design will be wider, and the conditional type I error rate and power of the unstratified design will fluctuate more wildly, depending on the m_1 value. Let's consider $(p_{01}, p_{02}) = (0.6, 0.8)$ and $\Delta_1 = \Delta_2 = 0.15$. Under $(\gamma_1, \alpha^*, 1 - \beta^*) = (0.5, 0.1, 0.9)$, the standard design will be the same as above, $(n, \bar{a}) = (53, 41)$, but the stratified rejection value $a(m_1)$ decreases from 47 to 37 as m_1 increases from 0 to 53. Figure 5.1(b) displays the conditional type I error rate and power of the unstratified and stratified designs. Comparing Figures 5.1(a) and (b), we observe that the stratified design controls its conditional type I error rate and power closely to their nominal levels regardless of $|p_{01} - p_{02}|$ value, but those of the standard design change farther away from their specified levels with the larger difference between subpopulations. We also observe that with a larger $|p_{01} - p_{02}|$ value, the conditional type I error and power of the stratified design fluctuate more often because the conditional critical value changes more frequently see Figure 5.1(b).

Let's investigate the impact of an erroneously specified prevalence on the study design. Suppose that the true prevalence is $\gamma_1 = 0.3$, but the study is designed under a wrong specification of $\gamma_1 = 0.5$. Let's assume $(p_{01}, p_{02}) = (0.65, 0.75)$, $\Delta_1 = \Delta_2 = 0.15$, and $(\alpha^*, 1 - \beta^*) = (0.1, 0.9)$ as above. Under the erroneously specified prevalence, the standard and stratified designs will be the same as above, as shown in Table 5.1. The standard design has marginal type I error and power $(\alpha, 1 - \beta) = (0.1530, 0.9631)$ and the stratified design has $(\alpha, 1 - \beta) = (0.0767, 0.9116)$. Under the true $\gamma_1 = 0.3$, $p_0 = \gamma_1 p_{01} + \gamma_2 p_{02} = 0.72$ and $p_1 = \gamma_1 p_{a1} + \gamma_2 p_{a2} = 0.87$ are farther away from $1/2$ than those under the specified $\gamma_1 = 0.5$, so that the marginal power for the stratified design is still larger than $1 - \beta^*$ even though the marginal type I error is much below $\alpha^* = 0.1$. The marginal type I error for the standard design is much larger than the specified $\alpha^* = 0.1$. Under a wrong projection of the prevalence, the type I error of a standard design can be heavily biased, but that of the stratified design will be always controlled below α^*.

Now, suppose that the true prevalence is $\gamma_1 = 0.7$, but the study is designed under an erroneously specified $\gamma_1 = 0.5$. In this case, the standard design has marginal type I error and power $(\alpha, 1 - \beta) = (0.0501, 0.8209)$ and the stratified design has $(\alpha, 1 - \beta) = (0.0768, 0.8762)$. The power for the stratified design is slightly smaller than $1 - \beta^*$ because of the conservative adjustment of conditional type I error. However, the power for the standard design is much smaller than $1 - \beta^*$. The impact of an erroneously specified prevalence on the bias of marginal type I error and power will be larger with a larger difference between p_{01} and p_{02}.

5.1.2 Two-Stage Designs

Because of ethical and economical issues, two-stage designs have been more popular for phase II cancer clinical trials than single-stage designs. We may stop a trial early when the RR of a study treatment turns out to be either too low or too high (e.g., London and Chang, 2005), but we consider the more popular design with an early stopping due to a low RR only here. If the experimental treatment is efficacious, we usually do not have a compelling ethical argument to stop the trial early and want to continue collecting more data to be used in designing a future phase III trial. Furthermore, this simplifies the computations and makes the statistical testing easier when the final sample size is different from a predetermined one. Under a two-stage design, we treat n_k patients during stage $k(= 1, 2)$. Let $n = n_1 + n_2$. For stage $k(= 1, 2)$ and subpopulation $j(= 1, 2)$, let M_{kj} and X_{kj} be random variables denoting the number of patients and the number of responders, respectively. Note that $n_k = m_{k1} + m_{k2}$.

5.1.2.1 Unstratified Testing

An example standard (unstratified) two-stage design is demonstrated at the beginning of this chapter. Given $(\alpha^*, 1 - \beta^*)$, a standard design $(n_1, n_2, \bar{a}_1, \bar{a})$ is chosen among the two-stage designs satisfying $\alpha \leq \alpha^*$ and $1 - \beta \geq 1 - \beta^*$, where α and $1 - \beta$ are obtained assuming that $X_1 = X_{11} + X_{12}$ and $X_2 = X_{21} + X_{22}$ are independent binomial random variables with probability of success $p_0 (= \gamma_1 p_{01} + \gamma_2 p_{02})$ under H_0 and $p_a (= \gamma_1 p_{a1} + \gamma_2 p_{a2})$ under H_a as in Chapter 2. The unstratified analysis conducts statistical analysis ignoring the number of patients from each subpopulation.

5.1.2.2 Stratified Testing

Given $(M_{11}, M_{21}) = (m_{11}, m_{21})$, a design (n_1, n_2, a_1, a) has conditional type I error

$$
\begin{aligned}
\alpha(m_{11}, m_{21}) &= P(X_{11} + X_{12} > a_1, X_{11} + X_{12} + X_{21} + X_{22} > a \,|\, p_{01}, p_{02}) \\
&= \sum_{x_{11}=0}^{m_{11}} \sum_{x_{12}=0}^{n_1-m_{11}} \sum_{x_{21}=0}^{m_{21}} \sum_{x_{22}=0}^{n_2-m_{21}} I(x_{11} + x_{12} > a_1, x_{11} + x_{12} + x_{21} + x_{22} > a) \\
&\quad \times b(x_{11}|m_{11}, p_{01})b(x_{12}|n_1 - m_{11}, p_{02})b(x_{21}|m_{21}, p_{01}) \\
&\quad \times b(x_{22}|n_2 - m_{21}, p_{02})
\end{aligned}
$$

and power

$$
\begin{aligned}
1 - \beta(m_{11}, m_{21}) &= P(X_{11} + X_{12} > a_1, X_{11} + X_{12} + X_{21} + X_{22} > a \,|\, p_{a1}, p_{a2}) \\
&= \sum_{x_{11}=0}^{m_{11}} \sum_{x_{12}=0}^{n_1-m_{11}} \sum_{x_{21}=0}^{m_{21}} \sum_{x_{22}=0}^{n_2-m_{21}} I(x_{11} + x_{12} > a_1, x_{11} + x_{12} + x_{21} \\
&\quad + x_{22} > a)b(x_{11}|m_{11}, p_{a1})b(x_{12}|n_1 - m_{11}, p_{a2}) \\
&\quad \times b(x_{21}|m_{21}, p_{a1})b(x_{22}|n_2 - m_{21}, p_{a2}).
\end{aligned}
\tag{5.3}
$$

We want to find a two-stage stratified design $\{n_1, n_2, a_1(m_{11}), a(m_{11}, m_{21})\}$ whose conditional type I error is no larger than α^* for each combination of (m_{11}, m_{21}) for $m_{k1} \in [0, n_k]$. In order to simplify the computation associated with the search procedure, we fix (n_1, n_2) at the first- and second-stage sample sizes for a standard two-stage design based on a specified prevalence γ_1, such as Simon's (1989) minimax or optimal design, or admissible design by Jung et al. (2004). Given $M_{11} = m_{11}$, we also propose to fix $a_1 = a_1(m_{11})$ at $[m_{11}p_{01} + m_{12}p_{02}]$, where $[c]$ denotes the largest integer not exceeding c. In other words, we reject the experimental therapy after stage 1 if the observed number of responders from stage 1 is no larger than the expected number of responders under H_0. Now, the only design parameter we need to choose is a, the rejection value at stage 2. At stage 2, given $\{\alpha^*, n_1, n_2, m_{11}, m_{21}, a_1(m_{11})\}$, we choose the largest $a = a(m_{11}, m_{21})$ satisfying $\alpha(m_{11}, m_{21}) \leq \alpha^*$. Its conditional power, $1 - \beta(m_{11}, m_{21})$, is calculated by (5.3).

If the observed prevalence is close to the specified one (i.e., $m_{11}/n_1 \approx \gamma_1$ and $m_{21}/n_2 \approx \gamma_1$), then the conditional rejection values $\{a_1(m_{11}), a(m_{11}, m_{21})\}$ will be the same as the unstratified rejection values $(\bar{a}_1, \bar{a})$ of the unstratified two-stage design by Simon (1989) or Jung et al. (2004). As in single-stage designs, the conditional power may be smaller than $1 - \beta^*$ for some (m_{11}, m_{21}). If we want to satisfy $1 - \beta \geq 1 - \beta^*$ for all combinations of $\{(m_{11}, m_{21}), 0 \leq m_{11} \leq n_1, 0 \leq m_{21} \leq n_2\}$, then we have to choose a slightly larger n than that of a standard unstratified design.

If the true prevalence of subpopulation 1 is γ_1, M_{k1} for $k = 1, 2$ are independent random variables following $b(n_k, \gamma_1)$. Given $(M_{11}, M_{21}) = (m_{11}, m_{21})$, let $\alpha(m_{11}, m_{21})$ and $1 - \beta(m_{11}, m_{21})$ denote the conditional type I rate and power for conditional rejection values $\{a_1(m_{11}), a(m_{11}, m_{21})\}$, respectively. Then, the marginal (unconditional) type I error rate and power are obtained by

$$\alpha = \sum_{m_{11}=0}^{n_1} \sum_{m_{21}=0}^{n_2} \alpha(m_{11}, m_{21}) b(m_{11}|n_1, \gamma_1) b(m_{21}|n_2, \gamma_1)$$

$$1 - \beta = \sum_{m_{11}=0}^{n_1} \sum_{m_{21}=0}^{n_2} \{1 - \beta(m_{11}, m_{21})\} b(m_{11}|n_1, \gamma_1) b(m_{21}|n_2, \gamma_1),$$

respectively. In summary, a phase II trial with a stratified two-stage design is conducted as follows:

- Specify $(p_{01}, p_{02}, p_{a1}, p_{a2})$ and $(\alpha^*, 1 - \beta^*)$.
- Choose sample sizes for the two stages (n_1, n_2) as follows.

  (a) Specify γ_1, the prevalence for subpopulation 1.
  (b) For $p_0 = \gamma_1 p_{01} + \gamma_2 p_{02}$ and $p_a = \gamma_1 p_{a1} + \gamma_2 p_{a2}$, choose a standard (unstratified) two-stage design for testing

  $$H_0 : p = p_0 \quad \text{vs.} \quad H_a : p = p_a$$

  that satisfies the $(\alpha^*, 1 - \beta^*)$-condition. We use (n_1, n_2) for the chosen standard design as the stage 1 and 2 sample sizes of the stratified design.

- Conduct the trial.

  (a) *Stage 1:* Treat n_1 patients and observe m_{11}, x_{11}, x_{12}. Calculate $a_1 = a_1(m_{11}) = [m_{11} p_{01} + m_{12} p_{02}]$ based on the observed m_{11}. Reject the experimental therapy if $x_1 = x_{11} + x_{12}$ is smaller than or equal to $a_1(m_{11})$. Otherwise, we proceed to stage 2.
  (b) *Stage 2:* Treat n_2 patients and observe m_{21}, x_{21}, x_{22}. Choose the largest integer $a = a(m_{11}, m_{21})$ satisfying $\alpha(m_{11}, m_{21}) \leq \alpha^*$ conditioning on (m_{11}, m_{21}). Accept the therapy if $x = x_{11} + x_{12} + x_{21} + x_{22}$ is larger than $a(m_{11}, m_{21})$.

- The conditional power $1 - \beta(m_{11}, m_{21})$ for the two-stage trial with $(n_1, n_2, m_{11}, m_{21}, a_1, a)$ is calculated by (5.3).

In designing a two-stage phase II trial with stratified analysis, we should include the description of the whole procedure described above as well as the design parameter values in the study protocol.

Chang, Jung, and Wu (2012) propose to drop the subpopulations with low efficacy after stage 1 using interim futility testing.

Example 5.2

We consider the design setting of Example 5.1 with $(p_{01}, p_{02}, \Delta_1, \Delta_2) = (0.65, 0.75, 0.15, 0.15)$, $\gamma_1 = 0.5$, and $(\alpha^*, 1 - \beta^*) = (0.1, 0.9)$. For this setting, Simon's optimal two-stage design is given as $(n_1, n_2, \bar{a}_1, \bar{a}) = (20, 39, 14, 45)$. We choose $(n_1, n_2) = (20, 39)$ for our stratified two-stage design.

Suppose that the study observed $(m_{11}, m_{21}) = (14, 28)$ and $(x_1, x) = (15, 45)$. Note that much larger number of patients than expected are accrued from the high-risk group, subpopulation 1, that is, $m_{11}/n_1 = 0.70$ and $m_{21}/n_2 = 0.72$ compared to the specified $\gamma_1 = 0.5$. By Simon's design, $x = 45$ equals $\bar{a} = 45$, so that the therapy will be rejected. However, the stratified critical values for $(m_{11}, m_{21}) = (14, 28)$ are given as $(a_1, a) = (13, 44)$, so that, with observations $(x_1, x) = (15, 45)$, the therapy will be accepted for further investigation. Similarly, the unstratified Simon's design may falsely accept the therapy if the trial accrues too many patients from the low-risk group compared to the projected $\gamma_2 = 0.5$.

Figure 5.2(a) displays the conditional type I error and power of Simon's optimal design (marked as Unstratified) and the stratified design under the design settings. While the conditional type I error rate of the stratified design is closely controlled below α^*, that of the unstratified design wildly fluctuates between 0.0185 and 0.3110, depending on (m_{11}, m_{21}). Also, the conditional power of the stratified design is closely maintained around $1 - \beta^*$, but that of Simon's design widely changes between 0.6447 and 0.9876. In the x-axis of Figure 5.2(a) (Figure 5.2(b) also), only m_{11} values are marked, but actually m_{21} values run from 0 to $n_2 = 39$ between consecutive m_{11} values. Consequently, the conditional type I error rate and power, especially for the standard unstratified design, regularly fluctuate between consecutive m_{11} values.

Figure 5.2(b) displays the conditional type I error rate and power of the two designs when the two subpopulations have a larger difference in RR, $(p_{01}, p_{02}) = (0.6, 0.8)$, with other parameters fixed at the same values as above. Note that with $\gamma_1 = 0.5$, Simon's optimal design will be identical to that for $(p_{01}, p_{02}) = (0.65, 0.75)$, that is, $(n_1, n_2, \bar{a}_1, \bar{a}) = (20, 39, 14, 45)$. As in the single-stage design case (Figure 5.1(b)), we observe that the conditional type I error rate and power of the the unstratified design fluctuate more wildly than those with $(p_{01}, p_{02}) = (0.65, 0.75)$, whereas the performance of the stratified design is almost unaffected. In conclusion, unstratified analysis can be more problematic when the difference in response rates between subpopulations is large.

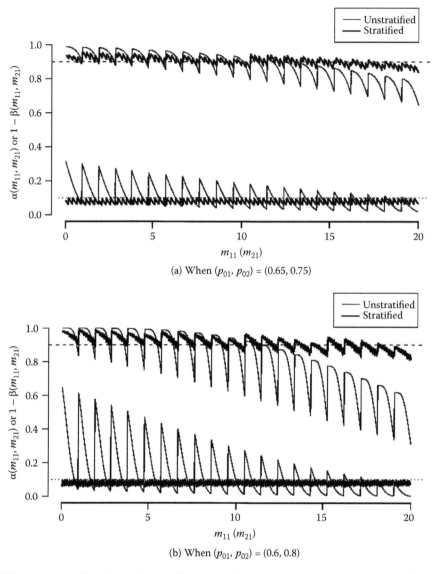

(a) When $(p_{01}, p_{02}) = (0.65, 0.75)$

(b) When $(p_{01}, p_{02}) = (0.6, 0.8)$

Figure 5.2 Conditional type I error and power of two-stage standard (un-stratified) and stratified designs under $(\alpha^*, 1 - \beta^*, \Delta) = (0.1, 0.9, 0.15)$. The unstratified design has $(n_1, n, \bar{a}_1, \bar{a}) = (20, 59, 14, 45)$. The upper lines are conditional powers and the lower lines are conditional type I error.

If the true prevalence is accurately specified, then Simon's optimal design has marginal type I error rate and power of $(\alpha, 1 - \beta) = (0.0954, 0.9010)$, and the stratified design has $(\alpha, 1 - \beta) = (0.0792, 0.9044)$ if $(p_{01}, p_{02}) = (0.65, 0.75)$ and $(\alpha, 1 - \beta) = (0.0788, 0.9159)$ if $(p_{01}, p_{02}) = (0.6, 0.8)$. Both designs using stratified analysis satisfy the condition of $(\alpha^*, 1 - \beta^*) = (0.1, 0.9)$. However, if the true prevalence of subpopulation 1 is $\gamma_1 = 0.3$ but $\gamma_1 = 0.5$ is specified in designing the study, then Simon's design based on unstratified analysis has $(\alpha, 1 - \beta) = (0.1618, 0.9521)$ if $(p_{01}, p_{02}) = (0.65, 0.75)$ and $(\alpha, 1 - \beta) = (0.2548, 0.9798)$ if $(p_{01}, p_{02}) = (0.6, 0.8)$. Note that Simon's design has a more biased marginal type I error rate when two subpopulations are more different in terms of RR. On the other hand, the stratified design always controls the marginal type I error below α^* and power close to $1 - \beta^*$ even under an erroneously specified prevalence, for example, $(\alpha, 1 - \beta) = (0.0776, 0.9203)$ if $(p_{01}, p_{02}) = (0.65, 0.75)$ and $(\alpha, 1 - \beta) = (0.0782, 0.9481)$ if $(p_{01}, p_{02}) = (0.6, 0.8)$.

5.1.3   Some Extensions

In this section, we present some extended concepts of stratified designs that are discussed above.

5.1.3.1   Conditional P-Value

In the previous sections, a stratified two-stage design is determined by the sample sizes (n_1, n_2) and the rejection value (a_1, a) conditioning on the number of patients from each subpopulation during each stage. When the trial is completed, however, the number of patients accrued to the study may be slightly different from the predetermined sample size. This happens since often some patients drop out or turn out to be ineligible after registration. Because of this, we usually accrue a slightly larger number of patients than the planned sample size, say, 5% more. As a result, the total number of eligible patients at the end of a trial tends to be different from the planned n. In this case, the sample size of a study is a random variable, and the rejection value chosen for the planned sample size may not be valid anymore if the realized sample size is different from that chosen at the design stage. As a flexible testing method for two-stage phase II trials, we propose to calculate the p-value conditioning on the observed sample size as well as the observed number of patients from each subpopulation, and to reject H_0 (or equivalently accept the experimental therapy) when the conditional p-value is smaller than the prespecified α^* level.

If a trial is stopped due to lack of efficacy after stage 1, then we usually are not interested in p-value calculation. Suppose that the trial has proceeded to stage 2 to observe (x_1, x) together with $(n_1, n_2, m_{11}, m_{21})$. Then, the interim testing after stage 1 will be conducted using the rejection value $a_1 = [m_{11}p_{01} + m_{12}p_{02}]$. Given m_{kj} $(m_{k1}+m_{k2} = n_k)$, X_{kj} is a $b(m_{kj}, p_{0j})$ random variable under H_0. Hence, the p-value for an observation $(x_{11}, x_{12}, x_{21}, x_{22})$ conditioning on

$(n_1, n_2, m_{11}, m_{21})$ is obtained by

$$\text{p-value} = \sum_{i_{11}=0}^{m_{11}} \sum_{i_{12}=0}^{m_{12}} \sum_{i_{21}=0}^{m_{21}} \sum_{i_{22}=0}^{m_{22}} I(i_{11} + i_{12} > a_1, i_{11} + i_{12} + i_{21} + i_{22} \geq x)$$

$$\times \prod_{j=1}^{2} \prod_{k=1}^{2} b(i_{kj} | m_{kj}, p_{0j}),$$

where $m_{k2} = n_k - m_{k1}$. We reject H_0 if p-value $< \alpha^*$. Note that the calculation of a conditional p-value does not require specification of the true prevalence. In order to avoid the informative sampling issue, the final sample size should be determined without looking at the response data from stage 2 patients.

Example 5.3

Let's revisit Example 5.2 with $(p_{01}, p_{02}) = (0.65, 0.75)$. Suppose that, at the design stage, we chose $(n_1, n_2) = (20, 39)$ based on Simon's optimal design, but the study accrued a slightly larger number of patients $(n_1, n_2) = (20, 40)$, among whom $(m_{11}, m_{21}) = (12, 25)$ were from subpopulation 1 and $(x_1, x) = (15, 46)$ responded. For the original sample size $(n_1, n_2) = (20, 39)$, the stratified rejection values are $(a_1, a) = (13, 45)$ with respect to $(m_{11}, m_{21}) = (12, 24)$ or $(12, 25)$. Hence, we could accept the therapy if the number of responders $(x_1, x) = (15, 46)$ was observed from the design as originally planned, $(n_1, n) = (20, 59)$. However, by having one more eligible patient from stage 2, it became unclear whether we should accept the therapy or not by the testing rule of the original design. To resolve this issue, we calculate the p-value for $(x_1, x) = (15, 46)$ conditioning on $(n_1, n_2) = (20, 40)$ and $(m_{11}, m_{21}) = (12, 25)$, p-value $= 0.1089$. The conditional p-value is marginally larger than $\alpha^* = 0.1$, so that we may consider accepting the therapy for further investigation.

5.1.3.2   When There Are More Than Two Subpopulations

Suppose that there are $J(\geq 2)$ subpopulations with RR p_j for subpopulation $j(= 1, \ldots, J)$. We consider two-stage designs here. We accrue n_1 and n_2 patients during stages 1 and 2, respectively. The response rates for J subpopulations are specified as $\mathbf{p}_0 = (p_{01}, \ldots, p_{0J})$ under H_0 and $\mathbf{p}_a = (p_{a1}, \ldots, p_{aJ})$ under H_a. Let $\mathbf{M}_k = (M_{k1}, \ldots, M_{kJ})$ denote the random vector representing the numbers of patients from the J subpopulations among n_k patients accrued during stage k ($\sum_{j=1}^{J} M_{kj} = n_k$, $k = 1, 2$), and $\mathbf{m}_k = (m_{k1}, \ldots, m_{kJ})$ denote their observed values. Let X_{kj} denote the number responders among M_{kj} patients from subpopulation j during stage k. Then, given m_{kj}, X_{kj} is a random variable with $b(m_{kj}, p_j)$.

Given $(\mathbf{m}_1, \mathbf{m}_2)$, the conditional type I error rate and power for chosen rejection values (a_1, a) are calculated as

$$\alpha(\mathbf{m}_1, \mathbf{m}_2) = P\left\{ \sum_{j=1}^{J} X_{1j} > a_1, \sum_{j=1}^{J}(X_{1j} + X_{2j}) > a | \mathbf{p}_0, \mathbf{m}_1, \mathbf{m}_2 \right\}$$

$$= \sum_{x_{11}=0}^{m_{11}} \cdots \sum_{x_{1J}=0}^{m_{1J}} \sum_{x_{21}=0}^{m_{21}} \cdots \sum_{x_{2J}=0}^{m_{2J}} I\left\{ \sum_{j=1}^{J} x_{1j} > a_1, \sum_{j=1}^{J}(x_{1j} + x_{2j}) > a \right\}$$

$$\times \prod_{j=1}^{J} b(x_{1j} | m_{1j}, p_{0j}) b(x_{2j} | m_{2j}, p_{0j})$$

and

$$1 - \beta(\mathbf{m}_1, \mathbf{m}_2) = P\left\{ \sum_{j=1}^{J} X_{1j} > a_1, \sum_{j=1}^{J}(X_{1j} + X_{2j}) > a | \mathbf{p}_a, \mathbf{m}_1, \mathbf{m}_2 \right\}$$

$$= \sum_{x_{11}=0}^{m_{11}} \cdots \sum_{x_{1J}=0}^{m_{1J}} \sum_{x_{21}=0}^{m_{21}} \cdots \sum_{x_{2J}=0}^{m_{2J}} I\left\{ \sum_{j=1}^{J} x_{1j} > a_1, \sum_{j=1}^{J}(x_{1j} + x_{2j}) > a \right\}$$

$$\times \prod_{j=1}^{J} b(x_{1j} | m_{1j}, p_{aj}) b(x_{2j} | m_{2j}, p_{aj}), \tag{5.4}$$

respectively. A phase II trial with a stratified two-stage design on a heterogeneous population with J subpopulations is conducted as follows:

- Specify $\mathbf{p}_0$, $\mathbf{p}_a$, and $(\alpha^*, 1 - \beta^*)$.
- Choose the sample sizes for two stages (n_1, n_2) as follows:

  (a) Specify the prevalence for each subpopulation, $(\gamma_1, \ldots, \gamma_J)$.

  (b) For $p_0 = \sum_{j=1}^{J} \gamma_j p_{0j}$ and $p_a = \sum_{j=1}^{J} \gamma_j p_{aj}$, choose a standard (unstratified) two-stage design for testing

  $$H_0 : p = p_0 \quad \text{vs.} \quad H_a : p = p_a$$

  that satisfies the $(\alpha^*, 1 - \beta^*)$ condition. We choose (n_1, n_2) for the standard design as the stage 1 and 2 sample sizes of our stratified design.

- Conduct the trial.

  (a) *Stage 1:* Treat n_1 patients and observe $(m_{11}, \ldots, m_{1J})$ and $(x_{11}, \ldots, x_{1J})$. Calculate $a_1 = [\sum_{j=1}^{J} m_{1j} p_{0j}]$. Reject the experimental therapy if $x_1 = \sum_{j=1}^{J} x_{1j}$ is smaller than or equal to a_1. Otherwise, proceed to stage 2.

(b) *Stage 2:* Treat n_2 patients and observe $(m_{21}, \ldots, m_{2J})$ and $(x_{21}, \ldots, x_{2J})$. Choose the largest integer a satisfying $\alpha(\mathbf{m}_1, \mathbf{m}_2) \leq \alpha^*$ conditioning on the observed $(\mathbf{m}_1, \mathbf{m}_2)$. Accept the experimental therapy for further investigation,if $x > a$ where $x = \sum_{k=1}^{2}\sum_{j=1}^{J} x_{1j}$.

- Calculate the conditional power $1 - \beta(\mathbf{m}_1, \mathbf{m}_2)$ for the two-stage testing with $(n_1, n_2, \mathbf{m}_1, \mathbf{m}_2, a_1, a)$ using (5.4).

Given sample sizes n_1 and n_2, $\mathbf{M}_1$ and $\mathbf{M}_2$ are independent multinomial random vectors with probabilities of "success" for the J subpopulations $(\gamma_1, \ldots, \gamma_J)$ and n_1 and n_2 independent trials, respectively. Hence, the marginal type I error rate and power can be calculated by taking the expectations of $\alpha(\mathbf{M}_1, \mathbf{M}_2)$ and $1 - \beta(\mathbf{M}_1, \mathbf{M}_2)$ with respect to $\mathbf{M}_1$ and $\mathbf{M}_2$.

5.2 Survival Outcome Case: Stratified One-Sample Log-Rank Test

In this section, we introduce a stratified analysis method for the one-sample log-rank test that was discussed in Section 4.3 and derive its sample size calculation method.

5.2.1 Statistical Testing

Suppose that there are J subpopulations, or strata, with different survival distributions because of different risk levels. For subpopulation $j(= 1, \ldots, J)$, let $\Lambda_{0j}(t)$ denote the cumulative hazard function of a selected historical control. Let $\Lambda_j(t)$ denote the cumulative hazard function of the experimental therapy for subpopulation j. We want to test

$$H_0 : \Lambda_j(t) = \Lambda_{0j}(t) \quad \text{for } j = 1, \ldots, J$$

against

$$H_1 : \Lambda_j(t) < \Lambda_{0j}(t) \quad \text{for } j = 1, \ldots, J.$$

Let n_j denote the number of patients from subpopulation j, and $n = \sum_{j=1}^{J} n_j$ the total sample size. For patient $i(= 1, \ldots, n_j)$ in subpopulation j, T_{ji} and C_{ji} denote the survival and censoring times, respectively. For $X_{ji} = \min(T_{ji}, C_{ji})$ and $\delta_{ji} = I(T_{ji} \leq C_{ji})$, we define $N_{ji}(t) = \delta_{ji} I(X_{ji} \leq t)$, $Y_{ji}(t) = I(X_{ji} \geq t)$, $N_j(t) = \sum_{i=1}^{n_j} N_{ji}(t)$ and $Y_j(t) = \sum_{i=1}^{n_j} Y_{ji}(t)$. Under H_0 for large n,

$$W = n^{-1/2} \sum_{j=1}^{J} \int_0^\infty \{dN_j(t) - Y_j(t)d\Lambda_{0j}(t)\}$$

is approximately normal with mean 0 and its variance can be consistently estimated by

$$\hat{\sigma}^2 = n^{-1} \sum_{j=1}^{J} \int_0^\infty Y_j(t) d\Lambda_{0j}(t).$$

Hence, we reject H_0 with one-sided α level if $Z = W/\hat{\sigma} < -z_{1-\alpha}$, where $z_{1-\alpha}$ denotes the $100(1 - \alpha)$ percentile of the standard normal distribution.

Note that we have the standardized test statistic is expressed as

$$W/\hat{\sigma} = \sum_{j=1}^{J} \frac{O_j - E_j}{\sqrt{E_j}},$$

where, for subpopulation j, $O_j = \int_0^\infty dN_j(t)$ is the observed number of events and $E_j = \int_0^\infty Y_j(t) d\Lambda_{0j}(t)$ is the expected number of events under H_0.

5.2.2   Sample Size Calculation

We calculate the required sample size $n = \sum_{j=1}^{J} n_j$ for a specified power under a specific alternative hypothesis $H_1 : \Lambda_j(t) = \Lambda_{1j}(t)$ for $j = 1, \dots, J$. Let $\gamma_j = n_j/n$ denote the expected prevalence of subpopulation j ($\gamma_j > 0$ and $\sum_{j=1}^{J} \gamma_j = 1$), $S_{1j}(t) = \exp\{-\Lambda_{1j}(t)\}$ denote the survivor function of T_{ji} under H_1, and $G(t)$ denote the survivor function of C_{ji}. Under H_1, $n^{-1}Y_j(t)$ uniformly converges to $\gamma_j G(t) S_{1j}(t)$, so that $\hat{\sigma}^2$ converges to

$$\sigma_0^2 = \sum_{j=1}^{J} \gamma_j \int_0^\infty G(t) S_{1j}(t) d\Lambda_{0j}(t).$$

Under H_1, W is approximately normal with mean

$$\sqrt{n}\omega \equiv \sqrt{n} \sum_{j=1}^{J} \gamma_j \int_0^\infty G(t) S_{1j}(t) d\{\Lambda_{1j}(t) - \Lambda_{0j}(t)\}$$

and variance

$$\sigma_1^2 = \sum_{j=1}^{J} \gamma_j \int_0^\infty G(t) S_{1j}(t) d\Lambda_{1j}(t) = -\sum_{j=1}^{J} \gamma_j \int_0^\infty G(t) dS_{1j}(t).$$

Note that σ_1^2 equals the probability that a patient has an event during the study period when H_1 is true, and $\omega = \sigma_1^2 - \sigma_0^2$.

Hence, we have the power function

$$1 - \beta = P(W/\hat{\sigma} < -z_{1-\alpha}|H_1) = P\left(\frac{W - \sqrt{n}\omega}{\sigma_1} \times \frac{\sigma_1}{\sigma_0} < -\frac{\sqrt{n}\omega}{\sigma_0} - z_{1-\alpha}|H_1\right).$$

By solving this equation and replacing $\omega = \sigma_1^2 - \sigma_0^2$, we obtain the required sample size

$$n = \frac{(\sigma_0 z_{1-\alpha} + \sigma_1 z_{1-\beta})^2}{(\sigma_1^2 - \sigma_0^2)^2}. \tag{5.5}$$

5.2.2.1   Under Uniform Accrual and Exponential Survival Models

Suppose that the survival distribution is exponential with hazard rate λ_{hj} under H_h for $h = 0, 1$. The survival and cumulative hazard functions are given as $S_{hj}(t) = \exp(-\lambda_{hj} t)$ and $\Lambda_{hj}(t) = \lambda_{hj} t$, respectively. Assuming patient accrual at a constant rate during period a and an additional follow-up period of b, the censoring distribution is $U(b, a+b)$ with a survival function $G(t) = P(C \geq t) = 1$ if $t \leq b$; $= (a+b)/a - t/a$ if $b \leq t \leq a+b$; $= 0$ otherwise. Under these assumptions, we have

$$\sigma_1^2 = 1 - \sum_{j=1}^{J} \gamma_j \frac{e^{-b\lambda_{1j}}}{a\lambda_{1j}} (1 - e^{-a\lambda_{1j}}). \tag{5.6}$$

Similarly, we can show that

$$\sigma_0^2 = \sum_{j=1}^{J} \gamma_j \frac{\lambda_{0j}}{\lambda_{1j}} \left\{ 1 - \frac{e^{-b\lambda_{1j}}}{a\lambda_{1j}} (1 - e^{-a\lambda_{1j}}) \right\}.$$

By plugging σ_0^2 and σ_1^2 in (5.5), we calculate a sample size under uniform accrual and exponential survival model.

If we expect similar efficacy improvement among subpopulations, we may assume a common hazard ratio $\Delta = \lambda_{0j}/\lambda_{1j}$. In this case, we have $\sigma_0^2 = \Delta \sigma_1^2$ and $\omega = \sigma_1^2 - \sigma_0^2 = (1 - \Delta)\sigma_1^2$. Hence, (5.5) is expressed as

$$n = \frac{(\sqrt{\Delta} z_{1-\alpha} + z_{1-\beta})^2}{\sigma_1^2 (\Delta - 1)^2}. \tag{5.7}$$

Since σ_1^2 is the probability of observing an event from each patient in the study, the required number of events $D = n\sigma_1^2$ is given as

$$D = \frac{(\sqrt{\Delta} z_{1-\alpha} + z_{1-\beta})^2}{(\Delta - 1)^2}. \tag{5.8}$$

5.2.2.2   When Accrual Rate Is Given

We assume (i) uniform accrual, (ii) exponential survival model, and (iii) constant a common hazard ratio $\Delta = \lambda_{01}/\lambda_{11} = \cdots = \lambda_{0J}/\lambda_{1J}$. Now, we further consider a sample size calculation when the accrual rate r is given instead of the accrual period a. From (5.6), $\sigma_1^2 = \sigma_1^2(a)$ is a function of an unknown variable a. By replacing n with $a \times r$ in the left side of (5.7), we obtain an equation on a,

$$a \times r \times \sigma_1^2(a) = \left(\frac{\sqrt{\Delta} z_{1-\alpha} + z_{1-\beta}}{\Delta - 1} \right)^2$$

or, simply

$$a \times r \times \sigma_1^2(a) = D \tag{5.9}$$

from $n\sigma_1^2 = D$. To use (5.9), we should calculate D by (5.8) first. We solve one of these equations using a numerical method such as the bisection method. Let a^* denote the solution to the equations. Then, the required sample size is obtained as $n = a^* \times r$.

References

Chang, M., Jung, S.H., and Wu, S.S. (2012). Two-stage designs with additional futility tests for phase II clinical trials with heterogeneous patient populations. *Sequential Analysis*, in press.

Jung, S.H., Chang, M., and Kang, S. (2012). Phase II cancer clinical trials with heterogeneous patient populations. *Journal of Biopharmaceutical Statistics*, 22, 312–328.

Jung, S.H., Lee, T.Y., Kim, K.M., and George, S. (2004). Admissible two-stage designs for phase II cancer clinical trials. *Statistics in Medicine*, 23, 561–569.

London, W.B. and Chang, M.N. (2005). One- and two-stage designs for stratified phase II clinical trials. *Statistics in Medicine*, 24, 2597–2611.

Simon, R. (1989). Optimal two-stage designs for phase II clinical trials. *Controlled Clinical Trials*, 10, 1–10.

Sposto, R. and Gaynon, P.S. (2009). An adjustment for for patient heterogeneity in the design of two-stage phase II trials. *Statistics in Medicine*, 28, 2566–2579.

Chapter 6

Randomized Phase II Trials for Selection: No Prospective Control Arms

Often, phase II protocols have multiple experimental therapies for efficacy screening with respect to the same patient population. Usually, the resources for clinical trials are limited, so that we may want to choose only a small number of therapies, ideally one therapy, to be compared with a standard therapy through a phase III trial. In this setting, we may take one of two approaches: (i) conduct multiple separate phase II trials, one for each experimental therapy, and evaluate them independently using a standard phase II trial design method for a single-arm phase II trial; (ii) conduct a single phase II trial with multiple experimental arms, randomize patients into the arms, and choose the best arm(s) using a selection method. The former approach requires more research resources due to the multiplicity of the studies. Also, the individual phase II trials may potentially have different patient characteristics, and the comparison among different therapies can be biased.

Because of these issues, the second approach is more attractive. However, the statistical approaches for analyzing randomized phase II trials are limited. Simon, Wittes, and Ellenberg (1985) consider randomizing n patients to each of K treatment arms through a single stage and picking the winner, the arm with the largest estimated response rate, among them. This approach is based on the statistical methods of ranking and selection, the basic concepts of which were introduced more than 50 years ago by Beckhofer (1954), with a substantial literature since that time. They show that, depending on the design setting, $n = 16$ to 70 patients per arm are required for a correct selection probability of 0.9 when there exists a difference of 0.15 in response rate among the K arms. Liu, LeBlanc, and Desai (1999) point out that this approach has a high selection probability even when the treatment arms have the same response rates. Sargent and Goldberg (2001) consider a similar approach by allowing selection based on other factors when the difference in observed response rates is small.

Palmer (1991) proposes a two-stage design for selection of the best of three treatments. In stage 1, cohorts of three patients are randomized to arms A,

B, and C, and a decision is made to continue to accrue the next cohort or to stop and choose the best two arms. In stage 2, cohorts of two patients are randomized to the two arms chosen at stage 1, and a decision is made to continue to accrue the next cohort or to stop and choose the winner. Given the maximum number of patients available for the study, the stopping time for each stage is chosen to minimize the number of future failures using a Bayesian approach. This method requires rapid determination of responses to be able to apply the sequential tests. As an extension of Palmer (1991), Cheung (2008) proposes a fully sequential approach that can accommodate more than three arms.

Steinberg and Venzon (2002) propose two-stage designs for a phase II trial with two experimental arms. In stage 1, n_1 patients are randomized to each arm. The trial is stopped after stage 1 if the difference in number of responders between the two arms are larger than d, which is chosen so that, when the two arms have a difference of 0.15 in response rate, the probability of selecting the inferior arm is controlled at a specified level. Otherwise, the trial proceeds to stage 2 to randomize an additional n_2 patients to each arm. After stage 2, the winner is chosen based on the cumulative responses through the two stages. Given $n = n_1 + n_2$, one can choose $n_1 = n_2 = n/2$ or to minimize the expected sample size for the specified response rates with 0.15 of difference. This approach does not control the overall error probabilities through the two-stage selection procedure.

Most of these existing methods do not accurately control the type I error and the power for the whole selection procedure. Furthermore, they do not allow unequal designs among different arms. In this chapter, we discuss Jung and George (2009). They propose exact and efficient methods for selecting a small number of experimental therapies for further investigation through a randomized phase II trial. If there exists a historical control, it is reasonable to choose an experimental arm that beats both the historical control and the other experimental arms. In this sense, at first, each of the parallel experimental arms is compared to a historical control by a single-arm phase II trial design called *independent evaluation*, and then between-arm comparisons are performed among the experimental arms that are accepted from the independent evaluation through single-arm phase II trial designs, called *between-arm comparison*. In a between-arm comparison, we use the uniformly minimum variance unbiased estimator (UMVUE) of response rate of each arm since, as shown in Chapter 3, for two-stage phase II trial designs, the maximum likelihood estimator (MLE) can be seriously biased, and the efficiency of UMVUE is comparable to that of MLE.

If there exists no historical control, we conduct between-arm comparisons at each stage, so that we can stop the trial early when a significant difference in efficacy is observed among the experimental arms.

6.1 With a Historical Control

We consider two-arm randomized phase II studies, each arm with a two-stage design for independent evaluation as the primary objective.

Example 6.1
Suppose that we randomize non-Hodgkin's lymphoma patients who relapsed from a rituximab-containing combination regimen to rituximab alone (Arm R, $n = 90$) or rituximab+lenalidomide (Arm R+L, $n = 45$) with 2-to-1 probability, each arm will go through independent evaluation with the following two-stage design:

   Arm R: $(a_1/n_1, a/n) = (10/57, 19/90)$ for 4% type I error at $p_0 = 0.15$
   and 95% power at $p_1 = 0.30$.

Arm R+L: $(a_1/n_1, a/n) = (4/21, 10/45)$ for 5% type I error at $p_0 = 0.15$ and
   89% power at $p_1 = 0.35$.

Arm R is a potential control arm for a future phase III trial in case Arm R+L is accepted in this trial, but it is included in this phase II trial because there is not enough historical data on the regimen. Twice as many patients will be accrued to Arm R than to Arm R+L to allow more precise estimation of the clinical parameters to be used in designing a future phase III trial. Arm R+L may not be investigated further if it does not seem to be more efficacious than Arm R. We want to compare the two arms accounting for the two-stage design for each arm.

   In general, we call the two arms arm x and arm y, respectively. For arm $k(= x, y)$, let $M_k(= 1$ or $2)$ denote the terminating stage and S_k the number of responders at stage M_k during independent evaluation. For an outcome (m_k, s_k), let $\hat{p}_k = \hat{p}_k(m_k, s_k)$ denote the UMVUE for the true response probabilities p_k; see Chapter 3.

6.1.1 When Both Arms Have Identical Two-Stage Designs

In this section, we assume that patients are randomized between two arms with the same two-stage design $(a_1/n_1, a/n)$ for independent evaluation, see Chapter 2.

6.1.1.1 One-Sided Test

Suppose that patients are randomized between two experimental arms, arm x and arm y, and consider selection of arm y compared to arm x. Usually, the selection procedure is bilateral, so that the associated test is two-sided. But we discuss one-sided test in this section, and expand the results to two-sided selection problems in the following section.

At first, each arm will be evaluated compared to a common historical control using a standard two-stage design for phase II trials. When such a trial is completed, we want to test whether the arm y is better than arm x or not. The hypotheses associated with this type of comparison are

$$H_0 : p_y \leq p_x \text{ vs. } H_a : p_y > p_x.$$

This is a one-sided test. So in this case, we usually would not want to accept the experimental arm y if it is not accepted in the independent evaluation. Thus, we want to select arm y for further investigation (or, reject H_0) if it is accepted in the independent evaluation, that is, $m_y = 2$ and $s_y > a$, and it has a higher response risponse rate than arm x, that is, $\hat{p}_y - \hat{p}_x \geq c$ for a chosen critical value c. Let $\hat{p}_k = \hat{p}(m_k, s_k)$ for given (M_k, S_k), and $\mathcal{D} = \{(m, s) : m = 1, 0 \leq s \leq a_1\} \cup \{(m, s) : m = 2, a_1 + 1 \leq s \leq n\}$ denote the sample space of each arm defined by the common two-stage design $(a_1/n_1, a/n)$. Given a true response rate $p_x = p_y = p$ under H_0, the probability of rejecting H_0 is

$$h(c|p) = P(\hat{p}_y - \hat{p}_x \geq c, m_y = 2, s_y > a|p)$$
$$= \sum_{(m_x, s_x) \in \mathcal{D}} \sum_{(m_y, s_y) \in \mathcal{D}} I\{\hat{p}(m_y, s_y) - \hat{p}(m_x, s_x) \geq c, m_y = 2, s_y > a\}$$
$$\times f(m_x, s_x|p) f(m_y, s_y|p), \tag{6.1}$$

where $I(\cdot)$ is the indicator function and $f(m, s|p)$ denotes the probability mass function of (M, S) under the common two-stage designs,

$$f(m, s|p)$$
$$= \begin{cases} p^s (1-p)^{n_1 - s} \binom{n_1}{s} & m = 1, \quad 0 \leq s \leq a_1 \\ p^s (1-p)^{n_1 + n_2 - s} \sum_{x_1 = a_1 + 1}^{n_1 \wedge s} \binom{n_1}{x_1} \binom{n_2}{s - x_1} & m = 2, \quad a_1 + 1 \leq s \leq n_1 + n_2 \end{cases}$$

for $(m, s) \in \mathcal{D}$, see Chapter 3. More generally, the probability of an event A in $\mathcal{D}^2$ is calculated by

$$P(A|p_x, p_y) = \sum_{(m_x, s_x) \in \mathcal{D}} \sum_{(m_y, s_y) \in \mathcal{D}} I\left[\{(m_x, s_x), (m_y, s_y)\} \in A\right]$$
$$\times f(m_x, s_x|p_x) f(m_y, s_y|p_y).$$

In contrast to asymptotic tests, such as the two-sample t-test, the operating characteristics of this exact test depend on the null response probability p, an unknown nuisance parameter. In order to remove the nuisance parameter, we control the type I error rate by maximizing the probability in (6.1) over the whole parameter space $p \in [0, 1]$, or over a subset of interest $\mathcal{I} \subset [0, 1]$. See Berger and Boos (1994) for the rationale for such an approach. Given α, we want to choose a critical value $c = c_\alpha$ so that the probability of accepting arm y is no larger than α under H_0, that is,

$$P\{\hat{p}(M_y, S_y) - \hat{p}(M_x, S_x) \geq c_\alpha, M_y = 2, S_y > a | H_0\}$$
$$= \max_{p \in \mathcal{I}} P\{\hat{p}(M_y, S_y) - \hat{p}(M_x, S_x) \geq c_\alpha, \quad M_y = 2, S_y > a | p_x = p_y = p\} \leq \alpha.$$

We will refer to probability (6.2) as the type I error rate. Let p_0 denote the response rate of a historical control. Then, we may choose a small interval around p_0, such as $\mathcal{I} = [p_0 - 0.2, p_0 + 0.2]$. If we want the type I error rate to be controlled under any true response rate value, we have to choose $\mathcal{I} = [0, 1]$. We use the latter in this chapter.

Let $H(c) = \max_{p \in \mathcal{I}} h(c|p)$. Obviously, $h(c|p)$ is monotone in c. Given c, however, $h(c|p)$ can have local maxima over $p \in \mathcal{I}$. For example, when both arms have the same design as that of Arm R+L in Example 6.1, $(a_1/n_1, a/n) = (4/21, 10/45)$, Figure 6.1 displays $h(c = 0.1|p)$ over $p \in [0, 1]$. Note that there are two local maxima, one around $p = 0.25$ and the other around 0.3. So, given α, calculation of the critical value c_α requires a two-stage numerical search procedure. For a given critical value c, $H(c)$ is calculated by the grid search for the maximum of $h(c|p)$ in the range of $p \in [0, 1]$. For any $p \in [0, 1]$, $h(c|p)$ is monotone in c, so that $H(c)$ is also monotone in c. Hence, the critical value $c = c_\alpha$ satisfying $H(c_\alpha) = \alpha$ can be obtained by the bisection method.

Let $\Delta(> 0)$ denote a clinically significant difference in response rate. Given p_x and $p_y = p_x + \Delta$, the probability of correct comparison, called the *power*, is calculated as

$$1 - \beta = P(\hat{p}_y - \hat{p}_x \geq c_\alpha, M_y = 2, S_y > a | p_x, p_y = p_x + \Delta).$$

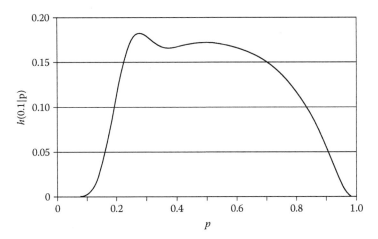

Figure 6.1 Plot of $h(c|p)$ for $c = 0.1$ and p between 0 and 1.

Suppose that arm y is accepted in the independent evaluation, and $\hat{c} = \hat{p}_y - \hat{p}_x$ denotes the observed difference from the data. Then, one may want to see how significant the evidence is against H_0. To this end, we propose to calculate a p-value by

$$\text{p-value} = \max_{0 \le p \le 1} P\{\hat{p}(M_y, S_y) - \hat{p}(M_x, S_x) \ge \hat{c}, M_y = 2, S_y > a | p_x = p_y = p\}.$$

Example 6.2

Suppose that we want to test if arm y has a higher response rate than arm x. The two arms have the same two-stage design $(a_1/n_1, a/n) = (4/21, 10/45)$ as in Arm R+L of Example 6.1. With $\alpha = 0.1$, we have $c_\alpha = 0.1520$, and the type I error rate is maximized at $p_x = p_y = 0.2692$. With $\Delta = 0.2$, the power is 0.669 for $(p_x, p_y) = (0.15, 0.35)$, 0.649 for $(p_x, p_y) = (0.2, 0.4)$, and 0.639 for $(p_x, p_y) = (0.25, 0.45)$. With $\Delta = 0.25$, the power is 0.809 for $(p_x, p_y) = (0.15, 0.4)$, 0.796 for $(p_x, p_y) = (0.2, 0.45)$, and 0.800 for $(p_x, p_y) = (0.25, 0.5)$. When we have $(m_x, s_x) = (2, 12)$ ($\hat{p}_x = 0.295$), we have p-value = 0.3064 if $(m_y, s_y) = (2, 15)$ ($\hat{p}_y = 0.342$); p-value = 0.1123 if $(m_y, s_y) = (2, 20)$ ($\hat{p}_y = 0.445$); and p-value = 0.0145 if $(m_y, s_y) = (2, 25)$ ($\hat{p}_y = 0.556$).

Note that the above comparison rule controls the type I error rate of selecting one experimental arm when both arms have an equal response rate. One may want to somewhat loosen the type I error control by allowing a selection of the inferior experimental arm whose response rate is smaller than the other only by a clinically negligible margin. Let $\delta(> 0)$ denote the maximum of clinically insignificant differences in response rate, for example, $\delta = 0.05$. Suppose that we do not care about falsely accepting arm y as far as p_y is within δ of p_x, that is, $p_y > p_x - \delta$. In this case, the hypotheses may be modified to

$$H_0 : p_y \le p_x - \delta \quad \text{vs.} \quad H_a : p_y > p_x - \delta.$$

We choose a critical value $c = c_\alpha$ satisfying

$$\max_{p_x, p_y \in \mathcal{I}} P\{\hat{p}(M_y, S_y) - \hat{p}(M_x, S_x) \ge c_\alpha, M_y = 2, S_y > a | p_x, p_y = p_x - \delta\} \le \alpha.$$

Given p_x and $p_y = p_x + \Delta$, the power is calculated as

$$1 - \beta = P\{\hat{p}(M_y, S_y) - \hat{p}(M_x, S_x) \ge c_\alpha, M_y = 2, S_y > a | p_x, p_y = p_x + \Delta\}.$$

For an observed difference $\hat{c} = \hat{p}_y - \hat{p}_x$, the p-value is calculated as

$$\text{p-value} = \max_{p_x, p_y \in \mathcal{I}} P\{\hat{p}(M_y, S_y) - \hat{p}(M_x, S_x) \ge \hat{c}, M_y = 2, S_y > a | p_x, p_y = p_x - \delta\}.$$

We will consider a selection procedure allowing the maximum clinically insignificant difference δ in the remainder of this chapter if not stated otherwise.

Example 6.3

Consider Example 6.2 with $\delta = 0.05$. With $\delta = 0.05$ and $\alpha = 0.1$, we have $c_\alpha = 0.0925$, and the Type I error rate is maximized at $(p_x, p_y) = (0.3138, 0.2638)$. With $\Delta = 0.2$, the power is 0.799 for $(p_x, p_y) = (0.15, 0.35)$, 0.820 for $(p_x, p_y) = (0.2, 0.4)$, and 0.827 for $(p_x, p_y) = (0.25, 0.45)$. If we observe $(m_x, s_x) = (2, 12)$, we have p-value $= 0.1640$ if $(m_y, s_y) = (2, 15)$; p-value $= 0.0529$ if $(m_y, s_y) = (2, 20)$; and p-value $= 0.0051$ if $(m_y, s_y) = (2, 25)$.

6.1.1.2 Two-Sided Test

We now want to compare two experimental arms and choose one that will be investigated further in a phase III trial. We would not care much if we select an inferior arm when its response rate is smaller than that of the other arm only by a clinically insignificant margin δ. In this case, the associated testing is two-sided. As in the one-sided case, we do not want to select an experimental arm if it is not accepted in the independent evaluation. That is, we want to select an experimental arm if it is accepted in the independent evaluation and its UMVUE is significantly larger than that of the other arm.

For arm $k(= x, y)$, let $\mathcal{A}_k = (M_k = 2, S_k > a)$ denote the event that arm k is accepted from an independent evaluation through a two-stage design. We select arm x if {arm x is accepted in the independent evaluation, but arm y is not} or {both arms are accepted in the independent evaluation and arm x has a significantly higher response rate than arm y}. That is, for a chosen critical value c, we select arm x if

$$S_x(c) = (\mathcal{A}_x \cap \bar{\mathcal{A}}_y) \cup \{\mathcal{A}_x \cap \mathcal{A}_y \cap (\hat{p}(M_x, S_x) - \hat{p}(M_y, S_y) \geq c)\}$$

is true, and arm y if

$$S_y(c) = (\bar{\mathcal{A}}_x \cap \mathcal{A}_y) \cup [\mathcal{A}_x \cap \mathcal{A}_y \cap \{\hat{p}(M_y, S_y) - \hat{p}(M_x, S_x) \geq c)\}]$$

is true, where $\bar{A}$ denotes the complement of event A. Since the two arms have the same two-stage design, $(a_1/n_1, a/n)$, the error probabilities $P(\mathcal{A}_x | p_x, p_y = p_x + \delta)$ and $P(\mathcal{A}_y | p_x, p_y = p_x - \delta)$ are identical. Hence, for specified p_x and p_y with $\delta = |p_x - p_y|$, the false selection probability is expressed as

$$\frac{1}{2}[P\{S_x(c)|p_y = p_x + \delta\} + P\{S_y(c)|p_x = p_y + \delta\}] = P\{S_y(c)|p_x = p_y + \delta\}.$$

Using this result, we obtain the critical value $c = c_\alpha$ so that the false selection probability under H_0, also called the type I error rate, does not exceed α, that is,

$$\max_{p_x, p_y \in \mathcal{I}} P\{S_y(c)|p_x, p_y = p_x - \delta\} \leq \alpha.$$

Noting that $\bar{\mathcal{A}}_x \cap \mathcal{A}_y \subset S_y(c)$ for any $c > 0$, so that we should choose an α larger than $\max_{p_x, p_y \in \mathcal{I}} P\{S_y(c)|p_x = p_y + \delta\}$. The probabilities of $S_x(c)$ and $S_y(c)$ will be unequal if the two arms have different designs. Cases with different designs will be discussed in the next section.

Given p_x and $p_y = p_x + \Delta$, the true selection probability, also called the power, is calculated as

$$1 - \beta = P\{\mathcal{S}_y(c_\alpha)|p_x, p_y = p_x + \Delta\}$$

with respect to a clinically significant difference Δ. Suppose that both arms are accepted in the independent evaluation and $\hat{c} = \hat{p}_y - \hat{p}_x(> 0)$ denotes the observed difference in UMVUE from a randomized phase II trial. Then, we calculate the p-value by

$$\text{p-value} = \max_{p_x, p_y = p_x - \delta \in \mathcal{I}} P[\bar{\mathcal{A}}_x \cap \mathcal{A}_y \cap \{\hat{p}(M_y, S_y) - \hat{p}(M_x, S_x) \geq \hat{c}\}|p_x, p_y = p_x - \delta].$$

We select neither arm if both arms are rejected in the independent evaluation, and select both arms if both arms are accepted in the independent evaluation and $|\hat{p}_x - \hat{p}_y| < c_\alpha$.

Example 6.4

Suppose that two experimental arms have the same two-stage design $(a_1/n_1, a/n) = (4/21, 10/45)$. With $\delta = 0.05$, we have $\max_{p_x, p_y \in \mathcal{I}} P\{\mathcal{S}_y(c)|p_x = p_y + \delta\} = 0.1333$. For $\alpha = 0.2$, we have $c_\alpha = 0.0444$ and the actual type I error rate is 0.1701, which is attained at $(p_x, p_y) = (0.567, 0.617)$, where the order is unimportant. With $\Delta = 0.15$, the power is 0.830 for $(p_x, p_y) = (0.25, 0.4)$, 0.827 for $(p_x, p_y) = (0.3, 0.45)$, and 0.822 for $(p_x, p_y) = (0.35, 0.5)$. When we observe $(m_x, s_x) = (2, 12)$, we have p-value = 0.1701 if $(m_y, s_y) = (2, 15)$; p-value = 0.1337 if $(m_y, s_y) = (2, 20)$; and p-value = 0.0013 if $(m_y, s_y) = (2, 25)$.

6.1.2   When Two Arms Have Different Two-Stage Designs

In a randomized phase II trial, we may want to use a different design for independent evaluation of each experimental arm. If we want to compare two experimental therapies evaluated by separate single-arm phase II trials, it is very likely that the two trials have different designs. In this section, we consider selection problems when two arms have different two-stage designs.

In the previous section, we have considered phase II trials randomizing patients to two arms with exactly the same two-stage designs for independent evaluation. In this case, we do not want to select an arm that is rejected in the independent evaluation. However, when the two arms have different two-stage designs, the probability of accepting an arm will be different from that of the other. So, a between-arm comparison incorporating the independent evaluation result may be unfair to the arm with a higher rejection probability.

As such, the selection rules in this section are based only on the comparison of the estimators of the response rates.

6.1.2.1   One-Sided Test

As before, we consider selection of arm y compared to arm x by testing

$$H_0 : p_y \leq p_x - \delta \quad \text{vs.} \quad H_a : p_y > p_x - \delta$$

for a maximal clinically negligible difference δ. We choose a critical value $c = c_\alpha$ satisfying

$$
\max_{0 \leq p_x < p_y \leq 1} P(\hat{p}_y - \hat{p}_x \geq c_\alpha | p_x = p_y + \delta)
$$

$$
= \max_{0 \leq p_x < p_y \leq 1} \sum_{(m_x, s_x) \in \mathcal{D}_x} \sum_{(m_y, s_y) \in \mathcal{D}_y} I\{\hat{p}_y(m_x, s_x) - \hat{p}_x(m_y, s_y) \geq c_\alpha\}
$$

$$
\times f_x(m_x, s_x | p_y + \delta) f_y(m_y, s_y | p_y) \leq \alpha,
$$

where $\mathcal{D}_k$, $\hat{p}_k(\cdot, \cdot)$, and $f_k(\cdot, \cdot | \cdot)$ are design-specific sample space, UMVUE of the response rate, and probability mass function of (M, S), respectively, for arm $k(= x, y)$.

The power for Δ and p_x ($p_y = p_x + \Delta$) is calculated by

$$
1 - \beta = P(\hat{p}_y - \hat{p}_x \geq c_\alpha | p_x, p_y = p_x + \Delta)
$$

$$
= \sum_{(m_x, s_x) \in \mathcal{D}_x} \sum_{(m_y, s_y) \in \mathcal{D}_y} I\{\hat{p}_y(m_x, s_x) - \hat{p}_x(m_y, s_y) \geq c_\alpha\} f_x(m_x, s_x | p_x)
$$

$$
\times f_y(m_y, s_y | p_x + \Delta).
$$

For an observed difference, $\hat{c} = \hat{p}_y - \hat{p}_x$, the p-value is calculated as

$$
\text{p-value} = \max_{0 \leq p_x, p_y \leq 1} P(\hat{p}_y - \hat{p}_x \geq \hat{c} | p_x = p_y + \delta)
$$

$$
= \max_{0 \leq p_x < p_y \leq 1} \sum_{(m_x, s_x) \in \mathcal{D}_x} \sum_{(m_y, s_y) \in \mathcal{D}_y} I\{\hat{p}_y(m_x, s_x) - \hat{p}_x(m_y, s_y) \geq \hat{c}\}
$$

$$
\times f_x(m_x, s_x | p_y + \delta) f_y(m_y, s_y | p_y).
$$

Example 6.5

Consider $\delta = 0.05$ in Example 6.1. Then with $\alpha = 0.1$, we have $c_\alpha = 0.0717$ and the type I error rate is maximized at $(p_x, p_y) = (0.2185, 0.1685)$. With $\Delta = 0.2$, the power is 0.933 for $(p_x, p_y) = (0.25, 0.45)$, 0.926 for $(p_x, p_y) = (0.30, 0.50)$, and 0.922 for $(p_x, p_y) = (0.35, 0.55)$. Table 6.1 displays p-values for this exact method.

Table 6.1   p-values for some chosen outcomes for comparing arm x (control) with $(a_1/n_1, a/n) = (10/57, 19/90)$ and arm y (experimental) with $(a_1/n_1, a/n) = (4/21, 10/45)$ at $\alpha = 0.1$ and $\delta = .05$

Arm x			Arm y			
m	s	$\hat{p}(m,s)$	m	s	$\hat{p}(m,s)$	**p-value**
2	20	0.230	2	11	0.283	0.1413
2	20	0.230	2	12	0.295	0.1169
2	20	0.230	2	13	0.309	0.0904
2	20	0.230	2	14	0.325	0.0675
2	20	0.230	2	15	0.342	0.0447
2	20	0.230	2	20	0.445	0.0017

6.1.2.2   Two-Sided Test

Suppose that two experimental arms have different two-stage designs for independent evaluation with respect to a historical control. We choose a critical value $c = c_\alpha$ satisfying

$$\max_{0 \le p_x, p_y \le 1} \{P(\hat{p}_y - \hat{p}_x \ge c_\alpha | p_x = p_y + \delta) + P(\hat{p}_x - \hat{p}_y \ge c_\alpha | p_y = p_x + \delta)\} \le \alpha. \quad (6.3)$$

Note that the two misselection errors in the left-hand side of (6.3) are not the same if the two arms have different designs. We fail to select one arm against the other if $|\hat{p}_x - \hat{p}_y| < c_\alpha$.

The power for Δ and p_x $(p_y = p_x + \Delta)$,

$$1 - \beta = P(\hat{p}_y - \hat{p}_x \ge c_\alpha | p_x, p_y = p_x + \Delta).$$

For an observed difference, $\hat{c} = |\hat{p}_x - \hat{p}_y|$, the p-value is calculated as

$$\text{p-value} = \max_{0 \le p_x, p_y \le 1} \{P(\hat{p}_y - \hat{p}_x \ge \hat{c} | p_x = p_y + \delta, p_y)$$
$$+ P(\hat{p}_x - \hat{p}_y \ge \hat{c} | p_x, p_y = p_x + \delta)\}.$$

Example 6.6

Suppose that both arms in Example 6.1 are experimental. Then with $\delta = 0.05$ and $\alpha = 0.1$, we have $c_\alpha = 0.1174$, and the type I error is maximized at $(p_x, p_y) = (0.2775, 0.2275)$, where the order is unimportant. With $\Delta = 0.2$, the power is 0.826 for $(p_x, p_y) = (0.25, 0.45)$, 0.831 for $(p_x, p_y) = (0.30, 0.50)$, and 0.838 for $(p_x, p_y) = (0.35, 0.55)$. Table 6.2 reports p-values for some chosen outcomes for the exact method.

Table 6.2 Shown are p-values for some chosen outcomes for comparing two experimental arms with two-stage designs $(a_1/n_1, a/n) = (10/57, 19/90)$ and $(a_1/n_1, a/n) = (4/21, 10/45)$ at $\alpha = 0.1$ and $\delta = .05$

	Arm x			Arm y		
m	s	$\hat{p}(m, s)$	m	s	$\hat{p}(m, s)$	**p-value**
2	33	0.333	2	20	0.407	0.2180
2	33	0.333	2	25	0.500	0.0277
2	33	0.333	2	30	0.600	0.0019
2	33	0.333	2	35	0.700	0.0001
2	33	0.333	2	40	0.800	0.0000

6.2 When No Historical Control Exists

In this section, we assume that there exist no historical control for comparison with experimental arms. In this case, we propose a two-stage design conducting a between-arm comparison at each stage. No independent evaluation of each experimental arm is conducted in this case.

Suppose that equal number of patients are randomized to each arm at each stage. During stage $l(= 1, 2)$, n_l patients are randomized to each arm, and X_l and Y_l denote the number of responders from arms x and y, respectively. Let $n = n_1 + n_2$, $X = X_1 + X_2$, and $Y = Y_1 + Y_2$. Given integers c_1 and c, we propose to select arm x if $X_1 - Y_1 > c_1$ or $X - Y > c$. The type I error probability for a clinically negligible difference δ is given as

$$\alpha = \max_{p_x, p_y \in (0,1)} P\{(X_1 - Y_1 > c_1) \cup (X - Y > c) | p_x = p_y - \delta\}$$
$$= P\{(X_1 - Y_1 > c_1) \cup (X - Y > c) | p_x = 0.5 - \delta/2, \, p_x = 0.5 + \delta/2\}$$

and the power for a clinically meaningful difference Δ is given as

$$1 - \beta = \min_{p_x, p_y \in (0,1)} P\{(X_1 - Y_1 > c_1) \cup (X - Y > c) | p_x = p_y + \Delta, p_y\}$$
$$= P\{(X_1 - Y_1 > c_1) \cup (X - Y > c) | p_x = 0.5 + \Delta/2, \, p_x = 0.5 - \Delta/2\}.$$

These probabilities are calculated using X_l and Y_l are independent $B(n_l, p_x)$ and $B(n_l, p_y)$ random variables, respectively.

Given type I error α^* and power $1 - \beta^*$, a candidate design (n_1, n, c_1, c) should satisfy

$$\alpha = P\{(X_1 - Y_1 > c_1) \cup (X - Y > c) | p_x = 0.5 - \delta/2, \, p_x = 0.5 + \delta/2\} \leq \alpha^*$$

and

$$1 - \beta = P\{(X_1 - Y_1 > c_1) \cup (X - Y > c) | p_x = 0.5 + \Delta/2, \, p_x = 0.5 - \Delta/2\} \geq 1 - \beta^*.$$

A search for a good two-stage selection design may be conducted to go through all combinations of (n_1, n, c_1, c). Among the candidate designs satisfying a $(\alpha^*, 1 - \beta^*)$-condition, the minimax design has the smallest n.

So far we assume that equal number of patients are randomized to each arm during each stage. If different numbers of patients are randomized between two arms, we may set up a selection rule based on the difference in sample proportions. Suppose that during stage $l(= 1, 2)$, m_l and n_l patients are randomized to arms x and y, respectively, and X_l and Y_l denote the numbers of responders from these arms. We select arm x if $X_1/ - Y_1 > c_1$ or $X - Y > c$. Let $m = m_1 + m_2$, $n = n_1 + n_2$, $X = X_1 + X_2$, and $Y = Y_1 + Y_2$. Given integers c_1 and c, we may select arm x if $X_1/m_1 - Y_1/n_1 > c_1$ or $X/m - Y/n > c$. The type I error rate and power are similarly calculated as in the balanced randomization case.

6.3   Extension to More Than Two Arms

In this section, we consider two-stage designs with balanced allocation. It can be easily extended to the cases with unbalanced allocation as in the two-arm cases. Suppose that, during stage $l(= 1, 2)$, we randomize n_l patients are randomized to each of K arms and observe the number of responders X_{kl} from arm $k(= 1, \ldots, K)$. Let $X_k = X_{k1} + X_{k2}$ and $n = n_1 + n_2$. Suppose that arm 1 has the highest response rate. We choose arm 1 if its response rate is significantly higher than that of the second best arm.

6.3.1   When a Historical Control Exists

When a historical control exists, each arm is independently evaluated compared to the common historical control at first. For arm $k(= 1, \ldots, K)$, let M_k and S_k denote the terminating stage and the cumulative number of responders at the terminating stage, respectively, that will be observed from a two-stage design $(a_1/n_1, a/n)$. By controlling the type I error rate accounting for the multiplicity of experimental arms, we choose a critical value $c = c_\alpha$ satisfying

$$\max_{p_1,\ldots,p_K \in (0,1)} P\{\hat{p}(M_1, S_1) - \max_{2 \leq k \leq K} \hat{p}(M_k, S_k) \geq c_\alpha,$$
$$M_1 = 2, S_1 > a | p_1 = p_2 - \delta, p_2 = \cdots = p_K\} \leq \alpha$$

with respect to a clinically negligible difference δ. Given p_1 and a clinically meaningful difference $\Delta(> \delta)$, the power is calculated as

$$1 - \beta = P\{\hat{p}(M_1, S_1) - \max_{2 \leq k \leq K} \hat{p}(M_k, S_k) \geq c_\alpha,$$
$$M_1 = 2, S_1 > a | p_1 = p_2 + \Delta, p_2 = \cdots = p_K\}.$$

6.3.2 When No Historical Control Exists

If there no historical control exists, there will be no independent evaluation of each experimental arm. A two-stage selection proceeds as follows. For chosen critical values (c_1, c), we select arm 1 if $X_{11} - \max_{2 \leq k \leq K} X_{k1} > c_1$ or $X_1 - \max_{2 \leq k \leq K} X_k > c$. Accounting for the multiplicity of experimental arms, we calculate the type I error rate for a clinically negligible difference δ by

$$\alpha = P\{(X_{11} - \max_{2 \leq k \leq K} X_{k1} > c_1) \cup (X_1 - \max_{2 \leq k \leq K} X_k > c) | p_1 = 0.5 - \delta/2,$$
$$p_2 = \cdots = p_K = 0.5 + \delta/2\}$$

and the power for a clinically meaningful difference Δ by

$$1 - \beta = P\{(X_{11} - \max_{2 \leq k \leq K} X_{k1} > c_1) \cup (X_1 - \max_{2 \leq k \leq K} X_k > c) | p_1 = 0.5 + \Delta/2,$$
$$p_2 = \cdots = p_K = 0.5 - \Delta/2\}.$$

Given $(\alpha^*, 1 - \beta^*)$, a candidate design (n_1, n, c_1, c) satisfies $\alpha \leq \alpha^*$ and $1 - \beta \geq 1 - \beta^*$. A search for the minimax design can be conducted as in the $K = 2$-arm case.

References

Beckhofer, R.E. (1954). A single-sample multiple decision procedure for ranking means of normal populations with known variances. *Annals of Mathematical Statistics*, 25, 16–39.

Berger, R. and Boos, D.D. (1994). P values maximized over a confidence set for the nuisance parameter. *Journal of American Statistical Association*, 89, 1012–1016.

Cheung, Y.K. (2008). Simple sequential boundaries for treatment selection in multi-armed randomized clinical trials with a control. *Biometrics*, 64, 940–949.

Jung, S.H. and George, S.L. (2009). Between-arm comparisons in randomized phase II trials. *Journal of Biopharmaceutical Statistics*, 19, 456–468.

Liu, P.Y., LeBlanc, M., and Desai, M. (1999). False positive rates of randomized phase II designs. *Controlled Clinical Trials*, 20, 343–352.

Palmer, C.R. (1991). A comparative phase II clinical trials procedure for choosing the best of three treatments. *Statistics in Medicine*, 20, 1051–1060.

Sargent, D.J. and Goldberg, R.M. (2001). A flexible design for multiple armed screening trials. *Statistics in Medicine*, 20, 1051–1060.

Simon, R., Wittes, R.E., Ellenberg, S.S. (1985). Randomized phase II clinical trials. *Cancer Treatment Reports*, 69, 1375–1381.

Steinberg, S.M. and Venzon, D.J. (2002). Early selection in a randomized phase II clinical trial. *Statistics in Medicine*, 21, 1711–1726.

Chapter 7

Randomized Phase II Cancer Clinical Trials with a Prospective Control on Binary Endpoints (I): Two-Sample Binomial Test

As an effort to speed the assessment of new therapies, a phase II clinical trial traditionally recruits a small number of patients only to the experimental therapy arm to be compared to a historical control. This implies that the traditional single-arm phase II trials are appropriate only when reliable and valid data for an existing standard therapy are available for the same patient population. Furthermore, the response assessment method used for the historical control should be identical to the one that will be used for a new study.

If no historical control data satisfying these conditions exist or the existing data are too small to represent the whole patient population, we have to consider a randomized phase II clinical trial with a prospective control to be compared with the experimental therapy under investigation. Pointing out that the success rate of phase III trials based on the outcomes from single-arm phase II trials is very low, Cannistra (2009) recommends a randomized phase II trial if a single-arm design is subject to any of these issues. Readers may refer to Gan et al. (2010) about more issues associated with which design to choose between a single-arm phase II trial and a randomized phase II trial.

In Chapter 6, we considered randomized phase II clinical trials with experimental arms only. In this chapter, we focus on randomized phase II trials for evaluating the efficacy of an experimental therapy compared to a prospective control. We discuss a statistical testing method for designing and analyzing randomized phase II clinical trials with a prospective control based on a two-sample binomial test (Jung, 2008). The following chapter discusses randomized phase II trials based on Fisher's (1935) exact test. Although we demonstrate these methods using tumor response as the endpoint, it can be applied to any binomial endpoint, for example, the proportion of patients progression-free at a fixed time point, say, 6 months, as in Section 4.5. Other types of randomized phase II trial designs have been proposed by many investigators, including Thall, Simon, and Ellenberg (1989), and Steinberg and

Venzon (2002). Rubinstein et al. (2005) discuss the strengths and weaknesses of some of these methods and propose a method for randomized phase II screening designs based on the usual large-sample approximation. The designs based on the large-sample theory usually do not control the type I error accurately with typically small sample sizes for phase II trials.

7.1 Two-Sample Binomial Test

7.1.1 Single-Stage Design

If patient accrual is fast or it takes long (say, longer than 6 months) for response assessment of each patient, we may consider using a single-stage design. Suppose that n patients are randomized to each arm, and let X and Y denote the number of responders in arms x (experimental) and y (control), respectively. Let p_x and p_y denote the true response rates for arms x and y, respectively. We want to test whether the experimental arm has a higher response rate than the control or not, that is, $H_0 : p_x \leq p_y$ against $H_1 : p_x > p_y$. A single-stage randomized phase II trial is conducted as follows.

- Randomize n patients to each arm, and observe the number of responders X and Y from arms x and y, respectively.

- Given a prespecified critical value a, accept the experimental arm x if $X - Y \geq a$.

In order to conduct a single-stage randomized phase II trial, we have to determine (n, a) at the design stage. Let p_0 denote the projected response rate for the historical control and Δ a clinically significant increase in response rate for arm x. For the purpose of type I and II error calculation, we specify a simple null hypothesis $H_0 : p_x = p_y = p_0$ and an alternative hypothesis $H_1 : p_x = p_0 + \Delta, p_y = p_0$. Given (n, a), the type I error rate and power of the single-stage design are calculated as

$$\alpha = P(X - Y \geq a | p_x = p_y = p_0)$$

and

$$1 - \beta = P(X - Y \geq a | p_x = p_0 + \Delta, p_y = p_0),$$

respectively. Let $B(n, p)$ denote the binomial distribution with n independent trials and a probability of success p for each trial. These probabilities are calculated assuming that $X \sim B(n, p_x)$ and $Y \sim B(n, p_y)$ are independent random variables. That is,

$$\alpha = \sum_{k_1=a_1}^{n_1} \sum_{y_1=\max(0,-k_1)}^{n_1-\max(0,k_1)} \sum_{k_2=a-k_1}^{n_2} \sum_{y_2=\max(0,-k_2)}^{n_2-\max(0,k_2)} b(y_1|n_1, p_0)b(k_1 + y_1|n_1, p_0)$$

$$\times b(y_2|n_2, p_0)b(k_2 + y_2|n_2, p_0)$$

and

$$1 - \beta = \sum_{k=a}^{n} \sum_{y=\max(0,-k)}^{n-\max(0,k)} b(y|n, p_0)b(k + y|n, p_x)b(y|n, p_0)b(k + y|n, p_x),$$

where $b(x|n, p) = \binom{n}{x} p^x (1 - p)^{n-x}$ for $x = 0, 1, \ldots, n$ denotes the probability mass function of the $B(n, p)$ distribution.

Suppose that we want to choose a single-stage design with type I error rate smaller than or equal to α^* and power larger than or equal to $1 - \beta^*$. There exist many single-stage designs satisfying the $(\alpha^*, 1-\beta^*)$-restriction. We choose design (n, a), which has the smallest n among those designs. Tables 7.1 to 7.9 list single-stage designs under various combinations of $(\alpha^*, 1 - \beta^*, \Delta)$.

7.1.2   Two-Stage Designs with Interim Futility Test

Because of ethical and economical reasons, clinical trials usually are conducted as a multistage design, so that we can terminate the trials when an experimental arm is believed to be significantly low (futility) or high (superiority) efficacy compared to the comparative control. Because of its small sample size, a typical phase II trial has two stages. In this section, we consider two-stage designs for randomized phase II trials between an experimental arm (arm x) and a control arm (arm y) with a futility stopping rule under balanced allocation. Trials with two or more experimental arms and a prospective control, with both futility and superiority stopping rules, or under unbalanced allocation will be investigated in the following sections. A two-stage randomized phase II trial with a futility stopping rule under balanced allocation will proceed as follows.

- *Stage 1*: Accrue n_1 patients to each arm, and observe X_1 and Y_1 denoting the number of responders among the n_1 first-stage patients for arms x and y, respectively.
  - (a) Proceed to the second stage if $X_1 - Y_1 \geq a_1$ for a chosen integer $a_1 \in [-n_1, n_1]$.
  - (b) Otherwise, we reject arm x (or fail to reject H_0) and stop the trial.
- *Stage 2*: Accrue an additional n_2 patients to each arm, and let X_2 and Y_2 denote the number of responders among the second-stage patients of arms x and y, respectively. Let $X = X_1 + X_2$ and $Y = Y_1 + Y_2$ denote the

Table 7.1 Minimax and optimal two-stage designs with a futility stopping value under $(\alpha^*, 1 - \beta^*) = (.1, .8)$ and balanced allocation $(\gamma = 1)$

		Single-Stage Design			Minimax Design				Optimal Design			
p_y	p_x	(n, a)	α	$1-\beta$	(n, n_1, a_1, a)	α	$1-\beta$	EN	(n, n_1, a_1, a)	α	$1-\beta$	EN
.05	.15	(63, 4)	.0740	.8009	(63, 47, 0, 4)	.0739	.8000	56.55	(74, 32, 1, 4)	.0789	.8010	48.01
	.2	(50, 4)	.0524	.8955	(45, 15, 1, 3)	.0799	.8078	24.49	(45, 15, 1, 3)	.0799	.8078	24.49
	.25	(50, 4)	.0524	.9734	(45, 9, 1, 3)	.0613	.8097	18.17	(45, 9, 1, 3)	.0613	.8097	18.17
.1	.25	(52, 5)	.0695	.8081	(47, 39, 3, 4)	.0986	.8033	40.36	(55, 29, 2, 4)	.0991	.8018	35.55
	.3	(50, 5)	.0656	.9231	(45, 18, 2, 3)	.0993	.8083	23.28	(45, 18, 2, 3)	.0993	.8083	23.28
.15	.3	(63, 6)	.0843	.8046	(61, 56, 5, 5)	.0994	.8013	56.58	(73, 27, 1, 6)	.0860	.8001	46.49
	.35	(50, 6)	.0610	.8576	(45, 17, 1, 5)	.0779	.8060	28.30	(46, 16, 1, 5)	.0779	.8026	28.01
.2	.35	(74, 7)	.0904	.8052	(74, 45, 0, 7)	.0894	.8005	61.03	(85, 31, 1, 7)	.0909	.8005	54.58
	.4	(50, 6)	.0840	.8431	(45, 31, 3, 5)	.0966	.8024	33.98	(48, 24, 2, 5)	.0991	.8025	31.03
.25	.4	(84, 8)	.0905	.8029	(83, 78, 7, 7)	.0992	.8025	78.57	(100, 41, 2, 8)	.0893	.8001	61.70
	.45	(53, 7)	.0720	.8039	(48, 28, 1, 6)	.0930	.8003	36.77	(53, 21, 1, 6)	.0940	.8014	34.73
.3	.45	(94, 9)	.0879	.8037	(89, 83, 7, 8)	.0996	.8003	83.81	(105, 50, 3, 8)	.0997	.8000	66.09
	.5	(54, 7)	.0859	.8063	(52, 49, 6, 6)	.0979	.8045	49.34	(62, 31, 3, 6)	.0999	.8006	38.56
.35	.5	(95, 9)	.0979	.8036	(95, 60, 0, 9)	.0968	.8002	78.83	(110, 46, 2, 9)	.0951	.8001	69.78
	.55	(54, 7)	.0947	.8025	(54, 35, 0, 7)	.0940	.8003	45.45	(62, 22, 1, 7)	.0938	.8000	39.49
.4	.55	(104, 10)	.0893	.8044	(99, 89, 7, 9)	.0999	.8017	90.60	(115, 53, 3, 9)	.0991	.8005	72.23
	.6	(61, 8)	.0827	.8078	(56, 31, 1, 7)	.0994	.8015	42.21	(64, 21, 1, 7)	.0996	.8003	39.81
.45	.6	(104, 10)	.0927	.8044	(102, 93, 8, 9)	.0997	.8021	94.21	(120, 47, 2, 10)	.0897	.8003	74.59
	.65	(60, 8)	.0842	.8008	(56, 52, 6, 7)	.0992	.8013	52.56	(68, 26, 2, 7)	.1000	.8014	40.20
.5	.65	(103, 10)	.0927	.8022	(101, 92, 8, 9)	.0996	.8000	93.21	(120, 46, 2, 10)	.0900	.8004	73.92
	.7	(60, 8)	.0853	.8046	(56, 48, 5, 7)	.0999	.8029	49.43	(66, 26, 2, 7)	.0995	.8013	39.56
.55	.7	(102, 10)	.0905	.8023	(98, 96, 9, 9)	.0998	.8037	96.22	(116, 50, 3, 9)	.0994	.8004	70.31
	.75	(59, 8)	.0825	.8025	(54, 25, 0, 7)	.0999	.8012	41.14	(60, 21, 1, 7)	.0982	.8005	38.10
.6	.75	(100, 10)	.0851	.8002	(95, 41, 0, 9)	.0982	.8000	70.42	(110, 41, 2, 9)	.0960	.8000	66.37
	.8	(52, 7)	.0965	.8043	(52, 29, 0, 7)	.0946	.8004	41.72	(60, 19, 1, 7)	.0930	.8025	36.81
.65	.8	(90, 9)	.0919	.8017	(88, 84, 8, 8)	.0990	.8025	84.45	(107, 39, 2, 9)	.0882	.8018	63.54
	.85	(51, 7)	.0884	.8083	(48, 41, 5, 6)	.0993	.8002	42.04	(60, 16, 1, 7)	.0843	.8006	34.77
.7	.85	(79, 8)	.0963	.8006	(79, 49, −1, 8)	.0958	.8000	67.89	(91, 28, 1, 8)	.0926	.8011	55.85
	.9	(50, 7)	.0777	.8175	(45, 20, 1, 6)	.0922	.8044	30.79	(49, 15, 1, 6)	.0908	.8012	29.31
.75	.9	(68, 7)	.0987	.8032	(68, 38, 0, 7)	.0967	.8003	54.58	(76, 25, 1, 7)	.0927	.8005	47.18
	.95	(50, 7)	.0663	.8474	(45, 11, 1, 5)	.0998	.8145	24.67	(46, 10, 1, 5)	.0982	.8008	24.30
.8	.95	(50, 7)	.0964	.8027	(56, 29, 0, 6)	.0940	.8003	44.27	(65, 18, 1, 6)	.0889	.8014	37.59
.85	.95	(101, 7)	.0996	.8043	(101, 51, 0, 7)	.0965	.8001	78.77	(116, 33, 1, 7)	.0922	.8008	68.77

Table 7.2 Minimax and optimal two-stage designs with a futility stopping value under $(\alpha^*, 1-\beta^*) = (.1, .85)$ and balanced allocation $(\gamma = 1)$

		Single-Stage Design			Minimax Design				Optimal Design			
p_y	p_x	(n, a)	α	$1-\beta$	(n, n_1, a_1, a)	α	$1-\beta$	EN	(n, n_1, a_1, a)	α	$1-\beta$	EN
.05	.15	(72, 4)	.0880	.8530	(72, 49, 0, 4)	.0876	.8502	62.67	(83, 39, 1, 4)	.0917	.8501	56.31
	.2	(40, 3)	.0952	.8909	(36, 21, 0, 3)	.0831	.8515	30.76	(46, 19, 1, 3)	.0897	.8510	28.18
	.25	(40, 3)	.0952	.9665	(35, 12, 1, 3)	.0604	.8507	18.69	(35, 12, 1, 3)	.0604	.8507	18.69
.1	.25	(58, 5)	.0806	.8532	(58, 38, 0, 5)	.0803	.8506	49.54	(67, 28, 1, 5)	.0843	.8512	43.99
	.3	(40, 4)	.0940	.9041	(35, 18, 0, 4)	.0784	.8517	28.43	(39, 18, 1, 4)	.0810	.8509	26.12
.15	.3	(71, 6)	.0974	.8540	(71, 45, 0, 6)	.0965	.8500	59.54	(82, 33, 1, 6)	.0988	.8503	54.12
	.35	(43, 5)	.0860	.8534	(43, 27, 0, 5)	.0855	.8501	36.22	(49, 21, 1, 5)	.0885	.8514	32.57
.2	.35	(92, 8)	.0831	.8544	(87, 75, 5, 7)	.0995	.8519	77.14	(105, 52, 3, 7)	.0986	.8502	66.28
	.4	(51, 6)	.0861	.8511	(51, 36, 0, 6)	.0859	.8502	44.38	(59, 23, 1, 6)	.0887	.8514	38.35
.25	.4	(103, 9)	.0855	.8526	(98, 87, 6, 8)	.0995	.8510	88.84	(114, 57, 3, 8)	.0994	.8502	73.76
	.45	(59, 7)	.0832	.8523	(56, 54, 6, 6)	.0997	.8536	54.22	(69, 24, 1, 7)	.0854	.8506	43.51
.3	.45	(114, 10)	.0848	.8537	(109, 59, 1, 9)	.0989	.8504	82.00	(122, 53, 2, 9)	.0985	.8504	78.89
	.5	(60, 7)	.0974	.8524	(60, 39, 0, 7)	.0967	.8500	50.53	(69, 26, 1, 7)	.0977	.8507	44.91
.35	.5	(115, 10)	.0944	.8521	(115, 76, 0, 10)	.0937	.8501	96.82	(133, 55, 2, 10)	.0930	.8500	84.81
	.55	(67, 8)	.0870	.8521	(64, 62, 7, 7)	.0996	.8522	62.22	(78, 26, 1, 8)	.0879	.8500	49.00
.4	.55	(124, 11)	.0867	.8512	(119, 66, 1, 10)	.0995	.8502	90.63	(134, 56, 2, 10)	.0989	.8507	86.13
	.6	(67, 8)	.0929	.8508	(67, 47, 0, 8)	.0926	.8500	57.84	(76, 28, 1, 8)	.0926	.8508	49.40
.45	.6	(124, 11)	.0900	.8512	(120, 109, 8, 10)	.0997	.8512	110.69	(137, 72, 4, 10)	.0984	.8501	90.13
	.65	(67, 8)	.0963	.8521	(67, 43, 0, 8)	.0955	.8501	56.03	(78, 26, 1, 8)	.0955	.8500	49.12
.5	.65	(123, 11)	.0902	.8502	(119, 108, 8, 10)	.0998	.8504	109.69	(137, 71, 4, 10)	.0985	.8505	89.38
	.7	(67, 8)	.0974	.8560	(67, 36, 0, 8)	.0950	.8500	52.95	(75, 27, 1, 8)	.0947	.8507	48.41
.55	.7	(122, 11)	.0883	.8518	(117, 78, 3, 10)	.0997	.8509	91.41	(132, 53, 2, 10)	.0991	.8502	83.41
	.75	(66, 8)	.0946	.8563	(66, 40, 1, 8)	.0918	.8501	51.84	(79, 30, 2, 8)	.0905	.8502	47.09
.6	.75	(111, 10)	.0965	.8504	(111, 76, −1, 10)	.0962	.8500	96.93	(127, 52, 2, 10)	.0934	.8504	80.65
	.8	(64, 8)	.0879	.8527	(61, 59, 7, 7)	.0997	.8541	59.22	(70, 35, 3, 7)	.0995	.8509	44.49
.65	.8	(109, 10)	.0886	.8542	(104, 67, 3, 9)	.0994	.8501	79.04	(118, 46, 2, 9)	.0990	.8501	72.75
	.85	(56, 7)	.0987	.8544	(56, 30, 0, 7)	.0964	.8505	44.40	(64, 21, 1, 7)	.0948	.8523	39.74
.7	.85	(96, 9)	.0902	.8503	(93, 90, 8, 8)	.1000	.8539	90.33	(109, 49, 3, 8)	.1000	.8509	66.44
	.9	(54, 7)	.0859	.8580	(50, 39, 4, 6)	.0991	.8508	41.13	(56, 24, 2, 6)	.0991	.8506	34.18
.75	.9	(84, 8)	.0905	.8552	(81, 64, 5, 7)	.0997	.8504	67.04	(93, 44, 3, 7)	.0993	.8506	57.17
	.95	(45, 6)	.0898	.8606	(44, 33, 4, 5)	.0989	.8502	34.75	(50, 15, 1, 6)	.0822	.8524	29.56
.8	.95	(70, 7)	.0844	.8543	(65, 27, 1, 6)	.0993	.8504	43.42	(70, 22, 1, 6)	.0986	.8501	42.39
.85	.95	(123, 8)	.0899	.8505	(118, 104, 6, 7)	.0995	.8508	105.99	(133, 65, 3, 7)	.0985	.8503	83.27

Table 7.3 Minimax and optimal two-stage designs with a futility stopping value under $(\alpha^*, 1-\beta^*) = (.1, .9)$ and balanced allocation $(\gamma = 1)$

		Single-Stage Design			Minimax Design				Optimal Design			
P_y	P_x	(n, a)	α	$1-\beta$	(n, n_1, a_1, a)	α	$1-\beta$	EN	(n, n_1, a_1, a)	α	$1-\beta$	EN
.05	.15	(98, 5)	.0688	.9018	(93, 86, 4, 4)	.0955	.9009	86.76	(112, 50, 1, 5)	.0740	.9007	75.20
	.2	(60, 4)	.0691	.9434	(55, 34, 2, 3)	.0971	.9032	38.06	(59, 33, 2, 3)	.0950	.9004	37.92
	.25	(60, 4)	.0691	.9896	(55, 22, 2, 2)	.0940	.9024	26.56	(55, 22, 2, 2)	.0940	.9024	26.56
.1	.25	(67, 5)	.0963	.9019	(67, 47, 0, 5)	.0960	.9002	58.38	(76, 36, 1, 5)	.0993	.9007	52.83
	.3	(60, 5)	.0842	.9621	(55, 27, 2, 4)	.0946	.9037	33.83	(55, 27, 2, 4)	.0946	.9037	33.83
.15	.3	(91, 7)	.0881	.9017	(91, 62, 0, 7)	.0877	.9001	77.96	(102, 44, 1, 7)	.0904	.9001	69.54
	.35	(60, 6)	.0791	.9205	(55, 40, 3, 5)	.0979	.9000	43.23	(62, 28, 1, 6)	.0754	.9004	42.45
.2	.35	(105, 8)	.0976	.9020	(105, 71, 0, 8)	.0969	.9001	89.42	(119, 49, 1, 8)	.0990	.9003	80.47
	.4	(66, 7)	.0782	.9037	(61, 60, 6, 6)	.0985	.9029	60.10	(73, 41, 3, 6)	.0977	.9009	48.82
.25	.4	(127, 10)	.0842	.9024	(122, 69, 1, 9)	.0996	.9006	93.42	(133, 64, 2, 9)	.0994	.9001	90.19
	.45	(68, 7)	.0987	.9037	(68, 42, 0, 7)	.0976	.9004	56.31	(75, 33, 1, 7)	.0985	.9001	51.62
.3	.45	(130, 10)	.0992	.9024	(130, 85, 0, 10)	.0982	.9001	109.00	(149, 66, 2, 10)	.0982	.9000	98.19
	.5	(76, 8)	.0920	.9031	(76, 47, 0, 8)	.0910	.9004	62.80	(85, 34, 1, 8)	.0924	.9002	56.81
.35	.5	(140, 11)	.0941	.9002	(140, 104, −1, 11)	.0940	.9000	125.11	(159, 70, 2, 11)	.0938	.9002	105.17
	.55	(83, 9)	.0832	.9010	(78, 63, 4, 8)	.0995	.9002	66.85	(85, 43, 2, 8)	.0996	.9000	58.43
.4	.55	(150, 12)	.0876	.9006	(145, 83, 1, 11)	.0999	.9002	112.04	(162, 70, 2, 11)	.1000	.9003	106.61
	.6	(84, 9)	.0902	.9039	(82, 74, 7, 8)	.0996	.9009	75.10	(95, 42, 2, 9)	.0885	.9001	61.57
.45	.6	(150, 12)	.0910	.9005	(146, 144, 11, 11)	.0994	.9018	144.21	(166, 75, 2, 12)	.0901	.9010	111.66
	.65	(83, 9)	.0923	.9010	(82, 78, 8, 8)	.0996	.9005	78.45	(96, 41, 2, 9)	.0912	.9003	61.33
.5	.65	(149, 12)	.0913	.9006	(145, 143, 11, 11)	.0997	.9019	143.21	(164, 86, 4, 11)	.0999	.9001	109.15
	.7	(82, 9)	.0921	.9004	(81, 77, 8, 8)	.0992	.9001	77.45	(95, 40, 2, 9)	.0907	.9002	60.28
.55	.7	(147, 12)	.0888	.9006	(142, 95, 3, 11)	.0998	.9004	111.81	(158, 67, 2, 11)	.0999	.9005	103.15
	.75	(81, 9)	.0896	.9023	(79, 76, 8, 8)	.0984	.9028	76.33	(94, 38, 2, 9)	.0876	.9001	58.43
.6	.75	(135, 11)	.0960	.9002	(135, 98, −1, 11)	.0959	.9000	119.70	(152, 65, 2, 11)	.0938	.9001	99.29
	.8	(79, 9)	.0836	.9027	(74, 34, 0, 8)	.0993	.9010	55.97	(81, 30, 1, 8)	.0986	.9001	52.83
.65	.8	(131, 11)	.0868	.9004	(126, 67, 1, 10)	.0990	.9003	94.37	(141, 58, 2, 10)	.0982	.9000	89.97
	.85	(70, 8)	.0918	.9039	(68, 64, 7, 7)	.0989	.9004	64.46	(78, 27, 1, 8)	.0887	.9006	49.61
.7	.85	(117, 10)	.0875	.9001	(112, 82, 4, 9)	.0997	.9007	90.26	(124, 53, 2, 9)	.0994	.9005	79.64
	.9	(60, 7)	.0974	.9033	(60, 31, 0, 7)	.0948	.9003	47.10	(67, 23, 1, 7)	.0927	.9002	42.19
.75	.9	(102, 9)	.0845	.9001	(97, 48, 1, 8)	.0988	.9011	70.20	(105, 37, 1, 8)	.0984	.9007	67.36
	.95	(60, 7)	.0850	.9307	(55, 19, 1, 6)	.0939	.9036	34.32	(56, 18, 1, 6)	.0937	.9016	34.09
.8	.95	(78, 7)	.0962	.9040	(78, 36, 0, 7)	.0924	.9003	59.47	(87, 28, 1, 7)	.0900	.9010	53.57
.85	.95	(151, 9)	.0851	.9020	(146, 61, 1, 8)	.0971	.9010	99.19	(154, 52, 1, 8)	.0970	.9004	97.40

Table 7.4 Minimax and optimal two-stage designs with a futility stopping value under $(\alpha^*, 1-\beta^*) = (.15, .8)$ and balanced allocation $(\gamma = 1)$.

p_y	p_x	Single-Stage Design			Minimax Design				Optimal Design			
		(n, a)	α	$1-\beta$	(n, n_1, a_1, a)	α	$1-\beta$	EN	(n, n_1, a_1, a)	α	$1-\beta$	EN
.05	.15	(50, 3)	.1211	.8018	(50, 38, 0, 3)	.1208	.8001	45.30	(59, 31, 1, 3)	.1232	.8011	41.62
	.2	(31, 3)	.0685	.8025	(26, 17, 1, 2)	.1417	.8071	19.96	(27, 16, 1, 2)	.1395	.8015	19.55
	.25	(30, 3)	.0654	.9096	(25, 10, 1, 2)	.1068	.8143	14.02	(25, 10, 1, 2)	.1068	.8143	14.02
.1	.25	(43, 4)	.1022	.8041	(38, 30, 2, 3)	.1479	.8022	32.04	(56, 17, 1, 3)	.1499	.8007	31.94
	.3	(30, 3)	.1375	.8796	(25, 17, 1, 3)	.1107	.8016	20.07	(28, 14, 1, 3)	.1118	.8006	19.18
.15	.3	(54, 5)	.1117	.8010	(49, 30, 1, 4)	.1484	.8001	38.12	(51, 28, 1, 4)	.1479	.8004	37.78
	.35	(32, 4)	.1086	.8060	(30, 27, 3, 3)	.1460	.8115	27.50	(32, 21, 2, 3)	.1461	.8025	23.81
.2	.35	(57, 5)	.1454	.8060	(57, 38, 0, 5)	.1436	.8006	48.59	(66, 30, 1, 5)	.1407	.8006	45.68
	.4	(33, 4)	.1397	.8040	(33, 23, 0, 4)	.1388	.8009	28.74	(39, 18, 1, 4)	.1369	.8024	26.75
.25	.4	(67, 6)	.1360	.8027	(66, 61, 5, 5)	.1499	.8033	61.87	(78, 33, 1, 6)	.1324	.8004	52.95
	.45	(41, 5)	.1250	.8100	(37, 35, 4, 4)	.1488	.8017	35.33	(43, 24, 2, 4)	.1486	.8013	29.85
.3	.45	(77, 7)	.1263	.8029	(72, 36, 0, 6)	.1497	.8011	55.84	(77, 37, 1, 6)	.1468	.8002	54.98
	.5	(41, 5)	.1388	.8034	(41, 28, 0, 5)	.1376	.8002	35.25	(46, 22, 1, 5)	.1345	.8004	32.43
.35	.5	(78, 7)	.1375	.8032	(76, 72, 6, 6)	.1488	.8026	72.67	(95, 39, 2, 6)	.1497	.8005	59.21
	.55	(48, 6)	.1194	.8052	(43, 22, 0, 5)	.1474	.8015	33.82	(50, 20, 1, 5)	.1429	.8001	33.03
.4	.55	(78, 7)	.1440	.8008	(78, 57, -1, 7)	.1437	.8001	69.87	(90, 38, 1, 7)	.1387	.8001	61.58
	.6	(48, 6)	.1258	.8040	(44, 43, 5, 5)	.1494	.8068	43.16	(49, 21, 1, 5)	.1489	.8010	33.25
.45	.6	(78, 7)	.1477	.8008	(78, 57, -1, 7)	.1474	.8001	69.83	(90, 38, 1, 7)	.1416	.8001	61.62
	.65	(48, 6)	.1295	.8052	(44, 39, 4, 5)	.1498	.8005	40.06	(49, 27, 2, 5)	.1476	.8007	34.50
.5	.65	(78, 7)	.1490	.8032	(78, 48, -1, 7)	.1472	.8000	66.61	(90, 37, 1, 7)	.1416	.8003	61.05
	.7	(48, 6)	.1307	.8090	(45, 34, 3, 5)	.1493	.8026	37.00	(53, 18, 1, 5)	.1497	.8011	33.19
.55	.7	(77, 7)	.1462	.8029	(77, 48, -1, 7)	.1447	.8003	66.00	(90, 35, 1, 7)	.1386	.8007	59.87
	.75	(47, 6)	.1270	.8063	(42, 38, 4, 5)	.1483	.8002	38.84	(48, 19, 1, 5)	.1465	.8001	31.63
.6	.75	(76, 7)	.1409	.8053	(73, 69, 6, 6)	.1496	.8002	69.68	(89, 37, 2, 6)	.1496	.8004	55.77
	.8	(46, 6)	.1208	.8064	(41, 18, 0, 5)	.1451	.8005	31.05	(45, 19, 1, 5)	.1404	.8002	30.29
.65	.8	(74, 7)	.1312	.8052	(69, 38, 1, 6)	.1492	.8010	52.02	(75, 31, 1, 6)	.1460	.8004	50.67
	.85	(38, 5)	.1394	.8014	(38, 26, 0, 5)	.1382	.8001	32.69	(44, 17, 1, 5)	.1300	.8007	28.57
.7	.85	(63, 6)	.1423	.8046	(62, 56, 5, 5)	.1499	.8009	57.06	(73, 27, 1, 6)	.1321	.8001	47.28
	.9	(37, 5)	.1265	.8087	(33, 22, 2, 4)	.1490	.8003	25.42	(36, 14, 1, 4)	.1475	.8003	23.20
.75	.9	(60, 6)	.1228	.8049	(55, 19, 0, 5)	.1447	.8030	39.68	(60, 23, 1, 5)	.1400	.8021	38.99
	.95	(30, 4)	.1477	.8279	(29, 11, 0, 4)	.1340	.8003	21.76	(33, 12, 1, 4)	.1268	.8008	20.53
.8	.95	(48, 5)	.1248	.8042	(43, 10, 0, 4)	.1495	.8027	30.19	(46, 18, 1, 4)	.1449	.8014	29.67
.85	.95	(89, 6)	.1235	.8058	(84, 36, 1, 5)	.1395	.8004	56.83	(89, 32, 1, 5)	.1379	.8003	56.50

Table 7.5 Minimax and optimal two-stage designs with a futility stopping value under $(\alpha^*, 1-\beta^*) = (.15, .85)$ and balanced allocation $(\gamma = 1)$

Py	Px	Single-Stage Design (n, a)	α	$1-\beta$	Minimax Design (n, n_1, a_1, a)	α	$1-\beta$	EN	Optimal Design (n, n_1, a_1, a)	α	$1-\beta$	EN
.05	.15	(58, 3)	.1391	.8518	(58, 45, 0, 3)	.1388	.8502	52.79	(69, 37, 1, 3)	.1399	.8502	49.49
	.2	(36, 3)	.0837	.8581	(31, 27, 2, 2)	.1469	.8519	27.66	(31, 27, 2, 2)	.1469	.8519	27.66
	.25	(30, 3)	.0654	.9096	(25, 13, 1, 2)	.1232	.8627	16.60	(26, 12, 1, 2)	.1195	.8520	16.07
.1	.25	(49, 4)	.1173	.8527	(49, 35, 0, 4)	.1169	.8505	43.12	(59, 32, 2, 3)	.1499	.8500	39.09
	.3	(30, 3)	.1375	.8796	(28, 17, 0, 3)	.1276	.8516	23.78	(32, 17, 1, 3)	.1276	.8500	22.75
.15	.3	(62, 5)	.1280	.8534	(61, 55, 4, 4)	.1487	.8527	56.04	(73, 32, 1, 5)	.1271	.8503	49.63
	.35	(36, 4)	.1225	.8502	(36, 30, 0, 4)	.1225	.8501	33.43	(44, 19, 1, 4)	.1238	.8502	29.22
.2	.35	(74, 6)	.1287	.8523	(70, 67, 5, 5)	.1489	.8515	67.50	(89, 41, 2, 5)	.1493	.8506	57.26
	.4	(45, 5)	.1171	.8557	(41, 35, 3, 4)	.1484	.8513	36.36	(45, 28, 2, 4)	.1466	.8501	33.22
.25	.4	(85, 7)	.1246	.8502	(80, 51, 1, 6)	.1496	.8512	64.18	(87, 42, 1, 6)	.1477	.8504	62.24
	.45	(46, 5)	.1388	.8533	(46, 32, 0, 5)	.1378	.8506	39.81	(52, 25, 1, 5)	.1354	.8500	36.74
.3	.45	(87, 7)	.1410	.8504	(87, 66, -1, 7)	.1408	.8500	78.86	(98, 46, 1, 7)	.1377	.8502	69.64
	.5	(54, 6)	.1238	.8561	(49, 45, 4, 5)	.1496	.8533	45.84	(55, 25, 1, 5)	.1495	.8510	38.16
.35	.5	(98, 8)	.1306	.8537	(93, 56, 1, 7)	.1493	.8502	73.04	(103, 45, 1, 7)	.1475	.8505	71.45
	.55	(54, 6)	.1334	.8522	(53, 49, 5, 5)	.1472	.8517	49.68	(63, 26, 1, 6)	.1298	.8503	42.36
.4	.55	(98, 8)	.1370	.8512	(95, 87, 6, 7)	.1500	.8508	88.58	(112, 51, 2, 7)	.1498	.8504	74.24
	.6	(54, 6)	.1399	.8510	(54, 37, -1, 6)	.1395	.8502	47.86	(61, 28, 1, 6)	.1356	.8507	42.71
.45	.6	(98, 8)	.1408	.8512	(97, 92, 7, 7)	.1482	.8505	92.84	(109, 61, 3, 7)	.1499	.8503	76.58
	.65	(54, 6)	.1437	.8522	(54, 33, -1, 6)	.1425	.8501	46.54	(63, 26, 1, 6)	.1378	.8503	42.45
.5	.65	(98, 8)	.1420	.8537	(97, 92, 7, 7)	.1493	.8532	92.84	(109, 60, 3, 7)	.1496	.8504	75.88
	.7	(54, 6)	.1449	.8561	(54, 33, 0, 6)	.1416	.8506	44.53	(60, 27, 1, 6)	.1373	.8502	41.72
.55	.7	(96, 8)	.1383	.8511	(93, 90, 7, 7)	.1497	.8524	90.50	(107, 50, 2, 7)	.1499	.8512	71.75
	.75	(53, 6)	.1414	.8559	(53, 32, 0, 6)	.1381	.8508	43.55	(60, 25, 1, 6)	.1336	.8507	40.53
.6	.75	(94, 8)	.1320	.8511	(89, 53, 1, 7)	.1499	.8507	69.58	(99, 41, 1, 7)	.1468	.8506	67.40
	.8	(51, 6)	.1331	.8511	(49, 46, 5, 5)	.1484	.8528	46.51	(55, 28, 2, 5)	.1499	.8520	37.22
.65	.8	(83, 7)	.1450	.8531	(83, 48, -1, 7)	.1428	.8502	69.91	(94, 39, 1, 7)	.1371	.8506	63.90
	.85	(50, 6)	.1243	.8576	(45, 19, 0, 5)	.1482	.8515	33.75	(49, 21, 1, 5)	.1439	.8514	33.20
.7	.85	(79, 7)	.1294	.8502	(74, 33, 0, 6)	.1500	.8502	55.69	(82, 33, 1, 6)	.1458	.8503	54.88
	.9	(41, 5)	.1388	.8551	(41, 22, 0, 5)	.1342	.8501	32.74	(47, 18, 1, 5)	.1283	.8525	30.40
.75	.9	(67, 6)	.1360	.8551	(64, 53, 4, 5)	.1489	.8505	55.37	(69, 36, 2, 5)	.1494	.8510	47.26
	.95	(38, 5)	.1161	.8517	(33, 11, 0, 4)	.1451	.8525	24.15	(37, 14, 1, 4)	.1385	.8505	23.50
.8	.95	(53, 5)	.1366	.8524	(53, 31, 0, 5)	.1334	.8503	43.39	(60, 28, 2, 4)	.1495	.8510	37.83
.85	.95	(98, 6)	.1350	.8516	(93, 78, 4, 5)	.1494	.8512	81.23	(103, 51, 2, 5)	.1469	.8503	68.57

Table 7.6 Minimax and optimal two-stage designs with a futility stopping value under $(\alpha^*, 1-\beta^*) = (.15, .9)$ and balanced allocation $(\gamma = 1)$

		Single-Stage Design			Minimax Design				Optimal Design			
p_y	p_x	(n, a)	α	$1-\beta$	(n, n_1, a_1, a)	α	$1-\beta$	EN	(n, n_1, a_1, a)	α	$1-\beta$	EN
.05	.15	(84, 4)	.1052	.9017	(79, 72, 3, 3)	.1469	.9021	73.16	(87, 59, 2, 3)	.1496	.9005	66.24
	.2	(50, 3)	.1211	.9430	(45, 29, 1, 3)	.1024	.9014	34.99	(47, 27, 1, 3)	.1034	.9004	34.39
	.25	(50, 3)	.1211	.9874	(45, 14, 1, 2)	.1412	.9003	23.57	(45, 14, 1, 2)	.1412	.9003	23.57
.1	.25	(58, 4)	.1376	.9036	(58, 40, 0, 4)	.1365	.9001	50.35	(66, 35, 1, 4)	.1369	.9002	48.01
	.3	(50, 4)	.1197	.9541	(45, 19, 1, 3)	.1487	.9004	29.14	(45, 19, 1, 3)	.1487	.9004	29.14
.15	.3	(73, 5)	.1477	.9034	(73, 51, 0, 5)	.1463	.9001	63.22	(82, 43, 1, 5)	.1452	.9004	60.14
	.35	(50, 5)	.1028	.9043	(45, 23, 0, 4)	.1438	.9011	35.82	(47, 27, 1, 4)	.1415	.9001	35.47
.2	.35	(86, 6)	.1468	.9000	(86, 69, −2, 6)	.1468	.9000	80.95	(99, 48, 1, 6)	.1449	.9001	70.90
	.4	(52, 5)	.1343	.9019	(52, 32, −1, 5)	.1337	.9000	45.62	(58, 30, 1, 5)	.1330	.9003	42.20
.25	.4	(99, 7)	.1428	.9002	(99, 79, −1, 7)	.1427	.9000	91.17	(111, 55, 1, 7)	.1406	.9002	80.54
	.45	(61, 6)	.1247	.9029	(57, 51, 4, 5)	.1491	.9002	52.27	(66, 36, 2, 5)	.1484	.9000	46.24
.3	.45	(111, 8)	.1359	.9002	(108, 105, 7, 7)	.1498	.9018	105.49	(120, 73, 3, 7)	.1497	.9001	88.31
	.5	(62, 6)	.1404	.9013	(62, 41, −1, 6)	.1397	.9001	54.47	(71, 33, 1, 6)	.1377	.9006	49.97
.35	.5	(113, 8)	.1477	.9006	(113, 79, −2, 8)	.1474	.9000	101.50	(129, 59, 1, 8)	.1440	.9001	91.31
	.55	(70, 7)	.1246	.9028	(65, 36, 0, 6)	.1497	.9004	51.93	(68, 30, 0, 6)	.1494	.9003	51.04
.4	.55	(123, 9)	.1343	.9003	(119, 95, 4, 8)	.1497	.9000	102.25	(133, 68, 2, 8)	.1480	.9001	93.77
	.6	(70, 7)	.1310	.9016	(67, 61, 5, 6)	.1497	.9021	62.22	(75, 40, 2, 6)	.1495	.9009	52.81
.45	.6	(123, 9)	.1380	.9003	(120, 112, 7, 8)	.1497	.9006	113.53	(136, 76, 3, 8)	.1480	.9003	96.51
	.65	(70, 7)	.1347	.9028	(68, 60, 5, 6)	.1489	.9007	61.64	(80, 34, 1, 7)	.1307	.9009	54.77
.5	.65	(122, 9)	.1382	.9001	(119, 111, 7, 8)	.1497	.9006	112.53	(135, 75, 3, 8)	.1479	.9004	95.50
	.7	(69, 7)	.1342	.9020	(67, 59, 5, 6)	.1481	.9001	60.63	(82, 36, 2, 6)	.1494	.9001	52.65
.55	.7	(121, 9)	.1360	.9024	(116, 92, 4, 8)	.1498	.9002	99.25	(123, 60, 1, 8)	.1500	.9001	89.20
	.75	(68, 7)	.1312	.9037	(64, 54, 4, 6)	.1496	.9016	56.49	(67, 40, 2, 6)	.1485	.9000	49.94
.6	.75	(109, 8)	.1499	.9024	(109, 68, −1, 8)	.1479	.9002	92.74	(123, 54, 1, 8)	.1431	.9004	85.80
	.8	(66, 7)	.1240	.9037	(61, 30, 0, 6)	.1461	.9007	47.12	(66, 30, 1, 6)	.1428	.9003	46.11
.65	.8	(105, 8)	.1389	.9020	(102, 98, 7, 7)	.1483	.9011	98.66	(122, 53, 2, 7)	.1499	.9005	79.22
	.85	(57, 6)	.1399	.9053	(56, 51, 5, 5)	.1495	.9025	51.88	(62, 28, 1, 6)	.1314	.9004	43.11
.7	.85	(91, 7)	.1464	.9017	(91, 55, −1, 7)	.1446	.9002	77.41	(102, 44, 1, 7)	.1385	.9001	70.31
	.9	(53, 6)	.1216	.9003	(48, 22, 0, 5)	.1482	.9010	36.70	(51, 24, 1, 5)	.1438	.9001	35.81
.75	.9	(85, 7)	.1246	.9017	(80, 33, 0, 6)	.1446	.9004	59.16	(85, 37, 1, 6)	.1415	.9003	58.43
	.95	(50, 5)	.1489	.9483	(45, 24, 2, 4)	.1491	.9040	30.47	(45, 24, 2, 4)	.1491	.9040	30.47
.8	.95	(69, 6)	.1204	.9022	(64, 21, 0, 5)	.1429	.9020	45.81	(66, 29, 1, 5)	.1394	.9001	45.08
.85	.95	(125, 7)	.1244	.9020	(120, 40, 0, 6)	.1418	.9002	85.01	(126, 51, 1, 6)	.1393	.9005	84.34

Table 7.7 Minimax and optimal two-stage designs with a futility stopping value under $(\alpha^*, 1-\beta^*) = (.2, .8)$ and balanced allocation $(\gamma = 1)$

		Single-Stage Design			Minimax Design				Optimal Design			
P_y	P_x	(n, a)	$1-\beta$	α	(n, n_1, a_1, a)	α	$1-\beta$	EN	(n, n_1, a_1, a)	α	$1-\beta$	EN
.05	.15	(50, 3)	.8018	.1211	(45, 28, 1, 2)	.1946	.8008	34.33	(45, 28, 1, 2)	.1946	.8008	34.33
	.2	(30, 2)	.8892	.1773	(25, 17, 1, 2)	.1397	.8018	19.63	(27, 16, 1, 2)	.1395	.8015	19.55
	.25	(30, 2)	.9586	.1773	(25, 9, 1, 1)	.1835	.8109	13.08	(25, 9, 1, 1)	.1835	.8109	13.08
.1	.25	(34, 3)	.8023	.1529	(34, 26, 0, 3)	.1524	.8004	30.75	(35, 27, 2, 2)	.1980	.8073	28.95
	.3	(30, 3)	.8796	.1375	(25, 12, 1, 2)	.1798	.8063	16.67	(25, 12, 1, 2)	.1798	.8063	16.67
.15	.3	(46, 4)	.8065	.1521	(41, 27, 1, 3)	.1991	.8031	32.93	(42, 26, 1, 3)	.1972	.8017	32.75
	.35	(30, 3)	.8589	.1810	(25, 18, −1, 3)	.1586	.8000	23.33	(28, 17, 1, 3)	.1566	.8002	21.44
.2	.35	(48, 4)	.8050	.1852	(48, 29, −1, 4)	.1835	.8005	42.10	(53, 23, 0, 4)	.1811	.8002	40.21
	.4	(33, 4)	.8040	.1397	(28, 15, 0, 3)	.1919	.8032	22.69	(29, 13, 0, 3)	.1912	.8021	22.57
.25	.4	(58, 5)	.8009	.1670	(53, 42, 2, 4)	.1998	.8016	45.88	(56, 33, 1, 4)	.1980	.8009	43.20
	.45	(34, 4)	.8052	.1629	(31, 29, 3, 3)	.2000	.8089	29.45	(35, 17, 1, 3)	.1992	.8001	24.58
.3	.45	(60, 5)	.8051	.1848	(60, 37, −1, 5)	.1825	.8002	51.91	(68, 38, 2, 4)	.1976	.8010	48.61
	.5	(35, 4)	.8090	.1804	(35, 23, 0, 4)	.1769	.8019	29.77	(41, 23, 2, 3)	.1947	.8013	28.66
.35	.5	(60, 5)	.8001	.1945	(60, 48, −2, 5)	.1944	.8000	56.44	(67, 30, 0, 5)	.1886	.8000	50.49
	.55	(35, 4)	.8052	.1901	(35, 20, −1, 4)	.1878	.8005	30.36	(38, 17, 0, 4)	.1843	.8012	29.00
.4	.55	(70, 6)	.8043	.1713	(65, 35, 0, 5)	.1968	.8013	51.46	(69, 29, 0, 5)	.1942	.8004	51.13
	.6	(35, 4)	.8040	.1966	(35, 21, −1, 4)	.1944	.8002	30.54	(39, 16, 0, 4)	.1895	.8013	29.14
.45	.6	(70, 6)	.8043	.1751	(65, 35, 0, 5)	.1997	.8013	51.43	(69, 29, 0, 5)	.1969	.8004	51.10
	.65	(42, 5)	.8092	.1618	(37, 19, 0, 4)	.1939	.8021	29.16	(38, 17, 0, 4)	.1924	.8012	28.93
.5	.65	(69, 6)	.8012	.1746	(64, 35, 0, 5)	.1998	.8006	50.88	(67, 30, 0, 5)	.1973	.8000	50.40
	.7	(41, 5)	.8034	.1601	(36, 20, 0, 4)	.1946	.8028	29.00	(38, 16, 0, 4)	.1916	.8021	28.54
.55	.7	(68, 6)	.8006	.1716	(63, 34, 0, 5)	.1968	.8010	49.90	(66, 29, 0, 5)	.1944	.8008	49.44
	.75	(34, 4)	.8052	.1969	(34, 18, −1, 4)	.1932	.8002	29.07	(37, 15, 0, 4)	.1872	.8002	27.60
.6	.75	(58, 5)	.8009	.1969	(58, 38, −2, 5)	.1961	.8001	52.42	(63, 29, 0, 5)	.1887	.8003	47.81
	.8	(33, 4)	.8040	.1896	(33, 18, −1, 4)	.1868	.8007	28.42	(36, 14, 0, 4)	.1807	.8023	26.68
.65	.8	(57, 5)	.8060	.1884	(56, 50, 4, 4)	.1974	.8016	51.39	(69, 24, 1, 4)	.1995	.8014	43.79
	.85	(32, 4)	.8060	.1794	(32, 21, 2, 3)	.1988	.8025	24.45	(38, 13, 1, 3)	.1981	.8005	23.47
.7	.85	(54, 5)	.8010	.1722	(49, 30, 1, 4)	.1987	.8001	38.44	(51, 19, 0, 4)	.1984	.8005	37.25
	.9	(31, 4)	.8129	.1657	(26, 16, 1, 3)	.1997	.8040	20.23	(28, 6, 0, 3)	.1976	.8016	19.73
.75	.9	(43, 4)	.8041	.1913	(43, 28, 0, 4)	.1867	.8001	36.42	(47, 16, 0, 4)	.1789	.8014	34.02
	.95	(30, 4)	.8279	.1477	(25, 5, 0, 3)	.1786	.8153	17.90	(26, 12, 1, 3)	.1716	.8055	17.69
.8	.95	(40, 4)	.8079	.1631	(35, 7, 0, 3)	.1927	.8013	24.76	(35, 7, 0, 3)	.1927	.8013	24.76
.85	.95	(63, 4)	.8009	.1903	(63, 39, −1, 4)	.1886	.8001	55.42	(69, 40, 2, 3)	.1994	.8006	49.23

Table 7.8 Minimax and optimal two-stage designs with a futility stopping value under $(\alpha^*, 1 - \beta^*) = (.2, .85)$ and balanced allocation $(\gamma = 1)$

p_y	p_x	Single-Stage Design (n, a)	$1 - \beta$	α	Minimax Design (n, n_1, a_1, a)	α	$1 - \beta$	EN	Optimal Design (n, n_1, a_1, a)	α	$1 - \beta$	EN
.05	.15	(58, 3)	.8518	.1391	(54, 46, 2, 2)	.1989	.8522	47.84	(54, 46, 2, 2)	.1989	.8522	47.84
	.2	(30, 2)	.8892	.1773	(26, 20, 0, 2)	.1588	.8502	23.93	(27, 16, 0, 2)	.1618	.8516	23.45
	.25	(30, 2)	.9586	.1773	(25, 13, 1, 2)	.1232	.8627	16.60	(26, 12, 1, 2)	.1195	.8520	16.07
.1	.25	(40, 3)	.8544	.1729	(40, 29, 0, 3)	.1717	.8505	35.47	(43, 21, 0, 3)	.1732	.8509	34.30
	.3	(30, 3)	.8796	.1375	(25, 22, 2, 2)	.1942	.8602	22.66	(27, 15, 1, 2)	.1981	.8500	19.50
.15	.3	(53, 4)	.8541	.1694	(52, 46, 3, 3)	.1980	.8547	47.39	(59, 37, 2, 3)	.1955	.8508	43.85
	.35	(30, 3)	.8589	.1810	(30, 20, 0, 3)	.1785	.8521	25.89	(32, 15, 0, 3)	.1787	.8512	25.25
.2	.35	(65, 5)	.8524	.1614	(60, 33, 0, 4)	.1999	.8519	48.16	(61, 31, 0, 4)	.1990	.8509	47.90
	.4	(38, 4)	.8537	.1569	(34, 32, 3, 3)	.1953	.8506	32.43	(40, 20, 1, 3)	.1988	.8523	28.42
.25	.4	(67, 5)	.8502	.1844	(67, 51, −2, 5)	.1843	.8500	62.46	(74, 35, 0, 5)	.1811	.8505	56.64
	.45	(39, 4)	.8518	.1795	(39, 26, −1, 4)	.1788	.8501	34.91	(43, 19, 0, 4)	.1769	.8504	32.79
.3	.45	(78, 6)	.8503	.1682	(73, 33, −1, 5)	.1985	.8501	59.26	(78, 35, 0, 5)	.1951	.8500	58.73
	.5	(40, 4)	.8529	.1963	(40, 26, −1, 4)	.1949	.8503	35.45	(45, 19, 0, 4)	.1909	.8504	33.83
.35	.5	(80, 6)	.8535	.1809	(76, 68, 4, 5)	.1995	.8506	70.12	(85, 42, 1, 5)	.1993	.8500	61.54
	.55	(47, 5)	.8501	.1651	(43, 34, 2, 4)	.1983	.8504	37.16	(45, 27, 1, 4)	.1971	.8500	34.98
.4	.55	(80, 6)	.8510	.1874	(79, 74, 5, 5)	.1988	.8510	75.13	(90, 50, 2, 5)	.1985	.8502	65.19
	.6	(48, 5)	.8558	.1742	(44, 42, 4, 4)	.1967	.8508	42.44	(49, 25, 1, 4)	.1995	.8516	35.62
.45	.6	(80, 6)	.8510	.1911	(80, 56, −2, 6)	.1905	.8502	72.38	(94, 49, 2, 5)	.1993	.8509	66.12
	.65	(47, 5)	.8501	.1754	(44, 42, 4, 4)	.1999	.8522	42.44	(53, 23, 1, 4)	.1988	.8519	36.24
.5	.65	(80, 6)	.8535	.1923	(80, 53, −1, 6)	.1898	.8503	69.59	(94, 48, 2, 5)	.1984	.8507	65.47
	.7	(47, 5)	.8539	.1767	(45, 37, 3, 4)	.1974	.8513	39.25	(50, 23, 1, 4)	.1984	.8503	34.92
.55	.7	(78, 6)	.8503	.1881	(77, 72, 5, 5)	.1988	.8510	73.13	(85, 49, 2, 5)	.1994	.8508	62.70
	.75	(46, 5)	.8533	.1728	(43, 37, 3, 4)	.1995	.8559	38.68	(45, 24, 1, 4)	.1976	.8500	33.29
.6	.75	(77, 6)	.8542	.1828	(73, 65, 4, 5)	.1999	.8525	67.12	(77, 41, 1, 5)	.1997	.8501	57.39
	.8	(45, 5)	.8557	.1664	(40, 20, 0, 4)	.1976	.8506	31.28	(41, 18, 0, 4)	.1959	.8500	31.05
.65	.8	(74, 6)	.8523	.1715	(69, 35, 0, 5)	.1953	.8504	53.69	(71, 32, 0, 5)	.1941	.8510	53.53
	.85	(36, 4)	.8502	.1935	(36, 27, −1, 4)	.1932	.8501	32.99	(39, 16, 0, 4)	.1844	.8504	29.19
.7	.85	(62, 5)	.8534	.1888	(62, 36, −1, 5)	.1854	.8502	52.91	(69, 38, 2, 4)	.1975	.8503	48.96
	.9	(34, 4)	.8503	.1769	(34, 29, 3, 3)	.1973	.8588	30.18	(42, 14, 1, 3)	.1978	.8500	25.71
.75	.9	(58, 5)	.8532	.1670	(53, 22, 0, 4)	.1948	.8518	39.65	(54, 20, 0, 4)	.1933	.8505	39.47
	.95	(32, 4)	.8568	.1555	(27, 8, 0, 3)	.1906	.8516	19.68	(27, 8, 0, 3)	.1906	.8516	19.68
.8	.95	(45, 4)	.8582	.1774	(42, 29, 2, 3)	.1976	.8506	33.03	(46, 19, 1, 3)	.1974	.8510	30.31
.85	.95	(85, 5)	.8515	.1662	(80, 26, 0, 4)	.1901	.8509	57.20	(80, 26, 0, 4)	.1901	.8509	57.20

Table 7.9 Minimax and optimal two-stage designs with a futility stopping value under $(\alpha^*, 1 - \beta^*) = (.2, .9)$ and balanced allocation $(\gamma = 1)$

p_y	p_x	Single-Stage Design			Minimax Design				Optimal Design			
		(n, a)	α	$1-\beta$	(n, n_1, a_1, a)	α	$1-\beta$	EN	(n, n_1, a_1, a)	α	$1-\beta$	EN
.05	.15	(70, 3)	.1623	.9034	(70, 52, 0, 3)	.1614	.9004	62.65	(74, 40, 0, 3)	.1636	.9004	60.58
	.2	(50, 3)	.1211	.9430	(45, 23, 1, 2)	.1786	.9011	30.85	(45, 23, 1, 2)	.1786	.9011	30.85
	.25	(50, 3)	.1211	.9874	(45, 14, 1, 2)	.1412	.9003	23.57	(45, 14, 1, 2)	.1412	.9003	23.57
.1	.25	(58, 4)	.1376	.9036	(53, 27, 0, 3)	.1959	.9021	42.38	(54, 25, 0, 3)	.1953	.9001	42.27
	.3	(50, 4)	.1197	.9541	(45, 19, 1, 3)	.1487	.9004	29.14	(45, 19, 1, 3)	.1487	.9004	29.14
.15	.3	(63, 4)	.1903	.9019	(63, 44, -1, 4)	.1895	.9002	56.80	(68, 36, 0, 4)	.1883	.9002	54.11
	.35	(50, 4)	.1623	.9386	(45, 24, 1, 3)	.1935	.9047	32.80	(46, 23, 1, 3)	.1912	.9013	32.59
.2	.35	(77, 5)	.1819	.9016	(77, 55, -1, 5)	.1811	.9001	69.08	(83, 43, 0, 5)	.1792	.9000	65.15
	.4	(50, 4)	.1901	.9266	(45, 29, -1, 4)	.1765	.9003	40.03	(48, 25, 0, 4)	.1758	.9006	38.12
.25	.4	(90, 6)	.1717	.9012	(85, 66, 2, 5)	.1993	.9003	73.25	(92, 52, 1, 5)	.1968	.9001	70.19
	.45	(54, 5)	.1583	.9027	(49, 29, 0, 4)	.1980	.9006	40.21	(50, 27, 0, 4)	.1972	.9002	39.94
.3	.45	(93, 6)	.1893	.9021	(93, 66, -1, 6)	.1879	.9002	82.53	(101, 51, 0, 6)	.1844	.9004	78.15
	.5	(55, 5)	.1744	.9013	(53, 50, 4, 4)	.1985	.9032	50.67	(57, 38, 2, 4)	.1997	.9014	44.72
.35	.5	(104, 7)	.1723	.9014	(99, 50, -1, 6)	.1972	.9000	80.55	(103, 53, 0, 6)	.1947	.9001	80.03
	.55	(56, 5)	.1863	.9024	(56, 37, -1, 5)	.1847	.9003	49.21	(61, 29, 0, 5)	.1815	.9006	46.75
.4	.55	(105, 7)	.1799	.9016	(100, 88, 4, 6)	.1987	.9002	91.54	(109, 49, 0, 6)	.2000	.9003	81.46
	.6	(56, 5)	.1927	.9013	(56, 40, -1, 5)	.1917	.9001	50.14	(60, 31, 0, 5)	.1876	.9003	46.99
.45	.6	(105, 7)	.1836	.9016	(101, 93, 5, 6)	.1988	.9002	95.03	(109, 59, 1, 6)	.1998	.9000	82.16
	.65	(56, 5)	.1964	.9024	(56, 37, -1, 5)	.1944	.9003	49.10	(61, 29, 0, 5)	.1896	.9006	46.68
.5	.65	(104, 7)	.1837	.9014	(100, 92, 5, 6)	.1986	.9001	94.03	(108, 58, 1, 6)	.1995	.9002	81.15
	.7	(55, 5)	.1955	.9013	(55, 38, -1, 5)	.1940	.9000	48.79	(60, 28, 0, 5)	.1885	.9002	45.70
.55	.7	(102, 7)	.1802	.9009	(97, 86, 4, 6)	.1999	.9017	89.25	(102, 50, 0, 6)	.1999	.9007	78.08
	.75	(54, 5)	.1921	.9028	(54, 33, -1, 5)	.1892	.9001	46.54	(59, 26, 0, 5)	.1842	.9008	44.33
.6	.75	(99, 7)	.1728	.9002	(94, 45, -1, 6)	.1962	.9005	75.70	(100, 45, 0, 6)	.1924	.9002	74.85
	.8	(52, 5)	.1839	.9019	(52, 32, -1, 5)	.1815	.9000	44.98	(58, 33, 2, 4)	.1974	.9007	41.83
.65	.8	(86, 6)	.1896	.9000	(86, 69, -2, 6)	.1895	.9000	80.43	(98, 53, 2, 5)	.1988	.9007	70.10
	.85	(50, 5)	.1726	.9043	(46, 28, 1, 4)	.2000	.9001	36.00	(47, 27, 1, 4)	.1984	.9001	35.87
.7	.85	(82, 6)	.1742	.9022	(77, 39, 0, 5)	.1980	.9003	59.87	(79, 36, 0, 5)	.1968	.9005	59.70
	.9	(50, 5)	.1628	.9231	(45, 14, 0, 4)	.1831	.9000	32.04	(45, 14, 0, 4)	.1831	.9000	32.04
.75	.9	(67, 5)	.1844	.9019	(64, 59, 4, 4)	.1995	.9000	60.14	(79, 30, 1, 4)	.2000	.9001	51.59
	.95	(50, 5)	.1489	.9483	(45, 15, 1, 3)	.1946	.9048	27.48	(45, 15, 1, 3)	.1946	.9048	27.48
.8	.95	(51, 4)	.1925	.9017	(51, 25, -1, 4)	.1882	.9000	43.28	(55, 19, 0, 4)	.1789	.9004	39.92
.85	.95	(98, 5)	.1834	.9018	(93, 86, 4, 4)	.1991	.9009	87.59	(103, 46, 1, 4)	.1999	.9009	71.17

total number of responders among the cumulative $n = n_1 + n_2$ patients for arms x and y, respectively.

(a) For an integer $a \in [a_1 - n_2, n]$, accept arm x (or reject H_0) for further investigation if $X - Y \geq a$.

(b) Otherwise, we reject arm x.

Now we discuss how to determine (n_1, n_2, a_1, a) using the exact two-sample binomial test for a randomized phase II clinical trial with a prospective control arm. Let p_0 denote the projected response rate for the historical control and Δ a clinically significant increase in response rate for arm x. For the purpose of type I and II error calculation, we specify a point null hypothesis $H_0 : p_x = p_y = p_0$ and an alternative hypothesis $H_1 : p_x = p_0 + \Delta, p_y = p_0$. For a two-stage design defined by (n_1, n, a_1, a), the type I error rate and power of the two-stage design are calculated as

$$\alpha = P(X_1 - Y_1 \geq a_1, X - Y \geq a | p_x = p_y = p_0)$$

and

$$1 - \beta = P(X_1 - Y_1 \geq a_1, X - Y \geq a | p_x = p_0 + \Delta, p_y = p_0),$$

respectively. These probabilities are calculated assuming that $X_1 \sim B(n_1, p_x)$, $X_2 \sim B(n_2, p_x)$, $Y_1 \sim B(n_1, p_y)$, and $Y_2 \sim B(n_2, p_y)$ are independent random variables. That is,

$$\alpha = \sum_{k_1=a_1}^{n_1} \sum_{y_1=\max(0,-k_1)}^{n_1-\max(0,k_1)} \sum_{k_2=a-k_1}^{n_2} \sum_{y_2=\max(0,-k_2)}^{n_2-\max(0,k_2)} b(y_1|n_1, p_0)b(k_1 + y_1|n_1, p_0)b(y_2|n_2, p_0)$$
$$\times b(k_2 + y_2|n_2, p_0)$$

and

$$1 - \beta = \sum_{k_1=a_1}^{n_1} \sum_{y_1=\max(0,-k_1)}^{n_1-\max(0,k_1)} \sum_{k_2=a-k_1}^{n_2} \sum_{y_2=\max(0,-k_2)}^{n_2-\max(0,k_2)} b(y_1|n_1, p_0)b(k_1 + y_1|n_1, p_x)$$
$$\times b(y_2|n_2, p_0)b(k_2 + y_2|n_2, p_x).$$

Suppose that we want to choose a two-stage design with type I error rate smaller than or equal to α^* and power larger than or equal to $1-\beta^*$. There exist many two-stage designs satisfying the $(\alpha^*, 1 - \beta^*)$-restriction. We next define two reasonable two-stage designs for a randomized phase II trial, mimicking the designs for single-arm trials by Simon (1989).

7.1.2.1 Optimal Design

We want to find the two-stage design with the smallest expected sample size when the experimental therapy has a low response rate specified under H_0.

The probability of early termination (PET) under $H_0 : p_x = p_y = p_0$ is calculated as

$$\text{PET} = P(X_1 - Y_1 < a_1|p_0) = \sum_{k_1=-n_1}^{a_1-1} \sum_{y_1=\max(0,-k_1)}^{n_1-\max(0,k_1)} b(y_1|n_1, p_0)b(k_1 + y_1|n_1, p_0).$$

Since under H_0 the sample size per arm is n_1 with probability PET and n with probability $1 - \text{PET}$, the expected sample size per arm under H_0 is obtained as

$$\text{EN} = n_1 \times \text{PET} + n \times (1 - \text{PET}).$$

Among the two-stage randomized phase II trial designs satisfying the $(\alpha^*, 1 - \beta^*)$-restriction, the *optimal design* is defined as the one with the smallest EN.

7.1.2.2 Minimax Design

Among the two-stage designs satisfying the $(\alpha^*, 1 - \beta^*)$-restriction, the *minimax design* is defined as the one with the smallest maximal sample size n per arm. For the chosen n, there may be more than one two-stage designs satisfying the (α^*, β^*)-restriction. In this case, we choose the design with the smallest EN as the minimax design.

Given n, the designs satisfying the $(\alpha^*, 1-\beta^*)$-restriction can be determined by an exhaustive enumeration of $(\alpha, 1 - \beta, \text{EN})$ by changing n_1, a_1, and a $(1 \leq n_1 \leq n - 1, -n_1 \leq a_1 \leq n_1, a_1 - n_2 \leq a \leq n)$. Among these designs, the one that minimizes EN is identified. For the given n, this design dominates all other designs in terms of EN. Let $D(n) = (n_1, n, a_1, a)$ denote the design with the smallest EN, denoted as $\text{EN}(n)$, among the designs with maximal sample size n while satisfying the $(\alpha^*, 1 - \beta^*)$-restriction. If n is too small, there may exist no designs satisfying the $(\alpha^*, 1 - \beta^*)$-restriction. The design $D(n)$ with the smallest n is the minimax design. If n exceeds a certain limit, the two-stage design practically becomes identical to the single-stage design in the sense that the critical value of the first stage of the two-stage design is the same as that of the corresponding single-stage designs and no decision is made in the second stage. Hence, as n increases beyond the limit, $\text{EN}(n)$ increases linearly. The search for the optimal design continues by checking $\text{EN}(n)$ until n becomes so large that $\text{EN}(n)$ starts to linearly increase in n.

Tables 7.1 to 7.9 report the minimax and optimal designs under $\alpha^* = 0.1$, 0.15, 0.2; $1 - \beta^* = 0.8, 0.85, 0.9$; $p_y = p_0 = 0.05 : 0.85(0.05)$; $\Delta = p_x - p_y = 0.1, 0.15, 0.2$ ($\Delta = 0.1$ also for $p_y = 0.05$ and 0.85). Note that the maximal sample size for $\alpha = 0.1$ or $1 - \beta = 0.9$ is too large, especially when combined with a small effect size $\Delta = 0.15$. Under each setting, the maximal sample size for the minimax design is smaller than or equal to the sample size of the single-stage design. Under some settings, the single-stage design requires more patients than the maximal sample size of the optimal design.

Example 7.1

We consider a randomized phase II trial to evaluate the antitumor activity of CD30 antibody, SGN-30, combined with GVD chemotherapy (arm x) compared with GVD plus placebo (arm y) in patients with relapsed/refractory classical Hodgkin's lymphoma. The primary objective of this study is for testing $H_0 : p_x \leq p_y$ against $H_1 : p_x > p_y$. For the purpose of type I error rate and power calculation, the hypotheses are specified as $H_0 : p_x = p_y = 0.7$ and $H_1 : p_x = 0.85, p_y = 0.7$, that is, $p_0 = 0.7$ and $\Delta = 0.15$. The design parameters are chosen based on a small study on GVD alone. Under $(\alpha^*, 1-\beta^*, p_0, p_x) = (0.15, 0.8, 0.7, 0.85)$, the minimax design is $(n_1, n, a_1, a) = (56, 62, 5, 5)$, which has $(\alpha, 1 - \beta, EN) = (0.1499, 0.8009, 57.06)$, and the optimal design is $(n_1, n, a_1, a) = (27, 73, 1, 6)$, which has $(\alpha, 1 - \beta, EN) = (0.1321, 0.8001, 47.28)$. Compared to the minimax design, the optimal design requires $11(= 73 - 62)$ more patients per arm in maximal sample size, but saves almost $10(\approx 57.06 - 47.28)$ patients per arm in expected sample size when arm x is inefficacious. When minimax and optimal designs are very different in terms of n and EN, we can find a compromise design that has n close to that of the minimax design and EN close to that of the optimal design. Under the design setting, the design $(n_1, n, a_1, a) = (29, 65, 0, 6)$, which has $(\alpha, 1 - \beta, EN) = (0.1367, 0.8007, 49.05)$, requires only $3(= 65 - 62)$ more maximal sample size than the minimax design and $1.77(= 49.05 - 47.28)$ more expected sample size under H_0 than the optimal design. The single-stage design under the same design parameters requires $n = 63$ patients to reject H_0 when $X - Y \geq 6$, for which $(\alpha, 1 - \beta) = (0.1423, 0.8046)$. Note that, compared to the sample size of this single-stage design, the compromise two-stage design requires a maximal sample size of only by 2, but its expected sample under H_0 is much smaller (49.05 vs. 63). If we slightly increase the type I error rate to $\alpha^* = 0.16$, the optimal design is given as $(n_1, n, a_1, a) = (27, 63, 1, 5)$, which has $(\alpha, 1 - \beta, EN) = (0.1593, 0.8006, 42.87)$. With an increase of 1% in α^*, we drastically reduce EN and n.

7.1.3 Extensions

So far, we have considered two-arm randomized phase II trials allocating an equal number of patients to each arm. Also, we have controlled type I and II error rates under point null and alternative hypotheses. In this section, we investigate some extensions from these standard design settings.

7.1.3.1 Unbalanced Randomized Trials

One may want to allocate more patients to one arm than the other for some reasons, for example, to collect more information on one arm than the other or to collect enough specimens for a correlative study on one arm. Suppose that we want to randomize a different number of patients between two arms.

Let m_l and n_l denote the sample sizes at stage $l(= 1, 2)$ of arms x and y, respectively ($m = m_1 + m_2, n = n_1 + n_2$). Also, let X_l and Y_l denote the number of responders among stage l patients of arms x and y, respectively ($X = X_1 + X_2, Y = Y_1 + Y_2$). If we want to assign γ times larger number of patients to arm x than to arm y, then we have $m_l = \gamma \times n_l$ and $m = \gamma \times n$. Note that a choice of $\gamma = 1$ corresponds to the balanced two-stage designs considered in the previous section. When $\gamma \neq 1$, it does not make sense to directly compare the numbers of responders between arms at each stage. We propose to compare the sample response rates between two arms in this case.

A two-stage design under an unbalanced allocation scheme proceeds as follows.

- *Stage 1*: Accrue m_1 patients to arm x and n_1 patients to arm y, and observe X_1 and Y_1.

  (a) Proceed to the second stage if $X_1/m_1 - Y_1/n_1 \geq a_1$ for a chosen constant $a_1 \in [-1, 1]$.
  (b) Otherwise, reject arm x (or fail to reject H_0) and stop the trial.

- *Stage 2*: Accrue an additional m_2 patients to arm x and n_2 patients to arm y, and observe X_2 and Y_2.

  (a) For a constant $a \in [-1, 1]$, accept arm x (or reject H_0) for further investigation if $X/m - Y/n \geq a$.
  (b) Otherwise, reject arm x.

Given $H_0 : p_x = p_y = p_0$ and $H_1 : (p_x, p_y) = (p_0 + \Delta, p_0)$, the type I error rate and power of a two-stage design, defined by $(m_1, n_1, m_2, n_2, a_1, a)$, are calculated as

$$\alpha = P(X_1/m_1 - Y_1/n_1 \geq a_1, X/m - Y/n \geq a | p_x = p_y = p_0)$$

and

$$1 - \beta = P(X_1/m_1 - Y_1/n_1 \geq a_1, X/m - Y/n \geq a | p_x = p_0 + \Delta, p_y = p_0),$$

respectively.

When H_0 is true, the probability of early termination and the expected sample size for arm x are calculated as

$$\text{PET} = P(X_1/m_1 - Y_1/n_1 < a_1 | p_0) = \sum_{x_1=0}^{m_1} \sum_{y_1=0}^{n_1} I(x_1/m_1 - y_1/n_1 < a_1)$$
$$\times b(x_1 | m_1, p_0) b(y_1 | n_1, p_0),$$

and

$$\text{EN}_x = m_1 \times \text{PET} + m \times (1 - \text{PET}),$$

respectively. Similarly, the expected sample size for arm y under H_0 is obtained as $\text{EN}_y = n - n_2 \times \text{PET}$. So, the expected total sample size is $\text{EN} = \text{EN}_x +$

$EN_y = (m+n) - (m_2+n_2) \times PET$, or approximately $EN = (\gamma+1)EN_y$. Among the two-stage designs satisfying the $(\alpha^*, 1-\beta^*)$-restriction, the *optimal design* is defined as the one with the smallest EN.

The *minimax design* is defined as the one with the smallest m (or $m+n$) among the two-stage designs satisfying the $(\alpha^*, 1-\beta^*)$-restriction.

Example 7.2

In Example 7.1, suppose that we want to assign twice as many patients to SGN-30 plus GVD arm (arm x), that is, $\gamma = 2$. Under the same design setting as in Example 7.1, $(p_0, p_x, \alpha^*, 1-\beta^*) = (0.7, 0.85, 0.15, 0.8)$, the minimax design is $(m_1, m, n_1, n, a_1, a) = (31, 93, 16, 47, -0.0081, 0.0721)$, which has $(\alpha, 1-\beta, EN) = (0.1463, 0.8014, 92.36)$, and the optimal design is $(m_1, m, n_1, n, a_1, a) = (35, 99, 18, 50, 0.0206, 0.0677)$, which has $(\alpha, 1-\beta, EN) = (0.1459, 0.8027, 92.21)$. Unbalanced designs usually require larger sample sizes than balanced designs. For example, for the minimax designs, the total maximal sample size for this unbalanced design, $m+n = 140$, is larger than that for the balanced design, 126 from Example 7.1. Since our search program for minimax and optimal designs goes through all possible combinations of $m = 2n$ and $m = 2n \pm 1$, we actually have $m \approx \gamma \times n$.

7.1.3.2 Strict Type I and II Error Control

So far, we have considered a simple null hypothesis $H_0 : p_x = p_y = p_0$ based on the response rate of a historical control, p_0. However, possibly due to a slightly different patient population or the variability of the estimated response rate for a historical control, the true response rate for the prospective control of a randomized trial may be different from p_0. In this case, the chosen critical values (a_1, a) under the point null hypothesis may not control the type I error rate accurately under the composite null hypothesis $H_0 : p_x = p_y$. In this section, we consider the balanced randomization case, but extension to the unbalanced case is straightforward. In order to protect the type I error rate accurately under the composite null hypothesis, we calculate type I error by

$$\alpha = \max_{p_0 \in [0,1]} P(X_1 - Y_1 \geq a_1, X - Y \geq a | p_x = p_y = p_0). \quad (7.1)$$

Because $B(n, p)$ has the largest variance with $p = 1/2$, the probability in (7.1) is maximized at $p_0 = 1/2$. Hence, (7.1) is simplified to

$$\alpha = P(X_1 - Y_1 \geq a_1, X - Y \geq a | p_x = p_y = 1/2).$$

We also have considered a simple alternative hypothesis for power calculation. So, a chosen two-stage design based on the point alternative hypothesis may be underpowered although the experimental arm really has a higher response rate than the control by Δ, that is, $H_1 : p_x = p_y + \Delta$. In order to guarantee a certain power level over the composite alternative hypothesis, we may calculate the power by

$$1 - \beta = \min_{p_0 \in [0, 1-\Delta]} P(X_1 - Y_1 \geq a_1, X - Y \geq a | p_x = p_0 + \Delta, p_y = p_0),$$

which can be simplified to

$$1 - \beta = P(X_1 - Y_1 \geq a_1, X - Y \geq a | p_x = 1/2 + \Delta/2, p_y = 1/2 - \Delta/2).$$

In summary, given Δ, if a design (n_1, n, a_1, a) has type I error α under H_0: $p_x = p_y = 1/2$ and power $1 - \beta$ under $H_1 : p_x = 1/2 + \Delta/2$, $p_y = 1/2 - \Delta/2$, its type I error and power are given as α and $1 - \beta$ under the composite hypotheses $H_0 : p_x = p_y$ and $H_1 : p_x = p_y + \Delta$.

Given $(\alpha^*, \beta^*, \Delta)$, the optimal and minimax designs are defined as in Section 7.1.2. We do not specify p_0 in designing a study controlling the type I error and power under composite hypotheses. For example, for $(\alpha^*, 1 - \beta^*, \Delta) = (0.15, 0.8, 0.15)$ as in Example 7.1, the minimax design is $(n_1, n, a_1, a) = (54, 78, -2, 7)$, which has $(\alpha, 1 - \beta, \text{EN}) = (0.1487, 0.8000, 70.43)$, and the optimal design is $(n_1, n, a_1, a) = (39, 89, 1, 7)$, which has $(\alpha, 1 - \beta, \text{EN}) = (0.1428, 0.8001, 61.75)$. Note that these sample sizes are larger than those in Example 7.1, which are calculated under point null and alternative hypotheses. Table 7.10 lists the minimax and the optimal designs when controlling the type I error rate and power over $p_0 \in [0, 1]$ for $\alpha^* = 0.15, 0.2, 1 - \beta^* = 0.8, 0.85$, and $\Delta = 0.15, 0.2$. Note that the minimax designs for some design settings have n_1 too close to n, for example, $(\alpha^*, 1 - \beta^*, \Delta) = (.1, .8, .2)$. They are not appropriate as two-stage designs.

7.1.3.3   Randomized Trials with One Control and K Experimental Arms

Suppose that there are $K (\geq 2)$ experimental arms and one control arm. We want to identify the experimental arms whose response rate is significantly higher than that of the control arm. We consider balanced allocations here, but the following results can be easily modified for an unbalanced allocation case.

In the first stage, we accrue n_1 patients to each of $K + 1$ arms. For stage 1, let X_{k1} denote the number of responders from experimental arm $k (= 1, \ldots, K)$ and Y_1 the number of responders from the control arm. For an integer $a_1 \in [-n_1, n_1]$, experimental arm k with $X_{k1} - Y_1 \geq a_1$ proceeds to the second stage together with the control. All experimental arms with $X_{k1} - Y_1 < a_1$ will be dropped because of lack of efficacy. If no experimental arm survives over stage 1, then the whole trial will be terminated after stage 1. In the second stage, patients are randomized to the experimental arms surviving over stage 1 and the control arm.

In the second stage, we accrue an additional n_2 patients to each of the control and the experimental arms that survived over the first stage. Let

Table 7.10 Minimax and optimal two-stage designs for binomial test with a futility stopping value for strict control of $(\alpha^*, 1-\beta^*)$ over $p_0 \in [0, 1]$ and balanced allocation $(\gamma = 1)$

α^*	$1-\beta^*$	Δ	Minimax Design				Optimal Design			
			(n, n_1, a_1, a)	α	$1-\beta$	EN	(n, n_1, a_1, a)	α	$1-\beta$	EN
.1	.8	.15	(104, 63, 0, 10)	.0925	.8003	84.95	(122, 46, 2, 10)	.0909	.8005	74.68
		.2	(56, 55, 7, 7)	.0997	.8007	55.11	(70, 32, 3, 7)	.0979	.8007	42.11
	.85	.15	(123, 102, 7, 10)	.0997	.8513	105.81	(144, 56, 2, 11)	.0898	.8502	90.19
		.2	(67, 47, 0, 8)	.0971	.8500	57.82	(76, 28, 1, 8)	.0964	.8508	49.45
	.9	.15	(150, 107, −1, 12)	.0919	.9000	131.99	(174, 69, 2, 12)	.0918	.9001	110.92
		.2	(84, 48, 0, 9)	.0930	.9000	67.46	(95, 42, 2, 9)	.0923	.9001	61.71
.15	.8	.15	(78, 54, −2, 7)	.1487	.8000	70.43	(89, 39, 1, 7)	.1428	.8001	61.75
		.2	(45, 39, 4, 5)	.1496	.8011	40.28	(52, 26, 2, 5)	.1473	.8009	34.81
	.85	.15	(97, 92, 7, 7)	.1493	.8502	92.84	(114, 46, 1, 8)	.1369	.8500	77.18
		.2	(54, 37, −1, 6)	.1444	.8502	47.82	(61, 28, 1, 6)	.1396	.8507	42.75
	.9	.15	(121, 112, 7, 8)	.1499	.9007	113.73	(134, 77, 3, 8)	.1495	.9002	96.58
		.2	(68, 65, 6, 6)	.1495	.9021	65.50	(79, 35, 1, 7)	.1318	.9002	54.91
.2	.8	.15	(65, 42, 1, 5)	.1991	.8002	52.50	(69, 29, 0, 5)	.1978	.8000	51.09
		.2	(40, 15, 0, 4)	.1930	.8023	29.31	(40, 15, 0, 4)	.1930	.8023	29.31
	.85	.15	(80, 62, −1, 6)	.1917	.8500	72.91	(89, 40, 0, 6)	.1854	.8504	66.68
		.2	(46, 43, 4, 4)	.1990	.8567	43.68	(53, 23, 1, 4)	.1996	.8503	36.24
	.9	.15	(101, 98, 6, 6)	.1982	.9003	98.65	(113, 57, 1, 6)	.1999	.9006	82.91
		.2	(56, 40, −1, 5)	.1965	.9001	50.10	(60, 31, 0, 5)	.1917	.9003	46.96

X_{k2} and Y_2 denote the number of responders from the second-stage patients of experimental arm k and the control, respectively. Note that the number of experimental arms in the second stage will be smaller than K if some experimental arms are rejected after stage 1. Also, let $X_k = X_{k1} + X_{k2}$ and $Y = Y_1 + Y_2$ denote the total number of responders from the cumulative $n = n_1 + n_2$ patients for experimental arm k and the control, respectively. For an integer $a \in [a_1 - n_2, n]$, we accept experimental arm k for further investigation if $X_k - Y \geq a$.

Let p_k denote the response rate for experimental arm $k (= 1, \ldots, K)$, and p_y that for the control arm. Also, let p_0 denote the response rate for a historical control. We consider the point null hypothesis $H_0 : p_1 = \cdots = p_K = p_y = p_0$. We propose to control the probability of erroneously accepting any inefficacious experimental arm, called the *family-wise error rate* (FWER),

$$
\begin{aligned}
\alpha &= \mathrm{P}\{\cup_{k=1}^K (X_{k1} - Y_1 \geq a_1, X_k - Y \geq a) | p_0\} \\
&= \sum_{y_1=0}^{n_1} \sum_{x_{11}=0}^{n_1} \cdots \sum_{x_{K1}=0}^{n_1} \sum_{y_2=0}^{n_2} \sum_{x_{12}=0}^{n_2} \cdots \sum_{x_{K2}=0}^{n_2} I\{\cup_{k=1}^K (x_{k1} - y_1 \geq a_1, x_{k1} \\
&\qquad + x_{k2} - y_1 - y_2 \geq a)\} b(y_1|n_1, p_0) b(y_2|n_2, p_0) \\
&\qquad \times \prod_{k=1}^K b(x_{k1}|n_1, p_0) b(x_{k2}|n_2, p_0).
\end{aligned}
\tag{7.2}
$$

The family-wise power under a specified alternative hypothesis

$$
H_1 : p_y = p_0, \, p_k = p_0 + \Delta \text{ for } k = 1, \ldots, K
$$

is calculated by

$$
\begin{aligned}
1 - \beta &= \mathrm{P}\{\cup_{k=1}^K (X_{k1} - Y_1 \geq a_1, X_k - Y \geq a) | p_1 = \cdots = p_K = p_0 + \Delta, p_y = p_0\} \\
&= \sum_{y_1=0}^{n_1} \sum_{x_{11}=0}^{n_1} \cdots \sum_{x_{K1}=0}^{n_1} \sum_{y_2=0}^{n_2} \sum_{x_{12}=0}^{n_2} \cdots \sum_{x_{K2}=0}^{n_2} I\{\cup_{k=1}^K (x_{k1} - y_1 \geq a_1, x_{k1} + x_{k2} - y_1 - y_2 \geq a)\} \\
&\qquad \times b(y_1|n_1, p_0) b(y_2|n_2, p_0) \prod_{k=1}^K b(x_{k1}|n_1, p_0 + \Delta) b(x_{k2}|n_2, p_0 + \Delta).
\end{aligned}
\tag{7.3}
$$

Given $(p_0, \Delta, \alpha^*, 1 - \beta^*)$, the optimal and minimax designs are defined as in a two-arm trial case. Let's consider the case where $K = 2$. There are two types of early termination: (i) when only one experimental arm is rejected, or (ii) when both experimental arms are rejected after stage 1. For type (i), the required sample size is $3n_1 + 2n_2$, and the probability of early termination under H_0 is

$$
\mathrm{PET}_1 = 2 \times \mathrm{P}(X_{11} - Y_1 < a_1, X_{21} - Y_1 \geq a_1 | p_0)
$$

and, for type (ii), the required sample size is $3n_1$ and the probability of early termination under H_0 is

$$\text{PET}_2 = P(X_{11} - Y_1 < a_1, X_{21} - Y_1 < a_1 | p_0).$$

Hence, the expected sample size under H_0 is obtained as

$$\begin{aligned} \text{EN} &= (3n_1 + 2n_2) \times \text{PET}_1 + 3n_1 \times \text{PET}_2 + 3n \times (1 - \text{PET}_1 - \text{PET}_2) \\ &= 3n - n_2 \times \text{PET}_1 - 3n_2 \times \text{PET}_2, \end{aligned}$$

and $1/3$ of which is the expected sample size per arm.

Even with $K = 2$, the search for the optimal and minimax designs requires heavy computations. For an expedited search, we may choose a reasonable n, for example, an integer slightly larger than that for a two-arm design, and find (n_1, a_1, a) satisfying the $(\alpha^*, 1 - \beta^*)$-condition in a narrow space, such as $n_1 \in [0.3n, 0.7n]$, $a_1 \in [-2, 2]$, and $a \in [n\Delta/2 - 2, n\Delta/2 + 2]$. This suggestion is based on our experience that an n_1 of around $n/2$ provides a convenient time schedule for the interim analysis, and, for reasonable two-stage designs, a_1 is chosen around 0 and a is chosen around $n\Delta/2$.

Example 7.3

Let's consider $(\alpha^*, 1 - \beta^*, p_0, \Delta) = (0.15, 0.8, 0.7, 0.15)$ and $K = 2$. We may choose $n = 70$ per arm, which is slightly larger than that for the minimax design for two-arm trials, 62 from Example 7.1, $n_1 \in [21, 49]$, $a_1 \in [-2, 2]$, and $a \in [3, 8]$. Within the range, we choose the design with the smallest EN among those satisfying the $(\alpha^*, 1 - \beta^*)$-condition. From the expedited search, we find design $(n_1, n, a_1, a) = (23, 70, 2, 7)$, which has operating characteristics $(\alpha, 1 - \beta) = (0.1382, 0.8003)$ and $\text{EN} = 40.01$ per arm.

In order to adjust for the multiplicity of statistical tests, we propose to control the FWER in testing and to choose a design satisfying the family-wise power $1 - \beta$ given in (7.3). However, one may want to choose a design satisfying the marginal power to accept each efficacious experimental therapy with a certain probability. Given (n_1, n), suppose that the critical values (a_1, a) are chosen to control the FWER given in (7.2) below α^* level. Then, the marginal power for experimental arm k with $p_k = p_0 + \Delta$ will be calculated as

$$\begin{aligned} 1 - \tilde{\beta} &= P(X_{k1} - Y_1 \geq a_1, X_k - Y \geq a | p_0, p_k) \\ &= \sum_{y_1=0}^{n_1} \sum_{x_{k1}=0}^{n_1} \sum_{y_2=0}^{n_2} \sum_{x_{k2}=0}^{n_2} I(x_{k1} - y_1 \geq a_1, x_{k1} + x_{k2} - y_1 - y_2 \geq a) \\ &\quad \times b(y_1 | n_1, p_0) b(y_2 | n_2, p_0) b(x_{k1} | n_1, p_k) b(x_{k2} | n_2, p_k) \end{aligned}$$

or

$$1 - \tilde{\beta} = \sum_{k_1=a_1}^{n_1} \sum_{y_1=\max(0,-k_1)}^{n_1-\max(0,k_1)} \sum_{k_2=a-k_1}^{n_2} \sum_{y_2=\max(0,-k_2)}^{n_2-\max(0,k_2)} b(y_1|n_1, p_0)b(k_1 + y_1|n_1, p_k)$$
$$\times\, b(y_2|n_2, p_0)b(k_2 + y_2|n_2, p_k).$$

In Example 7.3 with $K = 2$, the design $(n_1, n, a_1, a) = (23, 70, 2, 7)$ has a marginal power of $1 - \tilde{\beta} = 0.6654$ for $(p_0, \Delta) = (0.7, 0.15)$. Suppose that we want to control the marginal power at $1 - \tilde{\beta}^* = 0.8$ while controlling the FWER at $\alpha^* = 0.15$ for each experimental arm with $(p_0, \Delta) = (0.7, 0.15)$. Then we need a larger trial, such as $(n_1, n, a_1, a) = (44, 88, 0, 9)$, which has $(\alpha, 1 - \tilde{\beta}) = (0.1293, 0.8007)$.

7.2 Two-Stage Designs with Both Upper and Lower Stopping Values

In a regular multistage clinical trial, we have to consider stopping or continuing the trial depending on the outcome of the study therapy at each interim analysis. In a traditional single-arm phase II cancer trial, we usually consider stopping the trial early only for futility, but not for efficacy (also called *superiority*), since there are no ethical issues in treating future patients with an efficacious therapy. So far, we have considered early stopping for futility only. In a randomized phase II trial, however, we may also want to stop the trial early if the experimental therapy is shown to be more efficacious than the prospective control therapy. In this section, we investigate two-arm $(k = 1)$ two-stage randomized trials with both lower (futility) and upper (efficacy) early stopping values.

We consider balanced allocations, but an extension to unbalanced randomization can be easily derived. A two-stage phase II trial with design $\{(a_1, b_1)/n_1, a/n\}$ proceeds as follows:

> *Stage 1*: Randomize n_1 patients to each arm, and observe the number of responders X_1 and Y_1.
>
> (a) If $X_1 - Y_1 \leq a_1$, reject the experimental therapy and stop the trial.
> (b) If $X_1 - Y_1 \geq b_1$, accept the experimental therapy and stop the trial.
> (c) If $a_1 < X_1 - Y_1 < b_1$, continue to stage 2.
>
> *Stage 2*: Treat n_2 patients, and observe the number of responders X_2 and Y_2. Let $X = X_1 + X_2$ and $Y = Y_1 + Y_2$.
>
> (a) If $X - Y \leq a$, reject the experimental therapy.
> (b) If $X - Y > a$, accept the experimental therapy.

We want to test $H_0 : p_x = p_y$ against $H_0 : p_x > p_y$. For a two-stage design $\{(a_1, b_1)/n_1, a/n\}$, we reject the experimental therapy (or fail to reject H_0) if $(X_1 - Y_1 \le a_1)$ or $(a_1 < X_1 - Y_1 < b_1, X - Y \le a)$, the probability of which is calculated by

$$R(p_x, p_y) = \sum_{y_1=0}^{n_1-0\vee b_1} \sum_{x_1=0\vee(y_1+b_1)}^{n_1} b(x_1|n_1, p_x) b(y_1|n_1, p_y)$$

$$+ \sum_{y_1=0\vee(1-b_1)}^{n_1-0\vee(a_1+1)} \sum_{x_1=0\vee(y_1+a_1+1)}^{n_1\wedge(y_1+b_1-1)} \sum_{y_2=0}^{n_2-0\vee(a+1-x_1+y_1)}$$

$$\times \sum_{x_2=0\vee(y_2+a+1-x_1+y_1)}^{n_2} b(x_1|n_1, p_x) b(y_1|n_1, p_y) b(x_2|n_2, p_x) b(y_2|n_2, p_y)$$

for given p_x and p_y, where $a \wedge b = \min(a, b)$ and $a \vee b = \max(a, b)$. Under $H_0 : p_x = p_y = p_0$ and $H_1 : p_x = p_0 + \Delta$, $p_y = p_0$, the constraint on type I error probability and power is expressed as $R(p_x = p_y = p_0) \ge 1 - \alpha^*$ and $R(p_x = p_0 + \Delta, p_y = p_0) \le \beta^*$.

Given (p_0, Δ), there are many designs satisfying a type I error rate and power constraint $(\alpha^*, 1 - \beta^*)$. Among them, the *minimax design* minimizes the maximum number of patients $n = n_1 + n_2$. For a combination of response probabilities (p_x, p_y), the expected sample size per arm is given as

$$\text{EN}(p_x, p_y) = \text{PET}(p_x, p_y) \times n_1 + \{1 - \text{PET}(p_x, p_y)\} \times n,$$

where

$$\text{PET}(p_x, p_y) = 1 - P(a_1 < X_1 - Y_1 < b_1 | p_x, p_y)$$

$$= 1 - \sum_{y_1=0\vee(1-b_1)}^{n_1-0\vee(a_1+1)} \sum_{x_1=0\vee(y_1+a_1+1)}^{n_1\wedge(y_1+b_1-1)} b(x_1|n_1, p_x) b(y_1|n_1, p_y)$$

is the probability of early termination after stage 1. Let $\text{EN}_0 = \text{EN}(p_0, p_0)$ and $\text{EN}_1 = \text{EN}(p_0 + \Delta, p_0)$. The *optimal design* minimizes the average of the expected sample sizes for p_0 and Δ given as

$$\text{EN} = (\text{EN}_0 + \text{EN}_1)/2$$

among the designs satisfying the $(\alpha^*, 1 - \beta^*)$ condition. On the other hand, the minimax design minimizes the maximal sample size n.

Tables 7.11–7.19 list minimax and optimal two-stage designs with both upper and lower stopping values under various design settings of $(\alpha^*, 1 - \beta^*, p_x, p_y)$.

Table 7.11 Minimax and optimal two-stage designs with upper and lower early stopping values under $(\alpha^*, 1 - \beta^*) = (.1, .8)$ and balanced allocation $(\gamma = 1)$

		Minimax Design					Optimal Design				
P_y	P_x	(n, n_1, a_1, b_1, a)	α	$1-\beta$	EN_0	EN_1	(n, n_1, a_1, b_1, a)	α	$1-\beta$	EN_0	EN_1
.05	.15	(58, 29, −3, 3, 3)	.0993	.8007	54.39	41.49	(61, 27, −1, 3, 3)	.0994	.8001	46.54	40.86
	.2	(50, 23, 1, 3, 2)	.0802	.8065	25.72	27.11	(52, 15, 0, 2, 4)	.1000	.8017	23.25	21.87
	.25	(50, 9, 0, 2, 2)	.0923	.8149	17.50	19.14	(50, 9, 0, 2, 2)	.0923	.8149	17.50	19.14
.1	.25	(50, 29, 0, 4, 4)	.0933	.8040	36.36	35.26	(53, 25, 0, 4, 4)	.0898	.8006	34.99	35.02
	.3	(50, 18, 1, 3, 4)	.0956	.8046	21.74	22.36	(50, 18, 1, 3, 4)	.0956	.8046	21.74	22.36
.15	.3	(60, 27, −3, 5, 5)	.0994	.8004	53.06	44.97	(77, 35, 1, 5, 6)	.0972	.8015	45.14	46.60
	.35	(50, 22, 1, 4, 5)	.0920	.8062	27.39	28.26	(52, 21, 1, 4, 5)	.0896	.8005	26.96	28.35
.2	.35	(71, 48, −1, 7, 6)	.0998	.8001	59.56	57.14	(92, 38, 1, 6, 7)	.0997	.8016	52.91	56.44
	.4	(50, 25, 1, 5, 5)	.0970	.8032	31.05	32.52	(50, 25, 1, 5, 5)	.0970	.8032	31.05	32.52
.25	.4	(81, 73, 3, 8, 7)	.0998	.8025	74.41	74.41	(97, 45, 1, 7, 8)	.0991	.8005	60.65	63.72
	.45	(50, 29, 1, 7, 5)	.0962	.8013	35.31	38.70	(58, 20, 0, 5, 6)	.0989	.8008	34.37	36.94
.3	.45	(90, 73, 0, 9, 8)	.0981	.8002	79.83	78.08	(120, 44, 1, 7, 10)	.0999	.8008	66.69	71.45
	.5	(52, 23, −3, 6, 6)	.0993	.8013	44.81	40.12	(59, 22, 0, 6, 6)	.0996	.8014	36.80	41.29
.35	.5	(94, 61, −1, 11, 8)	.0998	.8001	77.99	79.47	(115, 51, 1, 8, 10)	.0988	.8001	71.37	75.27
	.55	(53, 38, −1, 8, 6)	.0989	.8001	45.69	44.87	(64, 24, 0, 6, 7)	.0991	.8016	39.70	43.05
.4	.55	(100, 73, −1, 10, 9)	.1000	.8002	85.95	83.11	(126, 50, 1, 8, 11)	.0991	.8006	74.10	79.30
	.6	(55, 38, 1, 10, 6)	.0998	.8003	43.95	48.06	(64, 31, 1, 7, 7)	.0973	.8006	41.01	44.71
.45	.6	(100, 95, 5, 10, 9)	.0995	.8001	95.64	95.71	(123, 56, 2, 9, 10)	.0999	.8011	73.72	81.20
	.65	(56, 52, 5, 9, 6)	.0998	.8020	52.37	52.75	(67, 29, 1, 7, 7)	.0998	.8025	40.54	46.01
.5	.65	(100, 96, 5, 10, 9)	.0997	.8014	96.51	96.56	(123, 55, 2, 9, 10)	.0999	.8004	72.99	81.28
	.7	(56, 48, 4, 11, 6)	.0999	.8029	49.31	51.48	(67, 28, 1, 7, 7)	.0989	.8009	39.85	46.29
.55	.7	(99, 88, 5, 10, 9)	.0999	.8001	89.40	89.83	(125, 48, 1, 8, 11)	.0997	.8001	72.45	79.69
	.75	(54, 31, 0, 11, 6)	.0998	.8015	41.25	49.84	(64, 34, 2, 7, 7)	.1000	.8018	40.45	44.03
.6	.75	(92, 62, −1, 14, 8)	.0999	.8002	77.90	84.91	(107, 55, 2, 9, 9)	.0997	.8001	68.76	75.86
	.8	(52, 31, 0, 8, 6)	.0991	.8004	39.88	43.37	(65, 29, 1, 6, 8)	.0996	.8006	38.87	41.93
.65	.8	(88, 85, 5, 9, 8)	.0989	.8022	85.31	85.38	(109, 49, 2, 8, 9)	.0996	.8019	63.55	71.80
	.85	(50, 30, 0, 7, 6)	.0964	.8001	38.15	40.28	(53, 21, 0, 6, 6)	.0995	.8004	33.76	40.06
.7	.85	(79, 39, −2, 9, 7)	.0997	.8003	64.08	68.87	(90, 36, 0, 7, 8)	.0999	.8007	57.70	65.41
	.9	(50, 26, 1, 6, 6)	.0908	.8011	32.66	36.87	(51, 18, 0, 5, 6)	.0986	.8003	30.47	36.61
.75	.9	(68, 43, 0, 9, 6)	.0985	.8001	53.84	60.10	(88, 36, 1, 6, 8)	.0999	.8026	50.28	57.19
	.95	(50, 18, 1, 5, 5)	.0926	.8078	25.69	34.82	(54, 23, 2, 5, 5)	.0983	.8004	27.17	32.54
.8	.95	(56, 35, 0, 7, 5)	.0987	.8007	43.71	48.64	(63, 28, 1, 6, 5)	.0987	.8017	37.62	48.43
.85	.95	(101, 62, 0, 9, 6)	.0988	.8005	78.91	90.18	(109, 39, 0, 7, 6)	.0998	.8018	68.20	91.51

Table 7.12 Minimax and optimal two-stage designs with upper and lower early stopping values under $(\alpha^*, 1 - \beta^*) = (.1, .85)$ and balanced allocation $(\gamma = 1)$

		Minimax Design					Optimal Design				
p_Y	p_X	(n, n_1, a_1, b_1, a)	α	$1-\beta$	EN_0	EN_1	(n, n_1, a_1, b_1, a)	α	$1-\beta$	EN_0	EN_1
.05	.15	(69, 48, −1, 4, 3)	.0959	.8502	59.48	54.30	(78, 40, 0, 4, 3)	.0995	.8507	53.66	53.02
	.2	(40, 21, 0, 3, 2)	.0953	.8551	26.94	26.47	(41, 20, 0, 3, 2)	.0949	.8514	26.54	26.43
	.25	(40, 12, 0, 2, 3)	.0838	.8576	18.16	16.95	(40, 12, 0, 2, 3)	.0838	.8576	18.16	16.95
.1	.25	(55, 25, −3, 4, 4)	.0993	.8512	50.10	38.68	(60, 22, −1, 4, 4)	.0997	.8519	43.43	40.06
	.3	(40, 17, 0, 4, 3)	.0891	.8542	25.30	26.71	(41, 18, 0, 3, 4)	.0988	.8511	25.09	23.27
.15	.3	(70, 39, −2, 7, 5)	.0997	.8505	59.61	56.05	(89, 37, 0, 5, 7)	.0996	.8514	55.95	52.95
	.35	(42, 25, −1, 5, 4)	.0943	.8511	34.23	31.79	(52, 21, 0, 4, 5)	.0980	.8516	31.84	30.62
.2	.35	(85, 80, 5, 9, 6)	.0995	.8501	80.46	80.71	(95, 44, 0, 7, 7)	.0986	.8503	64.69	65.39
	.4	(50, 34, 0, 6, 5)	.0966	.8508	40.28	39.06	(58, 27, 0, 5, 6)	.0973	.8526	38.47	36.97
.25	.4	(97, 87, 5, 11, 7)	.0999	.8500	88.35	89.29	(109, 47, 0, 8, 8)	.0998	.8511	72.78	75.90
	.45	(56, 54, 5, 8, 5)	.0997	.8536	54.13	54.22	(59, 27, −1, 6, 6)	.0996	.8517	43.68	41.88
.3	.45	(105, 68, −1, 13, 8)	.0999	.8501	87.53	91.34	(120, 59, 1, 9, 9)	.0997	.8511	79.61	82.94
	.5	(59, 53, 2, 8, 6)	.0998	.8501	54.45	54.28	(73, 32, 0, 6, 8)	.0995	.8536	47.56	46.00
.35	.5	(113, 67, −4, 11, 9)	.0999	.8501	99.59	90.99	(127, 56, 0, 9, 10)	.0999	.8503	85.44	87.38
	.55	(65, 47, 0, 8, 7)	.0979	.8500	54.29	52.60	(76, 37, 1, 7, 8)	.0959	.8506	48.74	49.93
.4	.55	(116, 91, 2, 17, 9)	.1000	.8500	99.66	106.42	(136, 57, 0, 9, 11)	.0997	.8504	89.40	91.00
	.6	(66, 48, −1, 9, 7)	.0983	.8501	57.06	54.99	(76, 32, 0, 7, 8)	.0983	.8502	49.65	51.34
.45	.6	(120, 109, 4, 11, 10)	.0999	.8505	111.13	110.74	(148, 61, 1, 9, 12)	.0998	.8506	89.86	93.19
	.65	(66, 59, 3, 9, 7)	.0996	.8500	60.41	60.44	(81, 38, 1, 7, 9)	.0995	.8504	50.82	51.71
.5	.65	(120, 112, 5, 11, 10)	.0998	.8521	113.21	113.06	(148, 60, 1, 9, 12)	.0999	.8511	89.22	93.44
	.7	(66, 43, −1, 10, 7)	.0981	.8501	55.03	55.80	(81, 37, 1, 7, 9)	.0989	.8507	50.14	51.69
.55	.7	(116, 80, 2, 17, 9)	.1000	.8503	92.29	105.65	(127, 55, 0, 10, 10)	.0996	.8501	85.80	93.53
	.75	(65, 42, 0, 9, 7)	.0981	.8501	51.79	52.90	(73, 32, 0, 7, 8)	.0994	.8512	48.37	50.46
.6	.75	(110, 104, 5, 11, 9)	.0996	.8503	104.90	104.94	(135, 64, 2, 9, 11)	.0999	.8505	82.72	87.28
	.8	(62, 50, 4, 12, 6)	.0999	.8520	52.04	56.24	(69, 26, 0, 7, 7)	.0994	.8520	43.69	51.02
.65	.8	(103, 76, 3, 15, 8)	.0999	.8508	83.27	93.36	(119, 50, 1, 9, 9)	.0998	.8504	73.43	84.67
	.85	(56, 35, 0, 9, 6)	.0984	.8509	44.11	48.27	(73, 29, 1, 6, 8)	.0987	.8507	41.11	45.36
.7	.85	(94, 78, 5, 12, 7)	.0998	.8508	80.34	83.94	(113, 54, 2, 8, 9)	.0986	.8504	68.30	74.62
	.9	(50, 39, 3, 9, 5)	.0996	.8509	40.93	44.27	(60, 25, 1, 6, 6)	.0988	.8502	34.71	41.62
.75	.9	(81, 64, 4, 11, 6)	.1000	.8504	66.77	72.05	(99, 48, 2, 7, 8)	.0988	.8501	58.97	64.70
	.95	(44, 27, 0, 6, 5)	.0980	.8502	33.73	35.49	(53, 24, 1, 5, 6)	.0989	.8543	31.02	34.96
.8	.95	(64, 45, 2, 10, 5)	.0996	.8517	49.72	59.04	(74, 35, 1, 6, 6)	.0993	.8517	45.79	53.17
.85	.95	(118, 104, 5, 10, 6)	.1000	.8509	105.54	108.15	(145, 71, 2, 7, 8)	.0988	.8501	86.90	96.44

Table 7.13 Minimax and optimal two-stage designs with upper and lower early stopping values under $(\alpha^*, 1-\beta^*) = (.1, .9)$ and balanced allocation ($\gamma = 1$)

		Minimax Design					Optimal Design				
p_y	p_x	(n, n_1, a_1, b_1, a)	α	$1-\beta$	EN_0	EN_1	(n, n_1, a_1, b_1, a)	α	$1-\beta$	EN_0	EN_1
.05	.15	(90, 67, −1, 4, 4)	.0980	.9000	78.50	70.64	(106, 49, 0, 4, 4)	.0950	.9003	69.23	63.63
	.2	(60, 25, 0, 3, 3)	.0870	.9048	36.00	32.81	(61, 24, 0, 3, 3)	.0855	.9008	35.62	32.80
	.25	(60, 15, 0, 2, 5)	.0966	.9045	25.04	20.67	(60, 15, 0, 2, 5)	.0966	.9045	25.04	20.67
.1	.25	(66, 41, −2, 6, 4)	.0982	.9000	58.27	51.35	(81, 37, 0, 5, 5)	.0873	.9001	53.82	50.93
	.3	(60, 27, 1, 4, 4)	.0909	.9046	33.25	32.54	(71, 19, 0, 3, 6)	.0992	.9012	34.89	29.99
.15	.3	(88, 63, −1, 7, 6)	.0988	.9002	75.45	69.13	(103, 47, 0, 6, 7)	.0969	.9003	68.66	63.71
	.35	(60, 28, 0, 5, 5)	.0946	.9030	40.16	37.91	(60, 28, 0, 5, 5)	.0946	.9030	40.16	37.91
.2	.35	(104, 66, −2, 10, 7)	.0992	.9001	89.14	83.30	(124, 56, 0, 7, 9)	.0995	.9001	82.59	76.11
	.4	(61, 52, 3, 9, 5)	.0992	.9001	53.59	54.44	(72, 36, 1, 6, 6)	.0995	.9003	45.96	45.31
.25	.4	(118, 77, −1, 14, 8)	.0998	.9000	98.78	102.17	(141, 59, 0, 8, 10)	.0997	.9006	92.01	87.22
	.45	(67, 43, −2, 9, 6)	.0992	.9000	58.10	54.47	(82, 36, 0, 6, 8)	.0999	.9014	53.44	49.15
.3	.45	(129, 76, −3, 13, 9)	.1000	.9001	110.86	105.84	(149, 69, 0, 9, 11)	.0998	.9006	101.48	95.36
	.5	(74, 70, 5, 8, 7)	.0990	.9012	70.29	70.23	(83, 40, 0, 7, 8)	.0998	.9000	57.00	53.76
.35	.5	(139, 74, −4, 12, 10)	.0998	.9003	119.71	107.67	(158, 66, 0, 10, 11)	.1000	.9009	104.86	104.86
	.55	(77, 72, 5, 11, 7)	.0999	.9000	72.68	72.93	(85, 42, 0, 8, 8)	.0992	.9006	59.70	58.26
.4	.55	(143, 105, 2, 18, 10)	.1000	.9002	118.51	126.39	(167, 68, 0, 10, 12)	.1000	.9010	109.30	107.93
	.6	(81, 73, 4, 9, 8)	.0994	.9004	74.19	73.85	(96, 44, 1, 8, 9)	.0974	.9005	60.70	61.11
.45	.6	(148, 76, −5, 12, 11)	.1000	.9001	129.15	112.02	(168, 85, 2, 11, 12)	.1000	.9001	110.39	110.39
	.65	(82, 56, −1, 10, 8)	.0984	.9002	69.06	65.27	(91, 43, 0, 8, 9)	.0998	.9010	62.45	60.46
.5	.65	(147, 102, −1, 13, 11)	.0988	.9001	123.96	116.90	(170, 82, 2, 11, 12)	.1000	.9005	108.21	110.72
	.7	(81, 59, −1, 10, 8)	.0986	.9001	69.93	66.00	(96, 42, 1, 8, 9)	.0997	.9003	59.35	61.29
.55	.7	(141, 111, 4, 17, 10)	.1000	.9004	118.77	124.38	(167, 78, 1, 10, 13)	.0995	.9000	108.41	105.67
	.75	(79, 72, 5, 9, 8)	.0986	.9003	72.71	72.63	(94, 47, 2, 8, 9)	.0995	.9004	58.40	59.75
.6	.75	(134, 109, 1, 13, 10)	.0999	.9000	118.40	115.77	(159, 79, 2, 10, 12)	.0998	.9001	101.49	102.03
	.8	(73, 44, 0, 12, 7)	.0995	.9001	57.07	64.73	(82, 42, 1, 8, 8)	.0994	.9016	54.88	56.59
.65	.8	(123, 100, 3, 17, 9)	.0999	.9000	106.78	112.93	(142, 63, 1, 10, 10)	.0999	.9011	90.80	98.48
	.85	(68, 65, 4, 8, 7)	.0989	.9005	65.36	65.26	(80, 37, 1, 7, 8)	.0991	.9016	49.95	52.01
.7	.85	(111, 90, 4, 15, 8)	.1000	.9002	94.68	100.94	(139, 59, 1, 8, 11)	.0994	.9002	84.27	85.50
	.9	(60, 31, −1, 8, 6)	.0996	.9012	46.57	49.94	(75, 33, 1, 6, 8)	.0996	.9005	44.51	46.12
.75	.9	(95, 62, 1, 12, 7)	.0999	.9004	74.19	84.25	(108, 51, 1, 8, 8)	.0983	.9000	69.40	75.83
	.95	(60, 27, 1, 6, 6)	.0902	.9009	36.14	42.36	(73, 24, 1, 5, 7)	.0997	.9012	35.86	42.51
.8	.95	(77, 67, 1, 8, 6)	.0998	.9001	70.20	69.39	(85, 39, 1, 7, 6)	.0998	.9006	52.92	63.73
.85	.95	(139, 81, 0, 12, 7)	.0997	.9001	107.12	127.33	(163, 83, 2, 8, 8)	.0996	.9005	102.33	111.77

Table 7.14 Minimax and optimal two-stage designs with upper and lower early stopping values under $(\alpha^*, 1-\beta^*) = (.15, .8)$ and balanced allocation ($\gamma = 1$)

p_y	p_x	Minimax Design					Optimal Design				
		(n, n_1, a_1, b_1, a)	α	$1-\beta$	EN_0	EN_1	(n, n_1, a_1, b_1, a)	α	$1-\beta$	EN_0	EN_1
.05	.15	(47, 10, −3, 2, 2)	.1457	.8035	44.69	34.57	(61, 18, −1, 2, 3)	.1499	.8015	41.71	33.23
	.2	(30, 17, 0, 2, 2)	.1245	.8041	19.89	19.07	(35, 15, 0, 2, 2)	.1214	.8016	19.46	18.71
	.25	(30, 9, 0, 2, 1)	.1199	.8076	13.36	14.19	(30, 9, 0, 2, 1)	.1199	.8076	13.36	14.19
.1	.25	(36, 35, 2, 4, 2)	.1495	.8047	35.08	35.10	(44, 22, 0, 3, 3)	.1447	.8012	28.54	27.45
	.3	(30, 9, −1, 2, 3)	.1422	.8168	20.69	16.41	(31, 12, 0, 3, 2)	.1253	.8010	18.02	18.99
.15	.3	(46, 36, 0, 8, 3)	.1500	.8006	40.27	42.48	(55, 28, 0, 4, 4)	.1472	.8001	36.95	35.99
	.35	(30, 15, −1, 3, 3)	.1482	.8040	22.58	20.23	(30, 15, −1, 3, 3)	.1482	.8040	22.58	20.23
.2	.35	(55, 42, −1, 6, 4)	.1496	.8001	48.35	46.86	(59, 35, 0, 6, 4)	.1499	.8014	44.38	45.26
	.4	(32, 12, −3, 4, 3)	.1488	.8010	29.32	25.55	(40, 20, 0, 4, 4)	.1336	.8014	26.78	26.38
.25	.4	(64, 57, 2, 6, 5)	.1493	.8011	58.24	58.10	(74, 33, 0, 6, 5)	.1500	.8000	48.78	50.97
	.45	(37, 35, 3, 6, 3)	.1488	.8017	35.20	35.33	(48, 20, 0, 4, 5)	.1438	.8001	29.18	28.72
.3	.45	(69, 60, 2, 11, 5)	.1499	.8001	62.62	64.53	(79, 32, −1, 6, 6)	.1497	.8001	54.94	54.89
	.5	(75, 70, 3, 7, 6)	.1496	.8035	70.71	70.65	(89, 33, −1, 6, 7)	.1497	.8025	59.53	59.17
.35	.5	(41, 33, 0, 7, 4)	.1500	.8001	36.22	36.39	(50, 23, 0, 5, 5)	.1478	.8018	32.64	33.15
	.55	(77, 52, −3, 9, 6)	.1486	.8001	68.18	65.31	(91, 48, 1, 7, 7)	.1484	.8002	60.46	61.80
.4	.55	(44, 39, 3, 7, 4)	.1480	.8004	39.72	40.10	(50, 18, −1, 5, 5)	.1493	.8021	34.17	35.07
	.6	(78, 49, −2, 10, 6)	.1493	.8001	66.20	67.35	(93, 40, 0, 7, 7)	.1494	.8016	60.33	63.10
.45	.6	(44, 39, 3, 9, 4)	.1498	.8005	39.93	41.01	(55, 24, 0, 5, 6)	.1469	.8015	34.75	35.12
	.65	(77, 70, 1, 9, 6)	.1498	.8000	72.27	72.12	(93, 39, 0, 7, 7)	.1492	.8012	59.77	63.29
.5	.65	(44, 42, 4, 6, 4)	.1480	.8015	42.10	42.13	(59, 26, 1, 5, 6)	.1499	.8005	33.69	35.05
	.7	(76, 41, −4, 9, 6)	.1499	.8000	67.32	65.21	(92, 45, 1, 7, 7)	.1487	.8004	58.69	61.56
.55	.7	(42, 38, 3, 7, 4)	.1492	.8008	38.57	38.94	(57, 26, 1, 5, 6)	.1468	.8016	33.24	34.65
	.75	(73, 69, 5, 9, 5)	.1496	.8002	69.40	69.72	(80, 30, −1, 7, 6)	.1497	.8003	55.47	61.45
.6	.75	(40, 26, 0, 7, 4)	.1489	.8004	31.76	34.15	(46, 23, 0, 5, 5)	.1492	.8012	31.12	32.10
	.8	(67, 66, 5, 7, 5)	.1486	.8006	66.04	66.06	(84, 42, 1, 6, 7)	.1496	.8002	53.00	54.74
.65	.8	(38, 22, −1, 6, 4)	.1447	.8005	30.36	31.81	(43, 17, 0, 5, 4)	.1480	.8006	26.79	31.42
	.85	(62, 40, −1, 7, 5)	.1497	.8006	50.84	51.35	(73, 26, 0, 6, 5)	.1489	.8000	44.44	53.33
.7	.85	(33, 22, 1, 7, 3)	.1495	.8004	25.24	29.34	(42, 14, 0, 4, 4)	.1492	.8001	23.65	28.23
	.9	(52, 35, 0, 8, 4)	.1486	.8009	42.24	46.98	(67, 31, 1, 5, 5)	.1493	.8000	39.53	43.30
.75	.9	(30, 15, 0, 5, 3)	.1364	.8010	20.82	25.60	(32, 13, 0, 4, 3)	.1483	.8072	19.74	24.33
	.95	(42, 22, 0, 7, 3)	.1499	.8013	30.36	38.84	(53, 19, 0, 4, 4)	.1487	.8024	30.65	36.87
.8	.95	(76, 48, −1, 9, 4)	.1497	.8003	63.39	72.32	(82, 38, 0, 6, 4)	.1500	.8013	55.50	66.80

Table 7.15 Minimax and optimal two-stage designs with upper and lower early stopping values under $(\alpha^*, 1 - \beta^*) = (.15, .85)$ and balanced allocation $(\gamma = 1)$

P_y	P_x	Minimax Design					Optimal Design				
		(n, n_1, a_1, b_1, a)	α	$1 - \beta$	EN_0	EN_1	(n, n_1, a_1, b_1, a)	α	$1 - \beta$	EN_0	EN_1
.05	.15	(55, 27, −5, 3, 2)	.1499	.8500	53.34	40.20	(57, 22, −2, 3, 2)	.1497	.8507	50.77	41.17
	.2	(30, 22, −1, 2, 2)	.1478	.8527	26.07	23.33	(37, 19, 0, 2, 2)	.1452	.8506	22.96	21.46
	.25	(30, 12, 0, 2, 1)	.1445	.8664	15.96	15.18	(31, 11, 0, 2, 1)	.1380	.8510	15.34	14.96
.1	.25	(46, 17, −3, 3, 3)	.1477	.8520	41.78	31.06	(66, 24, 0, 3, 4)	.1492	.8511	36.26	33.36
	.3	(30, 17, 0, 3, 2)	.1450	.8529	21.04	20.22	(30, 17, 0, 3, 2)	.1450	.8529	21.04	20.22
.15	.3	(59, 38, −2, 5, 4)	.1431	.8501	50.88	45.27	(69, 29, −1, 4, 5)	.1466	.8505	48.05	42.30
	.35	(35, 22, −1, 4, 3)	.1378	.8505	28.72	26.32	(41, 17, −1, 3, 4)	.1499	.8537	28.63	24.19
.2	.35	(70, 67, 4, 7, 4)	.1490	.8516	67.26	67.31	(85, 39, 0, 5, 6)	.1497	.8507	54.78	51.82
	.4	(41, 35, 2, 6, 3)	.1492	.8522	36.06	36.37	(45, 19, −1, 4, 4)	.1479	.8515	32.12	29.25
.25	.4	(78, 61, 1, 11, 5)	.1498	.8503	67.17	70.11	(90, 35, −1, 6, 6)	.1498	.8508	62.01	60.03
	.45	(44, 41, 2, 5, 4)	.1494	.8506	41.41	41.30	(57, 22, −1, 4, 6)	.1489	.8519	38.06	33.38
.3	.45	(85, 68, −1, 8, 6)	.1499	.8505	75.77	72.85	(91, 51, 0, 8, 6)	.1494	.8504	67.19	67.64
	.5	(49, 45, 3, 8, 4)	.1496	.8534	45.67	46.02	(55, 22, −1, 5, 5)	.1499	.8503	38.39	36.71
.35	.5	(90, 87, 5, 10, 6)	.1497	.8509	87.38	87.51	(110, 57, 1, 7, 8)	.1494	.8511	72.02	70.63
	.55	(52, 29, −4, 6, 5)	.1499	.8502	46.66	39.53	(56, 30, 0, 6, 5)	.1494	.8505	39.84	39.63
.4	.55	(95, 87, 5, 12, 6)	.1500	.8508	88.28	89.25	(112, 42, −1, 7, 8)	.1494	.8517	74.95	73.38
	.6	(53, 36, −2, 7, 5)	.1486	.8504	45.90	42.99	(73, 26, 0, 5, 7)	.1495	.8523	42.11	41.30
.45	.6	(95, 92, 4, 8, 7)	.1500	.8509	92.36	92.27	(104, 53, 0, 9, 7)	.1483	.8504	74.06	76.93
	.65	(53, 45, 1, 7, 5)	.1495	.8503	47.33	46.92	(56, 32, 0, 7, 5)	.1499	.8510	41.58	42.58
.5	.65	(95, 81, 0, 9, 7)	.1498	.8501	86.29	84.46	(102, 54, 0, 9, 7)	.1489	.8504	73.73	76.16
	.7	(53, 24, −3, 7, 5)	.1494	.8502	45.31	43.67	(57, 29, 0, 7, 5)	.1480	.8503	40.32	42.96
.55	.7	(93, 89, 4, 8, 7)	.1490	.8510	89.48	89.39	(113, 53, 0, 7, 9)	.1494	.8517	74.54	72.02
	.75	(52, 33, −1, 7, 5)	.1481	.8507	42.42	41.65	(68, 26, 0, 5, 7)	.1496	.8513	40.28	39.98
.6	.75	(88, 68, 2, 12, 6)	.1497	.8502	74.18	78.34	(105, 48, 0, 7, 8)	.1476	.8501	69.14	68.93
	.8	(49, 46, 4, 7, 4)	.1488	.8530	46.26	46.38	(61, 24, 0, 5, 6)	.1494	.8503	36.93	37.91
.65	.8	(82, 53, −2, 9, 6)	.1490	.8501	69.78	68.33	(98, 49, 1, 7, 7)	.1474	.8508	63.27	65.26
	.85	(44, 28, 0, 9, 4)	.1491	.8514	34.98	40.30	(53, 22, 0, 5, 5)	.1488	.8507	33.17	35.39
.7	.85	(73, 51, 1, 11, 5)	.1496	.8500	58.95	66.08	(92, 45, 1, 6, 7)	.1492	.8513	57.33	58.41
	.9	(40, 38, 3, 5, 4)	.1471	.8504	38.12	38.13	(44, 20, 0, 5, 4)	.1493	.8535	28.93	32.20
.75	.9	(64, 53, 3, 8, 4)	.1498	.8506	54.87	56.66	(80, 30, 0, 5, 6)	.1498	.8500	47.57	51.06
	.95	(32, 21, 0, 6, 3)	.1495	.8501	25.45	28.51	(39, 18, 0, 4, 4)	.1474	.8517	25.05	26.99
.8	.95	(52, 49, 2, 5, 4)	.1490	.8515	49.41	49.37	(54, 29, 0, 5, 4)	.1495	.8503	38.14	40.97
.85	.95	(92, 78, 3, 10, 4)	.1500	.8500	80.79	85.86	(101, 51, 0, 6, 5)	.1469	.8501	70.08	76.09

Table 7.16 Minimax and optimal two-stage designs with upper and lower early stopping values under $(\alpha^*, 1-\beta^*) = (.15, .9)$ and balanced allocation $(\gamma = 1)$

		Minimax Design					Optimal Design				
p_y	p_x	(n, n_1, a_1, b_1, a)	α	$1-\beta$	EN_0	EN_1	(n, n_1, a_1, b_1, a)	α	$1-\beta$	EN_0	EN_1
.05	.15	(76, 47, −3, 3, 3)	.1492	.9001	69.41	53.28	(82, 40, −1, 3, 3)	.1475	.9001	61.42	50.38
	.2	(50, 17, −1, 2, 3)	.1318	.9021	35.60	25.12	(50, 17, −1, 2, 3)	.1318	.9021	35.60	25.12
	.25	(50, 14, 0, 2, 2)	.1305	.9007	22.02	19.08	(50, 14, 0, 2, 2)	.1305	.9007	22.02	19.08
.1	.25	(55, 49, 0, 4, 3)	.1490	.9007	50.89	49.70	(77, 25, −1, 3, 5)	.1489	.9010	49.96	38.86
	.3	(50, 19, 0, 3, 3)	.1414	.9016	28.47	25.55	(50, 19, 0, 3, 3)	.1414	.9016	28.47	25.55
.15	.3	(72, 47, −2, 7, 4)	.1486	.9002	62.97	57.73	(88, 42, 0, 5, 5)	.1473	.9005	58.35	53.70
	.35	(50, 28, 0, 4, 4)	.1397	.9015	35.29	32.38	(54, 25, 0, 4, 4)	.1382	.9004	34.84	31.98
.2	.35	(86, 67, 0, 8, 5)	.1496	.9001	74.69	72.26	(105, 47, 0, 6, 6)	.1498	.9000	68.52	64.09
	.4	(50, 27, −4, 5, 4)	.1499	.9001	45.91	35.88	(64, 20, −1, 4, 5)	.1495	.9006	41.87	36.32
.25	.4	(97, 85, −1, 8, 6)	.1498	.9001	90.32	87.13	(114, 56, 0, 7, 7)	.1472	.9000	77.97	73.06
	.45	(57, 51, 3, 8, 4)	.1493	.9003	52.01	52.22	(69, 33, 0, 5, 6)	.1457	.9003	45.37	41.41
.3	.45	(109, 70, −3, 9, 7)	.1467	.9002	94.16	83.63	(120, 50, −2, 7, 8)	.1497	.9001	88.54	76.96
	.5	(60, 58, 3, 6, 5)	.1488	.9001	58.21	58.12	(76, 29, −1, 5, 7)	.1466	.9000	50.57	43.81
.35	.5	(113, 70, −3, 12, 7)	.1488	.9000	97.97	93.84	(140, 58, −1, 7, 10)	.1498	.9008	93.76	82.26
	.55	(64, 45, 0, 11, 5)	.1498	.9006	53.48	56.22	(75, 28, −1, 6, 6)	.1493	.9016	51.24	48.55
.4	.55	(118, 102, 4, 14, 7)	.1499	.9000	105.73	107.36	(135, 60, −1, 8, 9)	.1500	.9009	94.21	86.18
	.6	(67, 61, 4, 10, 5)	.1498	.9021	61.98	62.38	(82, 35, 0, 6, 7)	.1489	.9010	52.01	48.97
.45	.6	(121, 75, −3, 10, 8)	.1499	.9000	102.59	92.15	(145, 66, 0, 8, 10)	.1479	.9003	95.27	88.56
	.65	(67, 60, 1, 7, 6)	.1495	.9005	61.93	60.88	(77, 33, −1, 6, 7)	.1500	.9006	53.36	48.41
.5	.65	(120, 91, 0, 10, 8)	.1499	.9003	102.34	97.97	(144, 65, 0, 8, 10)	.1478	.9001	94.31	88.14
	.7	(67, 59, 3, 7, 6)	.1485	.9001	60.15	59.79	(73, 36, 0, 7, 6)	.1491	.9000	50.46	49.99
.55	.7	(115, 99, 4, 16, 7)	.1500	.9001	102.95	106.60	(141, 57, 0, 8, 9)	.1499	.9002	89.23	87.16
	.75	(64, 54, 3, 10, 5)	.1499	.9017	56.16	57.26	(77, 35, 0, 6, 7)	.1488	.9024	50.09	47.58
.6	.75	(108, 88, −2, 12, 7)	.1499	.9001	99.06	95.63	(124, 49, −1, 8, 8)	.1499	.9002	85.02	84.10
	.8	(59, 38, −1, 9, 5)	.1498	.9002	49.00	49.97	(70, 31, 0, 6, 6)	.1496	.9006	45.50	45.27
.65	.8	(103, 68, −2, 9, 7)	.1497	.9000	87.01	80.53	(133, 58, 1, 7, 9)	.1500	.9011	79.18	77.20
	.85	(55, 53, 3, 6, 5)	.1487	.9008	53.21	53.14	(71, 29, 0, 5, 7)	.1489	.9004	43.19	41.28
.7	.85	(90, 85, 3, 8, 6)	.1497	.9002	85.87	85.61	(103, 50, 0, 7, 7)	.1482	.9003	70.08	69.06
	.9	(50, 25, 0, 7, 4)	.1480	.9002	35.42	41.52	(57, 24, 0, 5, 5)	.1486	.9006	35.87	37.32
.75	.9	(76, 51, −1, 10, 5)	.1496	.9000	64.27	67.89	(91, 39, 0, 6, 6)	.1493	.9018	58.41	60.25
	.95	(50, 25, 1, 5, 4)	.1411	.9053	31.04	33.84	(52, 20, 0, 4, 5)	.1488	.9037	30.49	31.74
.8	.95	(60, 38, −1, 8, 4)	.1497	.9001	49.92	54.11	(76, 37, 1, 5, 5)	.1490	.9000	46.21	48.26
.85	.95	(112, 66, −1, 9, 5)	.1485	.9001	90.37	98.21	(129, 60, 0, 6, 6)	.1491	.9004	85.51	87.76

Table 7.17 Minimax and optimal two-stage designs with upper and lower early stopping values under $(\alpha^*, 1 - \beta^*) = (.2, .8)$ and balanced allocation $(\gamma = 1)$

		Minimax Design					Optimal Design				
P_y	P_x	(n, n_1, a_1, b_1, a)	α	$1-\beta$	EN_0	EN_1	(n, n_1, a_1, b_1, a)	α	$1-\beta$	EN_0	EN_1
.05	.15	(38, 37, 1, 3, 1)	.1982	.8024	37.12	37.13	(54, 26, 0, 2, 2)	.1941	.8003	31.81	30.13
	.2	(30, 14, 0, 2, 1)	.1579	.8019	17.56	17.21	(30, 14, 0, 2, 1)	.1579	.8019	17.56	17.21
	.25	(30, 9, 0, 2, 0)	.1824	.8148	13.36	14.19	(30, 9, 0, 2, 0)	.1824	.8148	13.36	14.19
.1	.25	(31, 8, −3, 2, 2)	.1948	.8032	28.37	21.37	(41, 13, −1, 2, 3)	.1972	.8041	26.46	21.79
	.3	(30, 12, 0, 2, 2)	.1863	.8153	15.86	14.91	(31, 11, 0, 2, 2)	.1790	.8012	15.37	14.57
.15	.3	(39, 34, 1, 6, 2)	.1998	.8036	35.37	36.02	(46, 18, −1, 3, 3)	.1993	.8017	31.31	28.40
	.35	(30, 15, 0, 3, 2)	.1840	.8102	19.50	19.12	(33, 8, −1, 2, 3)	.1970	.8061	20.60	17.26
.2	.35	(45, 41, 1, 4, 3)	.1992	.8002	41.69	41.52	(59, 29, 0, 4, 4)	.1873	.8012	38.31	37.20
	.4	(30, 17, 0, 4, 2)	.1931	.8003	21.54	21.94	(36, 16, 0, 3, 3)	.1908	.8000	21.58	20.91
.25	.4	(52, 47, 2, 7, 3)	.1993	.8005	48.08	48.47	(63, 29, −1, 4, 5)	.1986	.8001	43.17	39.82
	.45	(31, 29, 2, 5, 2)	.2000	.8089	29.28	29.36	(38, 15, −1, 3, 4)	.1959	.8000	25.11	22.65
.3	.45	(57, 52, 2, 5, 4)	.1994	.8013	52.64	52.55	(61, 33, −1, 6, 4)	.1934	.8008	46.56	46.25
	.5	(32, 26, −2, 4, 3)	.1994	.8003	29.19	27.69	(41, 18, 0, 4, 3)	.1992	.8021	25.52	25.85
.35	.5	(60, 37, −2, 7, 4)	.1996	.8004	50.49	49.42	(72, 29, −1, 5, 5)	.1999	.8016	48.24	46.92
	.55	(34, 20, −2, 5, 3)	.1980	.8002	28.73	27.31	(43, 21, 0, 4, 4)	.1928	.8018	27.76	27.32
.4	.55	(62, 41, −1, 9, 4)	.2000	.8002	51.87	54.23	(81, 36, 0, 5, 6)	.1992	.8003	50.07	49.11
	.6	(35, 19, −2, 6, 3)	.1978	.8010	29.50	29.71	(45, 20, 0, 4, 4)	.1995	.8013	27.67	27.55
.45	.6	(63, 55, 2, 9, 4)	.1993	.8003	57.12	58.07	(79, 31, −1, 5, 6)	.1995	.8010	51.42	49.67
	.65	(35, 27, 0, 6, 3)	.1987	.8002	30.04	30.37	(43, 16, −1, 4, 4)	.1990	.8032	28.52	28.09
.5	.65	(63, 49, 1, 9, 4)	.1995	.8001	53.74	55.70	(78, 31, −1, 5, 6)	.2000	.8004	50.93	49.38
	.7	(35, 21, −1, 6, 3)	.1992	.8004	28.24	29.30	(42, 16, −1, 4, 4)	.1985	.8015	28.02	27.76
.55	.7	(61, 45, 0, 9, 4)	.1999	.8014	51.76	54.02	(81, 34, 0, 5, 6)	.1991	.8003	48.82	48.83
	.75	(34, 22, −1, 6, 3)	.1966	.8010	28.15	28.94	(42, 20, 0, 4, 4)	.1996	.8014	26.69	26.85
.6	.75	(58, 39, −2, 8, 4)	.1981	.8004	50.29	50.77	(71, 26, −1, 5, 5)	.1996	.8027	46.48	47.41
	.8	(33, 19, −1, 5, 3)	.1960	.8002	25.97	26.53	(33, 19, −1, 5, 3)	.1960	.8002	25.97	26.53
.65	.8	(55, 37, −2, 6, 4)	.1995	.8001	46.95	45.32	(68, 32, 0, 5, 5)	.1920	.8010	43.84	44.74
	.85	(31, 25, 1, 4, 3)	.1978	.8008	26.07	26.12	(35, 17, 0, 4, 3)	.1970	.8039	22.85	24.15
.7	.85	(49, 30, 0, 8, 3)	.1993	.8002	38.11	43.76	(62, 23, −1, 4, 5)	.1985	.8005	39.94	39.76
	.9	(30, 19, 1, 4, 2)	.1995	.8020	21.10	22.14	(39, 14, 0, 3, 4)	.1972	.8003	20.69	21.87
.75	.9	(42, 41, 2, 4, 3)	.1998	.8019	41.08	41.08	(53, 25, 0, 4, 4)	.1919	.8006	33.66	35.02
	.95	(30, 13, 0, 3, 3)	.1862	.8021	17.81	19.43	(30, 13, 0, 3, 3)	.1862	.8021	17.81	19.43
.8	.95	(33, 12, −1, 5, 2)	.1997	.8032	24.43	30.73	(30, 16, 0, 4, 2)	.1984	.8010	24.10	29.62
.85	.95	(63, 39, −1, 5, 3)	.1983	.8003	50.71	52.36	(83, 27, 0, 4, 3)	.1997	.8008	45.71	55.08

Table 7.18 Minimax and optimal two-stage designs with upper and lower early stopping values under $(\alpha^*, 1 - \beta^*) = (.2, .85)$ and balanced allocation $(\gamma = 1)$

p_y	p_x	Minimax Design (n, n_1, a_1, b_1, a)	α	$1-\beta$	EN_0	EN_1	Optimal Design (n, n_1, a_1, b_1, a)	α	$1-\beta$	EN_0	EN_1
.05	.15	$(51, 22, -3, 2, 2)$	.1978	.8509	45.84	32.45	$(52, 22, -2, 2, 2)$	.1996	.8515	43.72	32.26
	.2	$(30, 19, 0, 2, 1)$	.1818	.8572	21.42	20.50	$(31, 18, 0, 2, 1)$	.1801	.8509	20.88	19.92
	.25	$(30, 12, 0, 2, 1)$	.1445	.8664	15.96	15.18	$(31, 11, 0, 2, 1)$	.1380	.8510	15.34	14.96
.1	.25	$(37, 25, -2, 3, 2)$	.1924	.8500	32.79	28.55	$(41, 19, -1, 3, 2)$	.1947	.8500	30.57	27.18
	.3	$(30, 10, -1, 2, 2)$	.1961	.8673	20.69	16.33	$(35, 15, 0, 2, 3)$	.1908	.8505	19.05	17.43
.15	.3	$(50, 30, -2, 4, 3)$	.1912	.8505	42.14	36.94	$(66, 20, -1, 3, 4)$	.1999	.8501	41.05	35.42
	.35	$(30, 10, -2, 3, 2)$	.1985	.8583	25.54	21.46	$(30, 10, -2, 3, 2)$	.1985	.8583	25.54	21.46
.2	.35	$(58, 43, 0, 8, 3)$	.1995	.8511	49.37	50.92	$(77, 35, 0, 4, 5)$	.1958	.8503	47.33	44.15
	.4	$(34, 32, 2, 4, 2)$	.1967	.8519	32.16	32.14	$(51, 19, 0, 3, 4)$	.1989	.8509	27.50	25.43
.25	.4	$(64, 60, 1, 5, 4)$	.1996	.8506	60.82	60.47	$(76, 37, -1, 5, 5)$	.1906	.8502	54.18	49.86
	.45	$(37, 32, 0, 4, 3)$	.1999	.8524	33.43	32.80	$(40, 14, -2, 4, 3)$	.1995	.8532	31.76	28.72
.3	.45	$(70, 50, -1, 10, 4)$	.1997	.8500	60.49	62.26	$(85, 40, -1, 5, 6)$	.1977	.8504	58.57	53.34
	.5	$(40, 23, -2, 6, 3)$	.1983	.8507	34.01	32.76	$(46, 22, -1, 4, 4)$	.1994	.8506	32.59	29.74
.35	.5	$(76, 68, 2, 6, 5)$	.1981	.8502	69.32	68.93	$(92, 38, -2, 5, 7)$	.1978	.8503	65.08	56.42
	.55	$(43, 34, 1, 7, 3)$	.1993	.8511	36.72	37.35	$(59, 24, 0, 4, 5)$	.1997	.8516	34.34	32.58
.4	.55	$(77, 74, 3, 6, 5)$	.1996	.8504	74.30	74.22	$(93, 47, 0, 6, 6)$	.1976	.8501	62.40	60.12
	.6	$(44, 38, 2, 7, 3)$	.1998	.8501	39.29	39.67	$(57, 19, -1, 4, 5)$	.1985	.8507	35.82	33.35
.45	.6	$(78, 70, 0, 7, 5)$	.1993	.8500	72.65	71.62	$(93, 40, -1, 6, 6)$	.1997	.8516	63.14	60.23
	.65	$(44, 42, 3, 6, 3)$	.1999	.8522	42.22	42.24	$(48, 24, -1, 5, 4)$	.1992	.8510	35.09	33.63
.5	.65	$(78, 52, -4, 8, 5)$	.1992	.8501	69.76	64.01	$(93, 39, -1, 6, 6)$	.1996	.8521	62.69	60.29
	.7	$(44, 37, 2, 7, 3)$	.1997	.8501	38.51	39.05	$(47, 24, -1, 5, 4)$	.1987	.8500	34.59	33.29
.55	.7	$(76, 64, -1, 7, 5)$	.1995	.8501	68.94	67.01	$(93, 44, 0, 6, 6)$	.1973	.8507	60.57	59.39
	.75	$(43, 36, 2, 6, 3)$	.1988	.8512	37.27	37.50	$(54, 19, -1, 4, 5)$	.1991	.8527	34.33	32.54
.6	.75	$(73, 65, 3, 10, 4)$	.1999	.8525	66.77	67.89	$(85, 31, -1, 6, 5)$	.1998	.8507	56.64	58.63
	.8	$(39, 28, 0, 8, 3)$	.1994	.8512	32.68	35.15	$(53, 23, 0, 4, 5)$	.1976	.8516	31.83	31.03
.65	.8	$(66, 49, 0, 9, 4)$	.1994	.8502	56.18	58.27	$(81, 36, -1, 5, 6)$	.1989	.8501	54.73	51.59
	.85	$(36, 22, -2, 6, 3)$	.1961	.8501	30.99	30.89	$(44, 22, 0, 4, 4)$	.1977	.8509	28.67	28.41
.7	.85	$(61, 41, -1, 6, 4)$	.1999	.8506	50.12	48.87	$(73, 36, 0, 5, 5)$	.1938	.8504	48.05	47.78
	.9	$(33, 29, 1, 4, 3)$	.1968	.8504	29.70	29.58	$(38, 18, 0, 4, 3)$	.1952	.8530	24.54	25.91
.75	.9	$(50, 29, -1, 8, 3)$	.1998	.8506	40.53	46.34	$(69, 29, 0, 4, 5)$	.1967	.8503	40.84	40.92
	.95	$(30, 14, 0, 4, 2)$	.1974	.8566	19.62	23.00	$(38, 13, 0, 3, 3)$	.1981	.8524	20.07	22.45
.8	.95	$(42, 29, 1, 6, 2)$	.1985	.8506	32.58	36.38	$(47, 24, 0, 4, 3)$	.1920	.8504	31.50	33.51
.85	.95	$(73, 42, -1, 7, 3)$	.1996	.8503	58.68	65.80	$(76, 46, 0, 6, 3)$	.1982	.8510	57.64	62.83

Table 7.19 Minimax and optimal two-stage designs with upper and lower early stopping values under $(\alpha^*, 1-\beta^*) = (.2, .9)$ and balanced allocation $(\gamma = 1)$

		Minimax Design					Optimal Design				
P_y	P_x	(n, n_1, a_1, b_1, a)	α	$1-\beta$	EN_0	EN_1	(n, n_1, a_1, b_1, a)	α	$1-\beta$	EN_0	EN_1
.05	.15	(65, 13, −4, 2, 2)	.1967	.9014	60.83	42.57	(70, 38, −1, 3, 2)	.1841	.9000	54.60	46.53
	.2	(50, 23, 0, 2, 2)	.1786	.9032	28.76	25.73	(54, 22, 0, 2, 2)	.1780	.9002	28.89	25.49
	.25	(50, 14, 0, 2, 1)	.1725	.9026	22.02	19.08	(50, 14, 0, 2, 1)	.1725	.9026	22.02	19.08
.1	.25	(50, 30, −1, 5, 2)	.1955	.9003	41.22	39.24	(57, 27, −1, 3, 3)	.1895	.9001	41.01	34.18
	.3	(50, 14, −1, 2, 4)	.1907	.9159	30.77	21.59	(75, 18, 0, 2, 7)	.1995	.9003	28.90	23.27
.15	.3	(61, 36, −4, 5, 3)	.1994	.9000	56.25	45.81	(73, 35, −1, 4, 4)	.1929	.9005	52.02	44.80
	.35	(50, 16, −1, 3, 3)	.1987	.9078	32.83	26.98	(52, 24, 0, 3, 4)	.1876	.9014	31.43	28.04
.2	.35	(73, 66, 0, 5, 4)	.2000	.9003	68.05	66.78	(92, 34, −2, 4, 6)	.1989	.9003	64.90	51.05
	.4	(50, 28, −1, 4, 4)	.1787	.9014	37.83	33.04	(52, 14, −2, 3, 4)	.1993	.9005	38.58	29.63
.25	.4	(83, 82, 4, 7, 4)	.1993	.9012	82.09	82.07	(107, 40, −1, 5, 6)	.1994	.9001	68.77	60.01
	.45	(50, 33, 0, 6, 3)	.2000	.9013	39.54	38.59	(54, 20, −2, 4, 4)	.1990	.9015	40.71	33.51
.3	.45	(90, 76, −1, 7, 5)	.1998	.9004	81.75	78.53	(104, 51, −1, 6, 6)	.1996	.9004	73.58	65.87
	.5	(52, 39, −3, 5, 4)	.1996	.9001	46.79	41.72	(57, 28, −1, 5, 4)	.1990	.9003	41.45	37.60
.35	.5	(95, 65, −2, 11, 5)	.1999	.9003	82.46	80.89	(118, 50, −1, 6, 7)	.1996	.9010	78.39	69.61
	.55	(54, 52, 2, 5, 4)	.1984	.9019	52.25	52.12	(63, 31, −1, 5, 5)	.1924	.9008	45.01	40.12
.4	.55	(100, 82, 2, 12, 5)	.1998	.9000	87.62	88.97	(124, 54, −1, 6, 8)	.1996	.9008	81.94	72.03
	.6	(55, 49, 0, 6, 4)	.2000	.9010	50.98	49.95	(64, 30, −1, 5, 5)	.1999	.9002	44.78	40.17
.45	.6	(101, 93, 4, 9, 5)	.2000	.9007	94.19	94.03	(122, 48, −2, 6, 8)	.1992	.9001	84.35	72.00
	.65	(55, 44, −3, 7, 4)	.1999	.9001	50.84	47.28	(69, 25, −1, 5, 5)	.1993	.9002	45.08	41.82
.5	.65	(100, 92, 4, 9, 5)	.1998	.9005	93.19	93.05	(116, 55, −1, 7, 7)	.1940	.9001	81.26	74.55
	.7	(55, 38, −1, 7, 4)	.1993	.9001	46.12	44.23	(66, 26, −1, 5, 5)	.1998	.9004	43.97	40.64
.55	.7	(97, 85, 3, 10, 5)	.1989	.9002	87.68	87.77	(121, 52, −1, 6, 8)	.1996	.9011	79.61	70.80
	.75	(53, 35, −5, 7, 4)	.1972	.9000	49.42	43.00	(61, 29, −1, 5, 5)	.1982	.9007	42.92	39.11
.6	.75	(90, 65, −2, 13, 5)	.1998	.9000	79.83	82.04	(111, 48, −1, 6, 7)	.1999	.9011	74.18	67.37
	.8	(50, 47, 1, 5, 4)	.1999	.9007	47.61	47.28	(69, 21, −1, 4, 6)	.1976	.9000	41.52	37.76
.65	.8	(85, 73, 1, 7, 5)	.1999	.9006	76.21	74.96	(102, 49, 0, 6, 6)	.1994	.9002	66.81	63.66
	.85	(50, 26, −1, 5, 4)	.1948	.9019	37.11	35.06	(58, 21, −1, 4, 5)	.1990	.9025	37.13	34.13
.7	.85	(75, 52, 0, 11, 4)	.1998	.9009	62.24	68.11	(93, 37, −1, 5, 6)	.1999	.9010	60.75	56.02
	.9	(50, 23, 0, 4, 4)	.1979	.9024	31.28	30.56	(51, 22, 0, 4, 4)	.1957	.9004	31.00	30.72
.75	.9	(64, 59, 3, 7, 3)	.1996	.9000	59.72	59.94	(87, 28, −1, 4, 6)	.1992	.9008	52.91	49.13
	.95	(50, 23, 1, 4, 3)	.1853	.9045	28.09	29.33	(54, 17, 0, 3, 5)	.1963	.9015	26.67	26.73
.8	.95	(51, 24, −2, 5, 3)	.1999	.9010	41.71	41.72	(64, 29, 0, 4, 4)	.1926	.9022	39.86	40.07
.85	.95	(93, 86, 3, 7, 3)	.1993	.9009	87.01	87.43	(112, 48, 0, 5, 4)	.1998	.9002	70.06	73.59

Table 7.20 Minimax and optimal two-stage designs for binomial test with a futility and a superiority stopping values for strict control of $(\alpha^*, 1 - \beta^*)$ over $p_0 \in [0, 1]$ and balanced allocation $(\gamma = 1)$

α^*	$1-\beta^*$	Δ	Minimax Design					Optimal Design				
			(n, n_1, a_1, b_1, a)	α	$1-\beta$	EN_0	EN_1	(n, n_1, a_1, b_1, a)	α	$1-\beta$	EN_0	EN_1
.1	.8	.15	(101, 98, 5, 10, 9)	.0997	.8025	98.39	98.40	(116, 54, 1, 9, 10)	.1000	.8002	74.86	80.61
		.2	(57, 48, 4, 12, 6)	.0999	.8006	49.50	52.57	(63, 27, 0, 7, 7)	.0996	.8015	41.75	46.04
	.85	.15	(122, 86, −1, 12, 10)	.0980	.8500	103.74	100.16	(143, 68, 2, 10, 11)	.0991	.8501	89.21	94.91
		.2	(67, 41, −1, 10, 7)	.0992	.8500	54.75	56.25	(84, 36, 1, 7, 9)	.0991	.8500	50.43	52.52
	.9	.15	(148, 103, −1, 13, 11)	.0997	.9000	125.01	117.63	(167, 79, 1, 11, 12)	.0999	.9012	110.62	111.04
		.2	(82, 65, 0, 10, 8)	.1000	.9003	72.14	69.27	(94, 40, 0, 8, 9)	.0997	.9015	62.22	61.99
.15	.8	.15	(78, 54, −2, 11, 6)	.1495	.8001	68.27	69.53	(94, 39, 0, 7, 7)	.1499	.8005	60.25	63.54
		.2	(45, 39, 3, 8, 4)	.1500	.8013	40.01	40.86	(55, 24, 0, 5, 6)	.1484	.8002	34.83	35.08
	.85	.15	(96, 85, 1, 9, 7)	.1496	.8507	88.46	87.35	(104, 53, 0, 9, 7)	.1496	.8501	74.10	76.91
		.2	(54, 36, −1, 8, 5)	.1479	.8506	45.23	44.87	(62, 31, 0, 6, 6)	.1462	.8503	42.53	41.97
	.9	.15	(121, 101, 1, 10, 8)	.1499	.9010	107.55	104.68	(145, 66, 0, 8, 10)	.1494	.9000	95.37	88.56
		.2	(68, 63, 3, 7, 6)	.1497	.9024	63.72	63.42	(79, 31, −1, 6, 7)	.1498	.9005	53.79	49.36
.2	.8	.15	(63, 59, 3, 8, 4)	.1997	.8003	59.70	59.96	(80, 30, −1, 5, 6)	.1997	.8003	51.60	50.05
		.2	(35, 20, −2, 7, 3)	.1998	.8000	30.03	31.25	(44, 15, −1, 4, 4)	.1981	.8013	28.87	28.68
	.85	.15	(78, 77, 4, 6, 5)	.1993	.8501	77.05	77.04	(95, 38, −1, 6, 6)	.1997	.8509	63.39	61.00
		.2	(45, 38, 0, 5, 4)	.1999	.8513	40.15	39.29	(52, 26, 0, 5, 4)	.1998	.8507	34.91	34.46
	.9	.15	(101, 98, 5, 9, 5)	.1982	.9003	98.31	98.28	(117, 56, −1, 7, 7)	.1957	.9001	82.30	75.01
		.2	(56, 37, −2, 8, 4)	.1987	.9002	48.43	46.27	(75, 33, 0, 5, 6)	.1934	.9003	46.49	42.79

7.2.1   Strict Control of Type I Error Rate and Power

The designs reported in Tables 7.11–7.19 are valid only when the response rate of the control arm, p_y, is accurately controlled. Now we consider a strict control of type I error rate and power to maintain type I error rate and power at the specified level regardless of the true p_y value. To this end, we control the type I error rate at $p_x = p_y = 0.5$ and calculate the power at $(p_x, p_y) = (0.5 - \Delta/2, 0.5 + \Delta/2)$ for given $H_1 : p_x - p_y = \Delta$. Table 7.20 lists minimax and optimal two-stage designs with both upper and lower stopping values under various design settings of $(\alpha^*, 1 - \beta^*, \Delta)$ when type I error rate and power are strictly controlled.

7.3   Discussions

While the number of randomized phase II trials is rapidly growing (Lee and Feng, 2005), we largely lack efficient design and analysis methods for them. This chapter proposes optimal and minimax designs for two-stage randomized phase II trials using two-sample binomial test. Given a design setting, the maximal sample size for the minimax two-stage design is usually smaller than or equal to the sample size for the single-stage design as in single-arm trial designs (Simon, 1989). The ratio of stage 1 sample size to the maximal size, n_1/n, for the minimax design is usually large, so that its operating characteristics and the maximal sample size are similar to those of the single-stage design. However, the ratio for the optimal design is usually small so that we can terminate the trial early and minimize the expected sample size when the experimental arm is inefficacious.

We have considered minimax and optimality criteria in this chapter. But often these two criteria conflict with each other, so that the minimax design may have an excessively large expected sample size under H_0 compared to the optimal design, and the optimal design may have an excessively large maximal sample size compared to the minimax design. In order to address this issue, we may combine these two criteria to derive a compromise design; refer to Jung, Carey, and Kim (2001) and Jung et al. (2004) for the single-arm design case. We have focused on two-stage designs, but the methods can be easily extended to designs with any number of stages.

A randomized phase II trial may look similar to a phase III trial in the sense that both include a prospective control and carry out statistical tests to compare between the control and an experimental arm. However, we do not want a phase II trial to be more than an efficacy screening study, while a phase III trial is to finalize scientific questions on an experimental regimen. As a result, we want phase II trials to be as simple as possible. In order to keep the sample size small and the study period short for a randomized phase II trial, we use a relatively large one-sided α, such as 15% or 20% (rather than the conventional two-sided $\alpha = 5\%$ level), and a moderate power, such as 80% or 85% (rather than 90%), and a short-term outcome variable as the primary endpoint, such as tumor response or time to progression (rather than overall survival). As shown in Tables 7.11–7.19 and 7.20, in most cases, the sample sizes for 10% α or 90% power are too big for a phase II trial.

It is claimed that a two-arm randomized phase II trial requires about four times the sample size of a single-arm phase II trial. This can be easily proved for single-stage trials by using normal approximation to binomial distributions. For a single-arm phase II trial with m patients, we will reject $H_0 : p_x = p_0$ (or accept the experimental therapy x) if

$$\frac{\hat{p}_x - p_0}{\sqrt{p_0(1 - p_0)/m}} > z_{1-\alpha},$$

where $z_{1-\alpha}$ denotes the $100(1 - \alpha)$ percentile of the standard normal distribution. Using the standard procedure for sample size calculation, it is easy to show that, for power $1 - \beta$ with respect to $H_1 : p_x = p_0 + \Delta$ using one-sided α, the required sample size is

$$m = \frac{p_0(1 - p_0)(z_{1-\alpha} + z_{1-\beta})^2}{\Delta^2}.$$

For a randomized trial with n patients per arm, we will reject $H_0 : p_x = p_y(= p_0)$ (or accept the experimental arm x) if

$$\frac{\hat{p}_x - \hat{p}_y}{\sqrt{2p_0(1 - p_0)/n}} > z_{1-\alpha}.$$

Similarly, we can show that, for power $1 - \beta$ with respect to $H_1 : p_x - p_y = \Delta$ using one-sided α, the required sample size per arm per arm is

$$n = \frac{2p_0(1 - p_0)(z_{1-\alpha} + z_{1-\beta})^2}{\Delta^2}.$$

So, the total sample size N for a randomized trial is

$$N = 2n = \frac{4p_0(1 - p_0)(z_{1-\alpha} + z_{1-\beta})^2}{\Delta^2} = 4m.$$

We also observe this by comparing the design tables in Chapter 2 and this chapter, for example, Table 2.4 and Table 7.3, especially for the designs with response rates around 50% for which the normal approximation holds well. The sample size of a typical single-arm phase II trial is about 50. So, if we want to design a two-arm randomized phase II trial with a total sample size of about 100, then we will have to increase α and lower the power. Otherwise, the required sample size for a randomized phase II trial will be around 200, which is too large for a phase II trial.

References

Cannistra, S.A. (2009). Phase II trials in *Journal of Clinical Oncology*. *Journal of Clinical Oncology*, 27 (19), 3073–3076.

Fisher, R.A. (1935). The logic of inductive inference (with discussion). *Journal of Royal Statistical Society*, 98, 39–82.

Gan, H.K., Grothey, A., Pond, G.P., Moore, M.J., Siu, L.L., and Sargent, D.J. (2010). Randomized phase II trials: Inevitable or inadvisable? *Journal of Clinical Oncology*, 28 (15), 2641–2647.

Jung, S.H. (2008). Randomized phase II trials with a prospective control. *Statistics in Medicine*, 27, 568–583.

Jung S.H., Carey, M., and Kim, K.M. (2001). Graphical search for two-stage designs for phase II clinical trials. *Control Clinical Trials*, 22, 367–372.

Jung, S.H., Lee, T.Y., Kim, K.M., and George, S. (2004). Admissible two-stage designs for phase II cancer clinical trials. *Statistics in Medicine*, 23, 561–569.

Lee, J.J. and Feng, L. (2005). Randomized phase II designs in cancer clinical trials: Current status and future directions. *Journal of Clinical Oncology*, 23 (19), 4450–4457.

Rubinstein, L.V., Korn, E.L., Freidlin, B., Hunsberger, S., Ivy, S.P., and Smith, M.A. (2005). Design issues of randomized phase II trials and a proposal for phase II screening trials. *Journal of Clinical Oncology*, 23 (28), 7199–7206.

Simon, R. (1989). Optimal two-stage designs for phase II clinical trials. *Controlled Clinical Trials*, 10, 1–10.

Steinberg, S.M. and Venzon, D.J. (2002). Early selection in a randomized phase II clinical trial. *Statistics in Medicine*, 21, 1711–1726.

Thall, P.F., Simon, R., and Ellenberg, S.S. (1989). A two-stage design for choosing among several experimental treatments and a control in clinical trials. *Biometrics*, 45, 537–547.

Chapter 8

Randomized Phase II Cancer Clinical Trials with a Prospective Control on Binary Endpoints (II): Fisher's Exact Test

In Chapter 7, we have considered randomized phase II trials for comparing the efficacy of an experimental therapy (arm x) with that of a prospective control (arm y) in terms of a binary endpoint, such as tumor response, using a two-sample binomial test. Let p_x and p_y denote the true response rates for arms x and y, respectively. We want to test whether the experimental arm has a higher response rate than the control or not, that is, $H_0 : p_x \leq p_y$ against $H_a : p_x > p_y$. The null distribution of the binomial test that was discussed in Chapter 7 depends on the common response probability $p_x = p_y (= p_0)$. Consequently, if the true response probabilities are different from the specified ones, the testing based on binomial distributions may not maintain the type I error rate close to the specified value. In order to avoid this issue, we have considered controlling the type I error rate over the whole range of $p_x = p_y$ values, that is, $[0, 1]$. This conservative control of the type I error rate is equivalent to controlling the type I error rate at $p_x = p_y = 1/2$. This results in an overly strong conservativeness when the true response probability is very different from 50%.

An alternative approach to avoiding specification of the nuisance parameter p_0 is to condition the null distribution of the two-sample binomial test on a sufficient statistic of p_0. This results in Fisher's (1935) exact test, which is derived by conditioning on the total number of responders from two arms. In this chapter, we investigate single-stage and two-stage randomized phase II trial designs using Fisher's exact test. Using some example designs, we show that Fisher's exact test accurately controls the type I error rate over a wide range of p_0 values, and is more powerful than the binomial test of Chapter 7 if the true response rates p_x and p_y are different from 50%. If we can project the true response rates accurately at the design stage, we can identify efficient designs by adopting Simon's (1989) optimal and minimax design concepts that were proposed for single-arm phase II trials.

8.1   Single-Stage Design

As was stated in the previous chapter, if patient accrual is fast or it takes long (say, longer than 6 months) for response assessment of each patient, we may consider using a single-stage design. Suppose that n patients are randomized to each arm, and let X and Y denote the number of responders in arms x (experimental) and y (control), respectively. Let $q_k = 1 - p_k$ for arm $k(= \text{x}, \text{y})$. Then the frequencies (and response probabilities in the parentheses) can be summarized as in Table 8.1.

At the design stage, n is determined. Fisher's exact test is based on the conditional distribution of X given the total number of responders $Z = X + Y$ with a probability mass function

$$f(x|z, \theta) = \frac{\binom{n}{x}\binom{n}{z-x}\theta^x}{\sum_{i=m_-}^{m_+} \binom{n}{i}\binom{n}{z-i}\theta^i}$$

for $m_- \leq x \leq m_+$, where $m_- = \max(0, z - n)$, $m_+ = \min(z, n)$, and $\theta = p_\text{x}q_\text{y}/(p_\text{y}q_\text{x})$ denotes the odds ratio. It is easy to show that $\sum_{i=m_-}^{m_+} \binom{n}{i}\binom{n}{z-i} = \binom{2n}{z}$.

Suppose that we want to control the type I error rate below α^*. Then, given $X + Y = z$, we reject $H_0 : p_\text{x} = p_\text{y} = p_0$ (that is, $\theta = 1$) in favor of $H_a : p_\text{x} > p_\text{y}$ (that is, $\theta > 1$) if $X - Y \geq a$, where a is the smallest integer satisfying

$$\alpha(z) \equiv \text{P}(X - Y \geq a|z, H_0) = \text{P}(2X \geq z + a|z, H_0) = \sum_{x=\langle(z+a)/2\rangle}^{m_+} f(x|z, \theta = 1) \leq \alpha^*,$$

where $\langle c \rangle$ is the round-up integer of c. Hence, the critical value a depends on the total number of responders z. However, the conditional type I error rate $\alpha(z)$ does not depend of the common response rate $p_\text{x} = p_\text{y}$ under H_0. Under $H_a : \theta = \theta_a(> 1)$, the conditional power on $X + Y = z$ is given by

$$1 - \beta(z) \equiv \text{P}(X - Y \geq a|z, H_a) = \sum_{x=\langle(z+a)/2\rangle}^{m_+} f(x|z, \theta_a).$$

Table 8.1   Frequencies (and response probabilities in the parentheses) of a single-stage randomized phase II trial

		Arm x	Arm y	Total
Response	Yes	$x\ (p_\text{x})$	$y\ (p_\text{y})$	z
	No	$n - x\ (q_\text{x})$	$n - y\ (q_\text{y})$	$2n - z$
Total		n	n	

We propose to choose n so that the marginal power is no smaller than a specified power level $1 - \beta^*$, that is,

$$E\{1 - \beta(Z)\} = \sum_{z=0}^{2n} \{1 - \beta(z)\} g(z) \geq 1 - \beta^*$$

where $g(z)$ is the probability mass function of $Z = X + Y$ under $H_a : p_x > p_y$ which is given by

$$g(z) = \sum_{x=m_-}^{m_+} \binom{n}{x} p_x^x q_x^{n-x} \binom{n}{z-x} p_y^{z-x} q_y^{n-z+x}$$

for $z = 0, 1, \ldots, 2n$. Since the conditional type I error rate is controlled below α^* for any z value, the marginal type I error rate

$$E\{\alpha(Z)\} = \sum_{z=0}^{2n} \alpha(z) g_0(z)$$

is controlled below α^* too. Here, $g_0(z)$ is the probability mass function $g(z)$ under $H_0 : p_x = p_y = p_0$, that is,

$$g_0(z) = p_0^z q_0^{2n-z} \sum_{x=m_-}^{m_+} \binom{n}{x} \binom{n}{z-x}.$$

Given the type I error rate α^*, power $1 - \beta^*$ and a specific alternative hypothesis $H_a : (p_x, p_y)$, we find a sample size n as follows.

8.1.1 Algorithm for Single-Stage Design

1. For $n = 1, 2, \ldots$,

   a. For $z = 0, 1, \ldots, 2n$, find the smallest integer $a = a(z)$ such that

   $$\alpha(z) = P(X - Y \geq a | z, \theta = 1) \leq \alpha^*$$

   and calculate the conditional power for the chosen $a = a(z)$

   $$1 - \beta(z) = P(X - Y \geq a | z, \theta_a).$$

   b. Calculate the marginal power $1 - \beta = E\{1 - \beta(Z)\}$.

2. Find the smallest integer n such that $1 - \beta \geq 1 - \beta^*$.

Fisher's test which is based on the conditional distribution of X given $Z = X + Y$, is valid under $\theta = 1$ (that is, controls the type I error rate exactly), and its conditional power depends only on the odds ratio θ_a under H_a. However, the marginal power, and hence the sample size n, depends on (p_x, p_y), so that we need to specify (p_x, p_y) at the design stage. If (p_x, p_y) are misspecified, the trial may be over- or underpowered, but the type I error rate in data analysis will always be appropriately controlled. Tables 8.2 to 8.10 list single-stage designs under various design settings.

8.2 Two-Stage Design

For ethical and economical reasons, clinical trials are often conducted using multiple stages. Phase II trials usually enter a small number of patients, so that practically the number of stages is two at the most.

Suppose that $n_l(l = 1, 2)$ patients are randomized to each arm during stage $l(= 1, 2)$. Let $n_1 + n_2 = n$ denote the maximal sample size for each arm, and let X_l and Y_l denote the number of responders during stage l in arms x and y, respectively ($X = X_1 + X_2$ and $Y = Y_1 + Y_2$).

We choose n_l at the design stage. Note that X_1 and X_2 are independent, and, given $X_l + Y_l = z_l$, X_l has the conditional probability mass function

$$f_l(x_l | z_l, \theta) = \frac{\binom{n_l}{x_l}\binom{n_l}{z_l - x_l}\theta^{x_l}}{\sum_{i=m_{l-}}^{m_{l+}} \binom{n_l}{i}\binom{n_l}{z_l - i}\theta^i}$$

for $m_{l-} \le x_l \le m_{l+}$, where $m_{l-} = \max(0, z_l - n_l)$ and $m_{l+} = \min(z_l, n_l)$.

8.2.1 Two-Stage Designs with a Futility Interim Test Only

At first, we consider designs with the same features as popular two-stage phase II trial designs with an early stopping rule when the experimental therapy has a low efficacy, that is, an interim futility test. The rejection values (a_1, a) are chosen conditional on z_1 and z_2 as follows:

Stage 1: Randomize n_1 patients to each arm, and observe $X_1 = x_1$ and $Y_1 = y_1$.

    a. Given $z_1(= x_1 + y_1)$, find a stopping value $a_1 = a_1(z_1)$.

    b. If $x_1 - y_1 \ge a_1$, proceed to stage 2. Otherwise, stop the trial.

Stage 2: Randomize n_2 patients to each arm, and observe x_2 and y_2 ($z_2 = x_2 + y_2$).

    a. Given (z_1, z_2), find a rejection value $a = a(z_1, z_2)$.

    b. Accept the experimental arm if $x - y \ge a$, where $x = x_1 + x_2$ and $y = y_1 + y_2$.

Now, we discuss how to choose the rejection values (a_1, a) conditioning on (z_1, z_2).

Table 8.2 Single-stage designs, and minimax and optimal two-stage designs for Fisher's exact test with $(\alpha^*, 1-\beta^*) = (.1, .8)$

p_y	p_x	θ	Single-Stage Design			Minimax Two-Stage Design				Optimal Two-Stage Design			
			n	α	$1-\beta$	(n,n_1)	α	$1-\beta$	EN	(n,n_1)	α	$1-\beta$	EN
.05	.15	3.353	95	.0500	.8021	(95, 49)	.0507	.8002	76.35	(99, 28)	.0538	.8003	72.58
	.2	4.750	54	.0318	.8033	(52, 23)	.0337	.8008	41.65	(53, 19)	.0354	.8008	41.44
	.25	6.333	50	.0299	.9261	(45, 1)	.0274	.8716	42.91	(45, 13)	.0312	.8861	35.39
.1	.25	3.000	68	.0563	.8022	(68, 30)	.0587	.8002	52.30	(70, 22)	.0615	.8001	50.90
	.3	3.857	50	.0564	.8545	(45, 11)	.0543	.8028	33.04	(45, 11)	.0543	.8028	33.04
.15	.3	2.429	81	.0670	.8020	(80, 79)	.0668	.8006	79.54	(85, 24)	.0709	.8005	59.45
	.35	3.051	50	.0636	.8026	(50, 26)	.0612	.8004	39.87	(52, 16)	.0623	.8020	37.59
.2	.35	2.154	91	.0709	.8021	(91, 46)	.0733	.8000	70.84	(96, 29)	.0749	.8004	66.89
	.4	2.667	57	.0679	.8071	(56, 28)	.0669	.8001	43.87	(58, 17)	.0683	.8009	41.01
.25	.4	2.000	100	.0768	.8025	(100, 60)	.0764	.8001	81.68	(107, 31)	.0780	.8004	73.44
	.45	2.455	59	.0701	.8033	(59, 34)	.0696	.8005	47.89	(64, 16)	.0720	.8010	43.90
.3	.45	1.909	106	.0777	.8014	(104, 52)	.0759	.8004	80.22	(111, 34)	.0780	.8007	76.56
	.5	2.333	61	.0700	.8023	(60, 34)	.0693	.8003	48.37	(64, 20)	.0713	.8007	45.02
.35	.5	1.857	111	.0769	.8013	(111, 73)	.0768	.8000	93.31	(120, 34)	.0813	.8000	81.35
	.55	2.270	66	.0704	.8001	(66, 46)	.0718	.8000	56.87	(69, 18)	.0770	.8004	47.04
.4	.55	1.833	112	.0762	.8033	(112, 67)	.0757	.8001	91.08	(122, 34)	.0788	.8000	82.33
	.6	2.250	67	.0683	.8066	(67, 34)	.0698	.8007	52.12	(69, 19)	.0767	.8003	47.28
.45	.6	1.833	112	.0792	.8033	(112, 67)	.0782	.8001	91.06	(122, 34)	.0791	.8000	82.26
	.65	2.270	66	.0685	.8001	(66, 46)	.0685	.8000	56.83	(69, 18)	.0769	.8004	46.89
.5	.65	1.857	111	.0793	.8013	(111, 73)	.0788	.8000	93.25	(120, 34)	.0785	.8000	81.15
	.7	2.333	61	.0654	.8023	(60, 34)	.0816	.8003	48.25	(64, 20)	.0756	.8007	44.76
.55	.7	1.909	106	.0737	.8014	(104, 52)	.0774	.8004	80.04	(111, 34)	.0810	.8007	76.23
	.75	2.455	59	.0825	.8033	(59, 34)	.0814	.8005	47.71	(64, 16)	.0804	.8010	43.38
.6	.75	2.000	100	.0830	.8025	(100, 60)	.0836	.8001	81.48	(109, 28)	.0828	.8001	72.89
	.8	2.667	57	.0757	.8071	(56, 28)	.0723	.8001	43.52	(58, 17)	.0717	.8009	40.34
.65	.8	2.154	91	.0723	.8021	(91, 46)	.0743	.8000	70.46	(98, 26)	.0783	.8005	66.16
	.85	3.051	50	.0649	.8026	(50, 26)	.0678	.8004	39.39	(54, 12)	.0728	.8016	36.56
.7	.85	2.429	81	.0734	.8020	(80, 79)	.0734	.8006	79.53	(85, 24)	.0751	.8005	58.32
	.9	3.857	50	.0685	.8545	(45, 11)	.0666	.8028	31.13	(45, 11)	.0666	.8028	31.13
.75	.9	3.000	68	.0712	.8022	(68, 30)	.0710	.8002	51.26	(72, 18)	.0724	.8010	49.14
	.95	6.333	50	.0671	.9261	(45, 1)	.0637	.8716	36.75	(45, 7)	.0676	.8683	30.66
.8	.95	4.750	54	.0659	.8033	(52, 23)	.0648	.8008	39.63	(54, 13)	.0664	.8005	37.52
.85	.95	3.353	95	.0707	.8021	(95, 49)	.0704	.8002	74.60	(101, 24)	.0724	.8005	68.74

Table 8.3 Single-stage designs, and minimax and optimal two-stage designs for Fisher's exact test with $(\alpha^*, 1-\beta^*) = (.1, .85)$

			Single-Stage Design			Minimax Two-Stage Design				Optimal Two-Stage Design			
p_y	p_x	θ	n	α	$1-\beta$	(n,n_1)	α	$1-\beta$	EN	(n,n_1)	α	$1-\beta$	EN
.05	.15	3.353	110	.0544	.8508	(110, 53)	.0549	.8504	86.67	(114, 36)	.0570	.8502	83.69
	.2	4.750	62	.0363	.8547	(60, 28)	.0376	.8502	48.09	(61, 21)	.0396	.8505	47.03
	.25	6.333	40	.0226	.8574	(39, 23)	.0251	.8501	33.29	(40, 13)	.0261	.8505	31.90
.1	.25	3.000	79	.0606	.8507	(79, 37)	.0613	.8501	61.28	(82, 25)	.0633	.8506	58.94
	.3	3.857	50	.0564	.8545	(50, 23)	.0549	.8508	39.19	(51, 17)	.0568	.8512	37.97
.15	.3	2.429	95	.0707	.8534	(94, 65)	.0705	.8501	80.92	(100, 30)	.0715	.8507	70.07
	.35	3.051	58	.0648	.8551	(58, 25)	.0650	.8503	44.12	(60, 19)	.0657	.8512	43.24
.2	.35	2.154	107	.0736	.8520	(107, 62)	.0748	.8500	86.52	(114, 35)	.0760	.8505	79.21
	.4	2.667	64	.0672	.8524	(64, 34)	.0685	.8502	50.82	(68, 20)	.0709	.8509	47.79
.25	.4	2.000	118	.0776	.8526	(117, 64)	.0768	.8503	92.66	(124, 39)	.0782	.8503	85.93
	.45	2.455	71	.0728	.8531	(71, 31)	.0724	.8503	53.34	(74, 22)	.0730	.8506	51.60
.3	.45	1.909	122	.0768	.8518	(122, 78)	.0770	.8501	101.53	(132, 41)	.0799	.8500	90.87
	.5	2.333	73	.0696	.8537	(73, 41)	.0728	.8505	58.54	(78, 23)	.0756	.8501	54.02
.35	.5	1.857	132	.0815	.8527	(128, 60)	.0813	.8502	96.59	(137, 44)	.0830	.8501	94.64
	.55	2.270	74	.0720	.8559	(74, 39)	.0719	.8504	58.15	(79, 24)	.0740	.8509	54.81
.4	.55	1.833	133	.0761	.8530	(133, 80)	.0769	.8502	108.20	(145, 42)	.0821	.8501	98.06
	.6	2.250	74	.0768	.8546	(74, 41)	.0756	.8504	58.98	(80, 23)	.0772	.8504	54.90
.45	.6	1.833	133	.0781	.8529	(133, 80)	.0773	.8502	108.18	(145, 42)	.0797	.8501	97.99
	.65	2.270	74	.0800	.8559	(74, 39)	.0783	.8504	58.08	(79, 24)	.0792	.8509	54.67
.5	.65	1.857	132	.0784	.8527	(128, 60)	.0821	.8502	96.47	(137, 44)	.0834	.8501	94.44
	.7	2.333	73	.0796	.8537	(73, 41)	.0784	.8505	58.41	(78, 23)	.0786	.8501	53.72
.55	.7	1.909	122	.0859	.8518	(122, 78)	.0874	.8501	101.41	(132, 41)	.0855	.8500	90.52
	.75	2.455	71	.0757	.8531	(71, 31)	.0728	.8503	53.03	(74, 22)	.0734	.8506	51.13
.6	.75	2.000	118	.0814	.8526	(117, 64)	.0790	.8503	92.40	(124, 39)	.0793	.8503	85.41
	.8	2.667	64	.0679	.8524	(64, 34)	.0729	.8502	50.48	(68, 20)	.0767	.8509	47.07
.65	.8	2.154	107	.0786	.8520	(107, 62)	.0810	.8500	86.19	(116, 32)	.0818	.8501	78.38
	.85	3.051	58	.0724	.8551	(58, 25)	.0705	.8503	43.44	(60, 19)	.0714	.8512	42.27
.7	.85	2.429	95	.0732	.8534	(94, 65)	.0753	.8501	80.61	(100, 30)	.0785	.8507	68.92
	.9	3.857	50	.0685	.8545	(50, 23)	.0720	.8508	38.23	(53, 13)	.0724	.8507	36.40
.75	.9	3.000	79	.0739	.8507	(79, 37)	.0740	.8501	60.25	(82, 25)	.0757	.8506	57.21
	.95	6.333	40	.0647	.8574	(39, 23)	.0641	.8501	32.08	(41, 10)	.0660	.8529	28.68
.8	.95	4.750	62	.0661	.8547	(60, 28)	.0686	.8502	46.13	(62, 17)	.0689	.8502	43.35
.85	.95	3.353	110	.0700	.8508	(110, 53)	.0731	.8504	84.60	(116, 32)	.0743	.8501	79.89

Table 8.4 Single-stage designs, and minimax and optimal two-stage designs for Fisher's exact test with $(\alpha^*, 1-\beta^*) = (.1, .9)$

			Single-Stage Design			Minimax Two-Stage Design				Optimal Two-Stage Design			
p_y	p_x	θ	n	α	$1-\beta$	(n,n_1)	α	$1-\beta$	EN	(n,n_1)	α	$1-\beta$	EN
.05	.15	3.353	130	.0596	.9005	(130, 72)	.0595	.9000	105.49	(135, 46)	.0611	.9002	99.20
	.2	4.750	72	.0412	.9036	(71, 43)	.0412	.9002	59.84	(73, 24)	.0450	.9001	55.34
	.25	6.333	60	.0352	.9549	(55, 1)	.0335	.9114	52.44	(55, 14)	.0373	.9279	42.35
.1	.25	3.000	93	.0650	.9007	(93, 54)	.0649	.9001	76.01	(98, 32)	.0665	.9002	70.55
	.3	3.857	60	.0525	.9037	(59, 27)	.0569	.9013	45.93	(61, 20)	.0587	.9002	44.90
.15	.3	2.429	112	.0705	.9001	(112, 64)	.0726	.9001	90.37	(118, 40)	.0745	.9003	83.89
	.35	3.051	69	.0643	.9029	(69, 35)	.0656	.9002	54.28	(74, 21)	.0682	.9002	52.10
.2	.35	2.154	128	.0754	.9012	(128, 66)	.0692	.9000	99.69	(135, 46)	.0779	.9001	95.13
	.4	2.667	77	.0689	.9002	(77, 54)	.0692	.9002	66.60	(82, 26)	.0724	.9009	57.88
.25	.4	2.000	140	.0768	.9015	(139, 76)	.0782	.9002	109.85	(146, 53)	.0794	.9001	103.66
	.45	2.455	81	.0709	.9009	(81, 50)	.0720	.9000	66.93	(88, 27)	.0752	.9001	61.32
.3	.45	1.909	147	.0789	.9007	(147, 102)	.0793	.9000	125.87	(160, 52)	.0820	.9000	110.60
	.5	2.333	89	.0769	.9029	(89, 48)	.0776	.9002	70.32	(95, 29)	.0788	.9001	65.76
.35	.5	1.857	158	.0835	.9016	(153, 78)	.0818	.9000	118.01	(163, 59)	.0838	.9002	115.00
	.55	2.270	90	.0736	.9027	(90, 52)	.0743	.9001	72.56	(98, 29)	.0771	.9003	67.28
.4	.55	1.833	159	.0783	.9011	(159, 106)	.0786	.9001	133.98	(172, 57)	.0827	.9001	118.88
	.6	2.250	90	.0744	.9015	(90, 56)	.0739	.9000	74.31	(97, 31)	.0761	.9002	67.40
.45	.6	1.833	159	.0794	.9010	(159, 106)	.0790	.9001	133.96	(172, 57)	.0806	.9001	118.81
	.65	2.270	90	.0772	.9027	(90, 52)	.0762	.9001	72.49	(98, 29)	.0781	.9003	67.12
.5	.65	1.857	158	.0798	.9016	(153, 78)	.0834	.9001	117.89	(163, 59)	.0847	.9002	114.81
	.7	2.333	89	.0771	.9029	(89, 48)	.0756	.9002	70.17	(95, 29)	.0765	.9001	65.44
.55	.7	1.909	147	.0888	.9007	(147, 102)	.0883	.9001	125.76	(160, 52)	.0863	.9000	110.24
	.75	2.455	81	.0697	.9009	(81, 50)	.0719	.9000	66.74	(88, 27)	.0792	.9001	60.81
.6	.75	2.000	140	.0803	.9015	(139, 76)	.0784	.9002	109.58	(146, 53)	.0795	.9001	103.17
	.8	2.667	77	.0809	.9002	(77, 54)	.0807	.9002	66.40	(82, 26)	.0803	.9009	57.15
.65	.8	2.154	128	.0827	.9012	(128, 66)	.0820	.9000	99.25	(135, 46)	.0826	.9001	94.37
	.85	3.051	69	.0686	.9029	(69, 35)	.0721	.9002	53.69	(74, 21)	.0751	.9002	50.90
.7	.85	2.429	112	.0788	.9001	(112, 64)	.0798	.9001	89.84	(118, 40)	.0805	.9003	82.79
	.9	3.857	60	.0687	.9037	(59, 27)	.0687	.9013	44.89	(61, 20)	.0703	.9002	43.31
.75	.9	3.000	93	.0748	.9007	(93, 54)	.0750	.9001	75.23	(98, 32)	.0763	.9002	68.80
	.95	6.333	60	.0656	.9549	(55, 1)	.0709	.9114	44.88	(55, 7)	.0702	.9061	36.89
.8	.95	4.750	72	.0707	.9036	(71, 43)	.0700	.9002	58.51	(76, 18)	.0712	.9002	51.83
.85	.95	3.353	130	.0742	.9005	(130, 72)	.0740	.9000	103.70	(136, 44)	.0755	.9002	95.49

Table 8.5 Single-stage designs, and minimax and optimal two-stage designs for Fisher's exact test with $(\alpha^*, 1-\beta^*) = (.15, .8)$

Py	Px	θ	Single-Stage Design			Minimax Two-Stage Design				Optimal Two-Stage Design			
			n	α	$1-\beta$	(n,n_1)	α	$1-\beta$	EN	(n,n_1)	α	$1-\beta$	EN
.05	.15	3.353	79	.0827	.8005	(78, 40)	.0823	.8001	63.00	(81, 26)	.0836	.8008	60.83
	.2	4.750	45	.0631	.8075	(44, 17)	.0620	.8033	35.11	(44, 17)	.0620	.8033	35.11
	.25	6.333	29	.0450	.8109	(29, 11)	.0448	.8014	23.96	(29, 11)	.0448	.8014	23.96
.1	.25	3.000	56	.0884	.8033	(56, 25)	.0896	.8003	43.46	(58, 19)	.0925	.8016	42.80
	.3	3.857	36	.0747	.8016	(36, 16)	.0783	.8009	28.41	(37, 12)	.0800	.8024	28.03
.15	.3	2.429	65	.1036	.8023	(65, 36)	.1036	.8004	52.42	(69, 22)	.1060	.8009	49.48
	.35	3.051	41	.0879	.8025	(41, 19)	.0919	.8010	32.01	(42, 14)	.0925	.8016	30.99
.2	.35	2.154	74	.1076	.8054	(74, 42)	.1097	.8001	59.74	(79, 26)	.1133	.8003	56.17
	.4	2.667	46	.0953	.8074	(46, 23)	.1016	.8007	36.19	(49, 14)	.1061	.8019	34.81
.25	.4	2.000	83	.1149	.8022	(81, 37)	.1147	.8005	61.35	(84, 30)	.1155	.8006	60.21
	.45	2.455	47	.0986	.8056	(47, 27)	.1007	.8005	38.25	(50, 17)	.1053	.8003	36.10
.3	.45	1.909	85	.1112	.8005	(85, 65)	.1115	.8000	75.76	(95, 27)	.1210	.8004	65.02
	.5	2.333	53	.1121	.8015	(49, 26)	.1100	.8007	38.88	(52, 19)	.1113	.8014	37.82
.35	.5	1.857	86	.1155	.8006	(86, 66)	.1153	.8000	76.73	(95, 32)	.1186	.8002	66.78
	.55	2.270	54	.1009	.8026	(54, 21)	.1169	.8016	39.62	(55, 19)	.1168	.8012	39.43
.4	.55	1.833	87	.1228	.8032	(87, 59)	.1216	.8004	74.05	(94, 35)	.1205	.8000	67.36
	.6	2.250	54	.1015	.8013	(54, 22)	.1150	.8017	39.95	(56, 18)	.1147	.8006	39.56
.45	.6	1.833	87	.1265	.8032	(87, 59)	.1252	.8004	74.03	(94, 35)	.1234	.8000	67.32
	.65	2.270	54	.1043	.8026	(54, 21)	.1151	.8016	39.53	(55, 19)	.1148	.8012	39.33
.5	.65	1.857	86	.1263	.8006	(86, 66)	.1260	.8000	76.69	(95, 32)	.1235	.8002	66.63
	.7	2.333	53	.1033	.8015	(49, 26)	.1147	.8007	38.77	(52, 19)	.1126	.8014	37.62
.55	.7	1.909	85	.1237	.8005	(85, 65)	.1234	.8000	75.70	(96, 26)	.1203	.8010	64.87
	.75	2.455	47	.1114	.8056	(47, 27)	.1240	.8005	38.09	(50, 17)	.1221	.8003	35.75
.6	.75	2.000	83	.1173	.8022	(81, 37)	.1134	.8005	61.08	(84, 30)	.1193	.8006	59.83
	.8	2.667	46	.1208	.8074	(46, 23)	.1163	.8007	35.87	(50, 12)	.1145	.8011	34.13
.65	.8	2.154	74	.1150	.8054	(74, 42)	.1214	.8001	59.46	(81, 23)	.1213	.8006	55.56
	.85	3.051	41	.1020	.8025	(41, 19)	.1004	.8010	31.48	(43, 12)	.1060	.8024	30.12
.7	.85	2.429	65	.1088	.8023	(65, 36)	.1083	.8004	51.98	(69, 22)	.1139	.8009	48.57
	.9	3.857	36	.1023	.8016	(36, 16)	.1068	.8009	27.53	(38, 9)	.1075	.8004	26.45
.75	.9	3.000	56	.1098	.8033	(56, 25)	.1099	.8003	42.52	(59, 17)	.1110	.8016	41.30
	.95	6.333	29	.0929	.8109	(29, 11)	.0919	.8014	21.76	(30, 7)	.0949	.8022	21.32
.8	.95	4.750	45	.0948	.8075	(44, 17)	.1036	.8033	32.81	(46, 11)	.1041	.8007	32.23
.85	.95	3.353	79	.1065	.8005	(78, 40)	.1071	.8001	61.38	(83, 22)	.1098	.8011	57.67

Table 8.6 Single-stage designs, and minimax and optimal two-stage designs for Fisher's exact test with $(\alpha^*, 1 - \beta^*) = (.15, .85)$

			Single-Stage Design			Minimax Two-Stage Design				Optimal Two-Stage Design			
py	px	θ	n	α	1−β	(n,n1)	α	1−β	EN	(n,n1)	α	1−β	EN
.05	.15	3.353	92	.0868	.8502	(92, 48)	.0870	.8500	74.20	(94, 35)	.0881	.8502	71.17
	.2	4.750	51	.0677	.8526	(51, 24)	.0676	.8506	41.27	(52, 18)	.0678	.8505	40.61
	.25	6.333	35	.0531	.8581	(34, 11)	.0516	.8506	27.56	(34, 11)	.0516	.8506	27.56
.1	.25	3.000	65	.0952	.8529	(65, 37)	.0950	.8502	53.18	(68, 24)	.0963	.8501	50.29
	.3	3.857	41	.0785	.8515	(41, 21)	.0823	.8500	33.09	(42, 16)	.0847	.8502	32.14
.15	.3	2.429	78	.1058	.8521	(78, 48)	.1067	.8502	64.71	(82, 29)	.1091	.8506	59.40
	.35	3.051	49	.0948	.8541	(49, 23)	.0976	.8506	38.15	(51, 17)	.1004	.8527	37.28
.2	.35	2.154	88	.1113	.8518	(88, 43)	.1120	.8502	67.92	(93, 32)	.1147	.8500	66.49
	.4	2.667	52	.0990	.8506	(52, 29)	.0992	.8506	42.01	(56, 18)	.1062	.8506	40.16
.25	.4	2.000	94	.1132	.8511	(94, 68)	.1133	.8502	82.03	(102, 37)	.1203	.8503	72.98
	.45	2.455	59	.1067	.8535	(59, 30)	.1122	.8503	46.22	(62, 19)	.1129	.8506	43.71
.3	.45	1.909	104	.1210	.8504	(100, 55)	.1200	.8501	79.37	(107, 39)	.1209	.8503	76.34
	.5	2.333	60	.1034	.8524	(60, 39)	.1062	.8501	50.53	(65, 22)	.1138	.8510	46.31
.35	.5	1.857	106	.1148	.8508	(106, 79)	.1148	.8501	93.40	(114, 39)	.1252	.8503	80.04
	.55	2.270	61	.1089	.8551	(61, 37)	.1082	.8507	50.16	(65, 24)	.1112	.8504	46.96
.4	.55	1.833	107	.1178	.8520	(107, 74)	.1170	.8500	91.60	(115, 45)	.1205	.8500	83.00
	.6	2.250	61	.1147	.8538	(61, 38)	.1132	.8500	50.57	(66, 23)	.1138	.8502	47.07
.45	.6	1.833	107	.1214	.8520	(107, 74)	.1203	.8500	91.59	(115, 45)	.1196	.8500	82.95
	.65	2.270	61	.1184	.8551	(61, 37)	.1163	.8507	50.11	(65, 24)	.1156	.8504	46.86
.5	.65	1.857	106	.1215	.8508	(106, 79)	.1210	.8501	93.36	(114, 39)	.1240	.8503	79.88
	.7	2.333	60	.1176	.8524	(60, 39)	.1163	.8501	50.45	(65, 22)	.1151	.8510	45.07
.55	.7	1.909	104	.1180	.8504	(100, 55)	.1159	.8501	79.22	(107, 39)	.1234	.8503	76.08
	.75	2.455	59	.1145	.8535	(59, 30)	.1104	.8503	46.00	(62, 19)	.1114	.8506	43.28
.6	.75	2.000	94	.1205	.8511	(94, 68)	.1256	.8502	81.91	(102, 37)	.1277	.8503	72.57
	.8	2.667	52	.0999	.8506	(52, 29)	.1071	.8506	41.72	(56, 18)	.1147	.8506	39.56
.65	.8	2.154	88	.1180	.8518	(88, 43)	.1146	.8502	67.52	(93, 32)	.1178	.8500	65.68
	.85	3.051	49	.1158	.8541	(49, 23)	.1160	.8506	37.60	(52, 15)	.1155	.8519	36.31
.7	.85	2.429	78	.1141	.8521	(78, 48)	.1190	.8502	64.33	(84, 26)	.1201	.8503	58.49
	.9	3.857	41	.0980	.8515	(41, 21)	.1000	.8500	32.34	(43, 14)	.1050	.8514	30.87
.75	.9	3.000	65	.1082	.8529	(65, 37)	.1102	.8502	52.50	(69, 22)	.1150	.8500	48.76
	.95	6.333	35	.1019	.8581	(34, 11)	.0997	.8506	24.75	(35, 7)	.1016	.8505	24.43
.8	.95	4.750	51	.0983	.8526	(51, 24)	.1021	.8506	39.45	(53, 15)	.1073	.8518	37.47
.85	.95	3.353	92	.1065	.8502	(92, 48)	.1101	.8500	72.52	(98, 27)	.1140	.8503	67.92

Table 8.7 Single-stage designs, and minimax and optimal two-stage designs for Fisher's exact test with $(\alpha^*, 1 - \beta^*) = (.15, .9)$

			Single-Stage Design			Minimax Two-Stage Design				Optimal Two-Stage Design			
p_y	p_x	θ	n	α	$1-\beta$	(n, n_1)	α	$1-\beta$	EN	(n, n_1)	α	$1-\beta$	EN
.05	.15	3.353	110	.0915	.9020	(110, 60)	.0919	.9002	89.25	(115, 42)	.0936	.9005	85.99
	.2	4.750	60	.0737	.9033	(60, 30)	.0735	.9001	48.69	(62, 23)	.0743	.9009	48.08
	.25	6.333	50	.0670	.9512	(45, 1)	.0627	.9019	42.91	(45, 13)	.0623	.9174	35.39
.1	.25	3.000	78	.0946	.9014	(78, 46)	.0988	.9000	64.23	(83, 29)	.1026	.9004	60.77
	.3	3.857	50	.0843	.9006	(50, 25)	.0855	.9007	39.89	(52, 17)	.0887	.9001	38.59
.15	.3	2.429	93	.1067	.9004	(93, 58)	.1082	.9001	77.32	(100, 36)	.1129	.9004	72.23
	.35	3.051	57	.1001	.9019	(57, 34)	.1000	.9002	47.06	(61, 21)	.1026	.9000	44.47
.2	.35	2.154	105	.1142	.9007	(105, 74)	.1143	.9001	90.77	(112, 45)	.1187	.9000	82.02
	.4	2.667	65	.1096	.9014	(65, 41)	.1094	.9000	54.32	(68, 26)	.1112	.9001	49.91
.25	.4	2.000	117	.1214	.9005	(117, 88)	.1212	.9000	103.51	(126, 47)	.1234	.9000	90.25
	.45	2.455	68	.1047	.9034	(68, 42)	.1079	.9004	56.31	(74, 26)	.1131	.9005	53.06
.3	.45	1.909	121	.1179	.9020	(121, 82)	.1179	.9002	102.82	(132, 51)	.1221	.9003	94.99
	.5	2.333	75	.1171	.9002	(72, 38)	.1152	.9003	56.69	(75, 31)	.1160	.9005	55.43
.35	.5	1.857	131	.1227	.9002	(130, 67)	.1279	.9001	100.77	(134, 58)	.1277	.9000	98.95
	.55	2.270	77	.1109	.9037	(77, 46)	.1151	.9001	62.85	(79, 31)	.1217	.9006	57.54
.4	.55	1.833	132	.1169	.9001	(132, 107)	.1171	.9000	120.19	(142, 53)	.1275	.9001	101.01
	.6	2.250	77	.1095	.9026	(77, 49)	.1093	.9000	64.15	(81, 29)	.1204	.9001	57.77
.45	.6	1.833	132	.1199	.9001	(132, 108)	.1198	.9000	120.65	(142, 53)	.1275	.9001	100.96
	.65	2.270	77	.1122	.9037	(77, 46)	.1103	.9001	62.79	(79, 31)	.1211	.9006	57.43
.5	.65	1.857	131	.1202	.9002	(130, 67)	.1261	.9001	100.67	(134, 58)	.1258	.9000	98.81
	.7	2.333	75	.1103	.9002	(72, 38)	.1186	.9003	56.55	(75, 31)	.1185	.9005	55.22
.55	.7	1.909	121	.1191	.9020	(121, 82)	.1315	.9002	102.72	(132, 51)	.1325	.9003	94.71
	.75	2.455	68	.1120	.9034	(68, 42)	.1268	.9004	56.13	(74, 26)	.1255	.9005	52.66
.6	.75	2.000	117	.1283	.9005	(117, 88)	.1278	.9000	103.39	(126, 47)	.1243	.9000	89.81
	.8	2.667	65	.1222	.9014	(65, 41)	.1204	.9000	54.08	(68, 26)	.1176	.9001	49.36
.65	.8	2.154	105	.1144	.9007	(105, 74)	.1156	.9001	90.56	(115, 41)	.1247	.9000	81.41
	.85	3.051	57	.1040	.9019	(57, 34)	.1048	.9002	46.66	(61, 21)	.1136	.9000	43.57
.7	.85	2.429	93	.1158	.9004	(93, 58)	.1150	.9001	76.91	(100, 36)	.1182	.9004	71.28
	.9	3.857	50	.1124	.9006	(50, 25)	.1111	.9007	39.03	(52, 17)	.1104	.9001	37.10
.75	.9	3.000	78	.1139	.9014	(78, 46)	.1135	.9000	63.54	(83, 29)	.1149	.9004	59.26
	.95	6.333	50	.1036	.9512	(45, 1)	.0977	.9019	36.75	(45, 8)	.1068	.9004	30.74
.8	.95	4.750	60	.1055	.9033	(60, 30)	.1058	.9001	46.93	(64, 19)	.1080	.9010	45.15
.85	.95	3.353	110	.1126	.9020	(110, 60)	.1121	.9002	87.55	(116, 40)	.1151	.9002	82.76

Table 8.8 Single-stage designs, and minimax and optimal two-stage designs for Fisher's exact test with $(\alpha^*, 1 - \beta^*) = (.2, .8)$

			Single-Stage Design			Minimax Two-Stage Design				Optimal Two-Stage Design			
p_y	p_x	θ	n	α	$1-\beta$	(n,n_1)	α	$1-\beta$	EN	(n,n_1)	α	$1-\beta$	EN
.05	.15	3.353	65	.1078	.8031	(65,36)	.1121	.8005	53.73	(68,24)	.1152	.8004	52.14
	.2	4.750	38	.0799	.8040	(38,15)	.0813	.8007	30.73	(38,15)	.0813	.8007	30.73
	.25	6.333	26	.0509	.8050	(25,10)	.0481	.8005	20.98	(25,10)	.0481	.8005	20.98
.1	.25	3.000	48	.1200	.8043	(47,19)	.1222	.8002	36.08	(47,19)	.1222	.8002	36.08
	.3	3.857	30	.0991	.8012	(30,19)	.1022	.8005	25.71	(31,13)	.1066	.8024	24.43
.15	.3	2.429	54	.1343	.8005	(54,40)	.1349	.8003	47.88	(60,18)	.1445	.8015	42.94
	.35	3.051	35	.1220	.8057	(34,15)	.1209	.8022	26.46	(35,13)	.1221	.8020	26.44
.2	.35	2.154	63	.1512	.8003	(62,29)	.1491	.8011	47.66	(65,23)	.1507	.8002	47.09
	.4	2.667	39	.1264	.8005	(39,26)	.1342	.8005	33.40	(40,14)	.1408	.8001	29.46
.25	.4	2.000	67	.1424	.8028	(67,47)	.1467	.8001	54.95	(73,24)	.1582	.8003	51.75
	.45	2.455	41	.1295	.8101	(40,35)	.1292	.8000	37.78	(45,12)	.1477	.8001	31.59
.3	.45	1.909	68	.1518	.8006	(68,55)	.1517	.8001	62.04	(75,30)	.1570	.8003	55.02
	.5	2.333	41	.1392	.8034	(41,28)	.1389	.8002	35.25	(45,16)	.1445	.8003	32.72
.35	.5	1.857	69	.1631	.8012	(69,54)	.1625	.8001	62.10	(76,32)	.1602	.8010	56.29
	.55	2.270	42	.1515	.8092	(42,25)	.1479	.8004	34.50	(46,16)	.1491	.8003	33.20
.4	.55	1.833	70	.1713	.8043	(70,50)	.1692	.8005	60.81	(77,32)	.1656	.8010	56.78
	.6	2.250	42	.1581	.8079	(42,26)	.1545	.8007	34.90	(45,18)	.1528	.8007	33.32
.45	.6	1.833	70	.1751	.8043	(70,50)	.1727	.8005	60.80	(77,32)	.1685	.8010	56.75
	.65	2.270	42	.1618	.8092	(42,25)	.1572	.8004	34.46	(46,16)	.1549	.8003	33.11
.5	.65	1.857	69	.1746	.8012	(69,54)	.1737	.8001	62.07	(76,32)	.1686	.8010	56.19
	.7	2.333	41	.1601	.8034	(41,28)	.1581	.8002	35.19	(45,16)	.1542	.8003	32.53
.55	.7	1.909	68	.1716	.8006	(68,55)	.1711	.8001	62.00	(77,28)	.1651	.8022	55.11
	.75	2.455	41	.1589	.8101	(41,23)	.1559	.8000	37.74	(45,12)	.1505	.8001	31.17
.6	.75	2.000	67	.1660	.8028	(67,47)	.1638	.8001	57.84	(73,24)	.1601	.8003	51.37
	.8	2.667	39	.1491	.8005	(39,26)	.1472	.8005	33.23	(40,14)	.1430	.8001	28.98
.65	.8	2.154	63	.1522	.8003	(62,29)	.1531	.8011	47.31	(65,23)	.1599	.8002	46.58
	.85	3.051	35	.1311	.8057	(34,15)	.1425	.8022	25.94	(36,11)	.1458	.8003	25.71
.7	.85	2.429	54	.1466	.8005	(54,40)	.1518	.8003	47.68	(60,18)	.1590	.8015	42.03
	.9	3.857	30	.1386	.8012	(30,19)	.1427	.8005	25.27	(33,7)	.1428	.8008	22.99
.75	.9	3.000	48	.1446	.8043	(47,19)	.1427	.8002	35.09	(48,17)	.1458	.8009	35.09
	.95	6.333	26	.1305	.8050	(25,10)	.1249	.8005	19.04	(26,6)	.1267	.8007	18.65
.8	.95	4.750	38	.1392	.8040	(38,15)	.1406	.8007	28.60	(40,9)	.1419	.8017	28.16
.85	.95	3.353	65	.1411	.8031	(65,36)	.1410	.8005	52.42	(70,20)	.1483	.8010	49.45

Table 8.9 Single-stage designs, and minimax and optimal two-stage designs for Fisher's exact test with $(\alpha^*, 1 - \beta^*) = (.2, .85)$

			Single-Stage Design			Minimax Two-Stage Design				Optimal Two-Stage Design			
Py	px	θ	n	α	1 − β	(n,n₁)	α	1 − β	EN	(n,n₁)	α	1 − β	EN
.05	.15	3.353	81	.1148	.8535	(78, 37)	.1197	.8503	62.00	(81, 29)	.1214	.8501	61.52
	.2	4.750	44	.0897	.8459	(44, 19)	.0924	.8504	35.50	(44, 19)	.0924	.8504	35.50
	.25	6.333	30	.0618	.8542	(30, 11)	.0621	.8519	24.68	(30, 11)	.0621	.8519	24.68
.1	.25	3.000	56	.1292	.8511	(56, 36)	.1301	.8501	47.58	(59, 21)	.1321	.8503	43.97
	.3	3.857	35	.1046	.8545	(35, 19)	.1097	.8521	28.76	(37, 12)	.1132	.8502	28.03
.15	.3	2.429	65	.1411	.8523	(65, 35)	.1411	.8506	52.01	(69, 26)	.1453	.8508	50.85
	.35	3.051	43	.1294	.8577	(42, 19)	.1344	.8508	32.60	(43, 16)	.1345	.8511	32.19
.2	.35	2.154	74	.1469	.8528	(74, 51)	.1497	.8502	63.64	(80, 30)	.1575	.8507	58.22
	.4	2.667	45	.1298	.8559	(45, 27)	.1349	.8501	37.22	(48, 18)	.1443	.8505	35.50
.25	.4	2.000	80	.1575	.8515	(78, 50)	.1530	.8500	65.29	(84, 36)	.1567	.8515	62.60
	.45	2.455	46	.1402	.8514	(46, 32)	.1398	.8501	39.81	(50, 20)	.1453	.8508	37.18
.3	.45	1.909	87	.1531	.8506	(87, 68)	.1561	.8501	78.21	(92, 36)	.1670	.8503	66.87
	.5	2.333	53	.1468	.8501	(50, 29)	.1568	.8510	40.70	(52, 21)	.1547	.8500	38.57
.35	.5	1.857	89	.1541	.8533	(89, 63)	.1537	.8502	76.97	(93, 40)	.1660	.8501	68.97
	.55	2.270	54	.1392	.8523	(53, 27)	.1589	.8503	41.47	(55, 23)	.1599	.8506	40.96
.4	.55	1.833	89	.1600	.8508	(89, 71)	.1595	.8501	80.61	(96, 39)	.1686	.8516	70.12
	.6	2.250	54	.1405	.8510	(53, 28)	.1569	.8501	41.85	(57, 21)	.1563	.8502	41.25
.45	.6	1.833	89	.1637	.8508	(89, 71)	.1632	.8501	80.60	(96, 39)	.1713	.8516	70.08
	.65	2.270	54	.1437	.8523	(53, 27)	.1564	.8503	41.41	(55, 23)	.1559	.8506	40.88
.5	.65	1.857	89	.1649	.8533	(89, 63)	.1627	.8502	76.92	(92, 50)	.1604	.8502	72.67
	.7	2.333	53	.1426	.8501	(50, 29)	.1548	.8510	40.60	(52, 21)	.1559	.8500	38.40
.55	.7	1.909	87	.1610	.8506	(87, 68)	.1603	.8501	78.15	(92, 36)	.1664	.8503	66.64
	.75	2.455	46	.1437	.8514	(46, 32)	.1616	.8501	39.70	(50, 20)	.1659	.8508	36.89
.6	.75	2.000	80	.1485	.8515	(78, 50)	.1621	.8500	65.14	(85, 34)	.1692	.8502	62.01
	.8	2.667	45	.1664	.8559	(45, 27)	.1615	.8501	36.99	(48, 18)	.1576	.8505	35.02
.65	.8	2.154	74	.1672	.8528	(74, 51)	.1679	.8502	63.45	(82, 27)	.1627	.8501	57.62
	.85	3.051	43	.1544	.8577	(42, 19)	.1439	.8508	32.05	(44, 14)	.1473	.8505	31.35
.7	.85	2.429	65	.1480	.8523	(65, 35)	.1503	.8506	51.56	(69, 26)	.1591	.8508	50.09
	.9	3.857	35	.1286	.8545	(35, 19)	.1362	.8521	28.13	(37, 12)	.1461	.8502	26.71
.75	.9	3.000	56	.1536	.8511	(56, 36)	.1545	.8501	47.08	(59, 21)	.1538	.8503	42.70
	.95	6.333	30	.1408	.8542	(30, 11)	.1373	.8519	22.36	(31, 7)	.1386	.8503	21.94
.8	.95	4.750	44	.1290	.8549	(44, 19)	.1429	.8504	33.53	(46, 14)	.1451	.8520	33.02
.85	.95	3.353	81	.1506	.8535	(78, 37)	.1496	.8503	60.17	(83, 26)	.1516	.8506	58.94

Table 8.10 Single-stage designs, and minimax and optimal two-stage designs for Fisher's exact test with $(\alpha^*, 1-\beta^*) = (.2, .9)$

			Single-Stage Design			Minimax Two-Stage Design				Optimal Two-Stage Design			
p_y	p_x	θ	n	α	$1-\beta$	(n,n_1)	α	$1-\beta$	EN	(n,n_1)	α	$1-\beta$	EN
.05	.15	3.353	96	.1209	.9006	(96, 55)	.1223	.9001	79.15	(101, 37)	.1262	.9000	76.02
	.2	4.750	52	.0987	.9037	(52, 26)	.1026	.9005	42.47	(53, 22)	.1040	.9001	42.05
	.25	6.333	50	.0968	.9698	(45, 1)	.0918	.9252	42.91	(45, 13)	.0934	.9379	35.39
.1	.25	3.000	67	.1370	.9004	(67, 43)	.1379	.9000	56.73	(71, 29)	.1397	.9001	53.71
	.3	3.857	50	.1225	.9299	(45, 17)	.1202	.9026	34.27	(45, 17)	.1202	.9026	34.27
.15	.3	2.429	81	.1506	.9012	(81, 58)	.1506	.9001	70.70	(87, 34)	.1541	.9003	64.10
	.35	3.051	50	.1330	.9045	(50, 30)	.1359	.9007	41.45	(54, 19)	.1432	.9001	39.69
.2	.35	2.154	93	.1555	.9014	(90, 56)	.1530	.9002	74.60	(96, 41)	.1567	.9002	71.53
	.4	2.667	56	.1446	.9022	(54, 33)	.1406	.9002	44.79	(58, 23)	.1456	.9004	43.08
.25	.4	2.000	99	.1522	.9002	(99, 82)	.1546	.9000	91.11	(110, 42)	.1668	.9000	79.41
	.45	2.455	61	.1471	.9032	(61, 39)	.1525	.9003	51.15	(64, 25)	.1579	.9004	47.04
.3	.45	1.909	102	.1604	.9008	(102, 81)	.1600	.9001	92.22	(110, 53)	.1621	.9000	83.91
	.5	2.333	62	.1440	.9013	(62, 46)	.1443	.9002	54.72	(68, 27)	.1581	.9002	49.92
.35	.5	1.857	113	.1630	.9007	(108, 63)	.1692	.9001	87.17	(113, 54)	.1684	.9000	85.87
	.55	2.270	63	.1522	.9023	(63, 45)	.1510	.9002	54.79	(68, 30)	.1541	.9003	51.04
.4	.55	1.833	114	.1560	.9008	(111, 60)	.1754	.9002	87.39	(115, 54)	.1747	.9002	86.88
	.6	2.250	63	.1586	.9011	(63, 48)	.1578	.9001	56.12	(68, 31)	.1561	.9007	51.41
.45	.6	1.833	114	.1590	.9008	(111, 60)	.1786	.9002	87.36	(115, 54)	.1777	.9002	86.85
	.65	2.270	63	.1623	.9023	(63, 45)	.1606	.9002	54.76	(68, 30)	.1580	.9003	50.96
.5	.65	1.857	113	.1592	.9007	(108, 63)	.1791	.9001	87.10	(113, 54)	.1775	.9000	85.76
	.7	2.333	62	.1616	.9013	(62, 46)	.1605	.9002	54.66	(68, 27)	.1566	.9002	49.72
.55	.7	1.909	102	.1710	.9008	(102, 81)	.1785	.9001	92.16	(114, 48)	.1735	.9001	83.69
	.75	2.455	61	.1584	.9032	(61, 39)	.1550	.9003	51.00	(64, 25)	.1548	.9004	46.70
.6	.75	2.000	99	.1728	.9002	(99, 82)	.1725	.9000	91.04	(110, 42)	.1659	.9000	79.01
	.8	2.667	56	.1446	.9022	(54, 33)	.1432	.9002	44.55	(58, 23)	.1573	.9004	42.59
.65	.8	2.154	93	.1589	.9014	(90, 56)	.1551	.9002	74.34	(96, 41)	.1663	.9002	71.03
	.85	3.051	50	.1445	.9045	(50, 30)	.1597	.9007	41.08	(54, 19)	.1608	.9001	38.86
.7	.85	2.429	81	.1591	.9012	(81, 58)	.1649	.9001	70.43	(87, 34)	.1638	.9003	63.29
	.9	3.857	50	.1537	.9299	(45, 17)	.1444	.9026	33.08	(46, 15)	.1474	.9008	32.95
.75	.9	3.000	67	.1424	.9004	(67, 43)	.1492	.9000	56.19	(71, 29)	.1576	.9001	52.54
	.95	6.333	50	.1484	.9698	(45, 1)	.1422	.9252	36.75	(45, 7)	.1439	.9172	30.66
.8	.95	4.750	52	.1385	.9037	(52, 26)	.1406	.9005	40.80	(55, 18)	.1466	.9003	39.58
.85	.95	3.353	96	.1465	.9006	(96, 55)	.1527	.9001	77.69	(101, 37)	.1577	.9000	73.17

8.2.1.1   Choice of a_1 and a

For now, we assume that n_1 and n_2 are given. We may consider different options of choosing a_1. For example,

- We may wish to stop the trial early if the experimental arm is worse than the control. In this case, we choose $a_1 = 0$. Note that this a_1 is constant with respect to z_1.

- We may choose a_1 so that the conditional probability of early termination given z_1 is no smaller than a prespecified level $\psi_0 (= 0.6 \text{ to } 0.8)$ under $H_0 : \theta = 1$, that is,

$$\text{PET}_0(z_1) = \text{P}(X_1 - Y_1 < a|z_1, H_0) = \sum_{x_1=m_{1-}}^{[(a_1+z_1)/2]-1} f_1(x_1|z_1, \theta = 1) \geq \psi_0,$$

  where $[c]$ denotes the largest integer not exceeding c.

- We may choose a_1 so that the conditional probability of early termination given z_1 is no larger than a prespecified level $\psi_1 (= 0.02 \text{ to } 0.1)$ under $H_a : \theta = \theta_a$, that is,

$$\text{PET}_1(z_1) = \text{P}(X_1 - Y_1 < a|z_1, H_a) = \sum_{x_1=m_{1-}}^{[(a_1+z_1)/2]-1} f_1(x_1|z_1, \theta_a) \leq \psi_1.$$

Most standard optimal two-stage phase II trials stop early when the observed response probability from stage 1 is no larger than the specified response probability under H_0; refer to Chapter 2 (Simon, 1989; Jung et al., 2004) for single-arm trial cases and Tables 7.1 to 7.9 for randomized trial cases based on binomial distributions. Based on this, we propose to use $a_1 = 0$ among the above three options. This option simplifies the computations for study design too.

With a_1 fixed at 0, we choose the second-stage rejection value a conditioning on (z_1, z_2). Given type I error rate α^*, $a = a(z_1, z_2)$ is chosen as the smallest integer satisfying

$$\alpha(z_1, z_2) \equiv \text{P}(X_1 - Y_1 \geq a_1, X - Y \geq a|z_1, z_2, \theta = 1) \leq \alpha^*.$$

We calculate $\alpha(z_1, z_2)$ by

$$\text{P}(X_1 \geq (a_1 + z_1)/2, X_1 + X_2 \geq (a + z_1 + z_2)/2|z_1, z_2, \theta = 1)$$
$$= \sum_{x_1=m_{1-}}^{m_{1+}} \sum_{x_2=m_{2-}}^{m_{2+}} I\{x_1 \geq (a_1 + z_1)/2, x_1 + x_2 \geq (a + z_1 + z_2)/2\}$$
$$\times f_1(x_1|z_1, 1) f_2(x_2|z_2, 1),$$

where $I(\cdot)$ is the indicator function.

Given z_1 and z_2, the conditional power under $H_a : \theta = \theta_a$ is obtained by

$$
\begin{aligned}
1 - \beta(z_1, z_2) &= P(X_1 - Y_1 \geq a_1, X - Y \geq a | z_1, z_2, \theta_a) \\
&= \sum_{x_1=m_{1-}}^{m_{1+}} \sum_{x_2=m_{2-}}^{m_{2+}} I\{x_1 \geq (a_1 + z_1)/2, x_1 + x_2 \geq (a + z_1 + z_2)/2\} \\
&\quad \times f_1(x_1 | z_1, \theta_a) f_2(x_2 | z_2, \theta_a).
\end{aligned}
$$

Note that, as in the single-stage case, the calculation of type I error rate $\alpha(z_1, z_2)$ and rejection values (a_1, a) does not require specification of the common response probability $p_x = p_y$ under H_0, and that the conditional power $1 - \beta(z_1, z_2)$ requires specification of the odds ratio θ_a under H_a, but not the response probabilities for the two arms, p_x and p_y.

8.2.1.2   Choice of n_1 and n_2

Now we discuss how to choose sample sizes n_1 and n_2 at the design stage based on some optimality criteria.

Given (α^*, β^*), we propose to choose n_1 and n_2 so that the marginal power is maintained above $1 - \beta^*$ while controlling the conditional type I error rates for any (z_1, z_2) below α^* as in the choice of (a_1, a). For stage $l(= 1, 2)$, the marginal distribution of $Z_l = X_l + Y_l$ has a probability mass function

$$
g_l(z_l) = \sum_{x_l=m_{l-}}^{m_{l+}} \binom{n_l}{x_l} p_x^{x_l} q_x^{n_l - x_l} \binom{n_l}{z_l - x_l} p_y^{z_l - x_l} q_y^{n_l - z_l + x_l}
$$

for $z_l = 0, \dots, 2n_l$. Under $H_0 : p_x = p_y = p_0$, this is expressed as

$$
g_{0l}(z_l) = p_0^{z_l} q_0^{2n_l - z_l} \sum_{x_l=m_{l-}}^{m_{l+}} \binom{n_l}{x_l} \binom{n_l}{z_l - x_l}.
$$

Furthermore, Z_1 and Z_2 are independent. Hence, we choose n_1 and n_2 so that the marginal power is no smaller than a specified level $1 - \beta^*$, that is,

$$
1 - \beta \equiv \sum_{z_1=0}^{2n_1} \sum_{z_2=0}^{2n_2} \{1 - \beta(z_1, z_2)\} g_1(z_1) g_2(z_2) \geq 1 - \beta^*.
$$

The marginal type I error rate for a chosen two-stage design is calculated by

$$
\alpha \equiv \sum_{z_1=0}^{2n_1} \sum_{z_2=0}^{2n_2} \alpha(z_1, z_2) g_{01}(z_1) g_{02}(z_2).
$$

Since the conditional type I error rate is controlled below α^* for any (z_1, z_2), the marginal type I error rate does not exceed α^*.

Although we do not have to specify any response rates for testing, we need to do so when choosing (n_1, n_2) at the design stage. If the specified response rates are different from the true ones, then the marginal power may be different from the expected one for the chosen sample sizes. But even in this case, the two-stage Fisher's test is still valid in the sense that it always controls both the conditional and marginal type I error rates below the specified level. Let $\mathrm{PET}_0 \equiv E\{\mathrm{PET}_0(Z_1)|H_0\} = \sum_{z_1=0}^{2n_1} \mathrm{PET}_0(z_1)g_{01}(z_1)$ denote the marginal probability of early termination under H_0. Then, among those (n_1, n_2) satisfying the $(\alpha^*, 1 - \beta^*)$-condition, the Simon-type (1989) minimax and the optimal designs can be chosen as follows:

- *Minimax design* has the smallest maximal sample size $n(= n_1 + n_2)$.
- *Optimal design* has the smallest marginal expected sample size EN under H_0, where

$$\mathrm{EN} = n_1 \times \mathrm{PET}_0 + n \times (1 - \mathrm{PET}_0).$$

Tables 8.2 to 8.10 report the sample sizes (n, n_1) of the minimax and optimal two-stage designs for $\alpha^* = 0.1, 0.15$, or 0.2, $1 - \beta^* = 0.8, 0.85$, or 0.9, and various combinations of (p_x, p_y) under H_a. For comparison, we also list the sample size n of the single-stage design under each setting. Note that the maximal sample size of the two-stage minimax is slightly smaller than or equal to the sample size of the single-stage design. If experimental therapy is inefficacious, however, the expected sample sizes of two-stage minimax and optimal designs are much smaller than the sample size of the single-stage design.

One of the popular approaches for randomized phase II trials is to use the asymptotic method. Given $(\alpha^*, p_y, n_1, n_2)$, we find c satisfying

$$\alpha = P\left(X_1 - Y_1 \geq 0, \frac{X - Y}{\sqrt{2n\hat{p}\hat{q}}} \geq c \,\middle|\, p_x = p_y\right)$$

using the normal approximation to binomial distributions, where $\hat{p} = (X + Y)/2n$ and $\hat{q} = 1 - \hat{p}$. For an approximate critical value c, the exact type I error rate is calculated by using the true binomial distribution. For a specified $p_x(\neq p_y)$, the exact power is calculated similarly. From Table 8.5, the minimax design under $(\alpha^*, 1 - \beta^*, p_x, p_y) = (0.15, 0.8, 0.5, 0.35)$ has $(n, n_1) = (86, 66)$, for which the asymptotic method has $\alpha = 0.157$ and $1 - \beta = 0.840$. Since the sample size is relatively large in this case, the asymptotic method controls the power close to the nominal $\alpha^* = 0.15$.

Now, we consider the minimax design $(n, n_1) = (29, 11)$ under $(\alpha^*, 1 - \beta^*, p_x, p_y) = (0.15, 0.8, 0.35, 0.05)$. In this case, the asymptotic method has $\alpha = 0.244$, which is far larger than the nominal $\alpha^* = 0.15$ because of the small sample size.

8.2.2 Two-Stage Designs with Both Superiority and Futility Interim Tests

So far, we have investigated two-stage designs with a futility stopping rule only. One may also want to stop the trial early when the experimental arm is significantly more efficacious than the control. In this section, we consider a two-stage randomized phase II trial with an interim look for both futility and superiority. A two-stage phase II trial with early stopping values (a_1, b_1) and a rejection value a at the second stage that are chosen conditional on z_1 and z_2 is conducted as follows:

Stage 1: Randomize n_1 patients to each arm; observe x_1 and y_1.

    a. Given $z_1(= x_1 + y_1)$, find stopping value $a_1 = a_1(z_1)$ and $b_1 = b_1(z_1)$.

    b. If $x_1 - y_1 \leq a_1$, then reject the experimental therapy and stop the trial.

    c. If $x_1 - y_1 \geq b_1$, then accept the experimental therapy and stop the trial.

    d. If $a_1 < x_1 - y_1 < b_1$, then proceed to the second stage.

Stage 2: Randomize n_2 patients to each arm; observe x_2 and y_2 ($z_2 = x_2 + y_2$).

    a. Given (z_1, z_2), find a rejection value $a = a(z_1, z_2)$.

    b. Accept the experimental arm if $x - y > a$, where $x = x_1 + x_2$ and $y = y_1 + y_2$.

At the design stage of a two-stage design, we have to determine (n_1, n_2) and (a_1, b_1, a) for all possible values of (z_1, z_2).

8.2.2.1 Choice of a_1, b_1, and a

Suppose that (n_1, n_2) are given. Then we have to choose the critical values (a_1, b_1, a) conditioning on (z_1, z_2). A complete search of optimal designs will go through all possible values of (a_1, b_1, a) for all (z_1, z_2) values. This is practically impossible due to its heavy computation. In the two-stage designs based on binomial test that were discussed in Chapter 7, the early stopping values for futility and superiority were determined around the expected differences under H_0 and under H_a, respectively. Based on this observation, we propose to use $a_1 = -1$ as in the designs with futility test only (note that equality sign is included in the lower stopping value here) and $b_1 = [n_1(p_x - p_y)] + 1$ for (p_x, p_y) that are specified under H_a for power calculation. Here, $[c]$ is the largest integer not exceeding c. Once (a_1, b_1) are chosen for stage 1, we choose $a = a(z_1, z_2)$ for given (z_1, z_2) after stage 2 as the smallest integer satisfying

$$\alpha(z_1, z_2) \equiv P(X_1 - Y_1 \geq b_1 | z_1, \theta = 1)$$
$$+ P(a_1 < X_1 - Y_1 < b_1, X - Y > a | z_1, z_2, \theta = 1) \leq \alpha^*,$$

where α^* denotes a prespecified type I error rate.

Given z_1 and z_2, the conditional power under $H_a : \theta = \theta_a$ is obtained by

$$1 - \beta(z_1, z_2) = P(X_1 - Y_1 \geq b_1 | z_1, \theta_a) + P(a_1 < X_1 - Y_1 < b_1, X - Y > a | z_1, z_2, \theta_a).$$

Note that, as in the single-stage case, the calculation of the type I error rate $\alpha(z_1, z_2)$ and critical values (a_1, b_1, a) does not require specification of the common response probability $p_x = p_y$ under H_0, and that the conditional power $1 - \beta(z_1, z_2)$ requires specification of the odds ratio θ_a under H_a, but not the response probabilities for the two arms, p_x and p_y.

8.2.2.2 Choice of n_1 and n_2

Now we discuss how to choose sample sizes n_1 and n_2 at the design stage based on some optimality criteria.

Given $(\alpha^*, 1 - \beta^*)$, we propose to choose n_1 and n_2 so that the marginal power is maintained above $1 - \beta^*$ while controlling the conditional type I error rates for any (z_1, z_2) below α^* as in the choice of (a_1, b_1, a). We choose n_1 and n_2 so that the marginal power is no smaller than a specified level $1 - \beta^*$, that is,

$$1 - \beta \equiv \sum_{z_1=0}^{2n_1} \sum_{z_2=0}^{2n_2} \{1 - \beta(z_1, z_2)\} g_1(z_1) g_2(z_2) \geq 1 - \beta^*.$$

The marginal type I error rate is calculated by

$$\alpha \equiv \sum_{z_1=0}^{2n_1} \sum_{z_2=0}^{2n_2} \alpha(z_1, z_2) g_{01}(z_1) g_{02}(z_2).$$

Since the conditional type I error rate is controlled below α^* for any (z_1, z_2), the marginal type I error rate does not exceed α^*.

Given z_1, the probability of early termination is calculated as

$$\text{PET}_h(z_1) = 1 - P(a_1 < x_1 - y_1 < b_1 | H_h)$$

under H_h $(h = 0, a)$. Let

$$\text{PET} \equiv \frac{1}{2} \left[E\{\text{PET}_0(Z_1) | H_0\} + E\{\text{PET}_1(Z_1) | H_a\} \right]$$

$$= \frac{1}{2} \left\{ \sum_{z_1=0}^{2n_1} \text{PET}_0(z_1) g_{01}(z_1) + \sum_{z_1=0}^{2n_1} \text{PET}_1(z_1) g_1(z_1) \right\}$$

denote the mean of the marginal probabilities of early termination under H_0 and H_a. Then, among those (n_1, n_2) satisfying the $(\alpha^*, 1 - \beta^*)$-condition, the Simon-type (1989) minimax and the optimal designs can be chosen as follows:

- *Minimax design* has the smallest maximal sample size $n(= n_1 + n_2)$.
- *Optimal design* has the smallest marginal expected sample size EN under H_0, where

$$\text{EN} = n_1 \times \text{PET} + n \times (1 - \text{PET}).$$

Tables 8.11 to 8.19 report the sample sizes (n, n_1) of the minimax and optimal two-stage designs for $\alpha^* = 0.1$, 0.15, or 0.2, $1 - \beta^* = 0.8$, 0.85, or 0.9, and various combinations of (p_x, p_y) under H_a.

8.3 Extensions

In this section, we investigate unbalanced two-stage designs with both futility and superiority tests and conditional p-values for two-stage designs based on Fisher's exact test.

8.3.1 Unbalanced Two-Stage Randomized Trials

One may want to accrue more patients to one arm than the other for some reasons, for example, to treat more patients by an experimental therapy than a control. In this case, the test statistic based on the difference in number of responders between two arms that has been considered so far is not appropriate. Let m_l and n_l denote the sample sizes at stage $l(= 1, 2)$ of arms x and y, respectively ($m = m_1 + m_2, n = n_1 + n_2$). Also, let X_l and Y_l denote the number of responders among stage l patients of arms x and y, respectively ($X = X_1 + X_2, Y = Y_1 + Y_2$). If we want to assign γ times larger number of patients to arm x than to arm y, then we have $m_l = \gamma \times n_l$ and $m = \gamma \times n$. Note that a choice of $\gamma = 1$ corresponds to the balanced two-stage designs considered in the previous section. When $\gamma \neq 1$, it does not make sense to directly compare the numbers of responders between arms at each stage. For the odds ratio, $\theta = (p_x q_y)/(q_x p_y)$, we want to design a study for $H_0 : \theta = 1$, $H_0 : \theta = \theta_a(> 1)$, where $q_k = 1 - p_k$.

With an interim look with both futility and superiority tests, we consider following two-stage design.

- *Stage 1*: Accrue m_1 patients to arm x and n_1 patients to arm y, and observe X_1 and Y_1. For $\hat{p}_{x,1} = X_1/m_1$, $\hat{p}_{y,1} = Y_1/n_1$, $\hat{q}_{k,1} = 1 - \hat{p}_{k,1}$, and $\hat{\theta}_1 = (\hat{p}_{x,1}\hat{q}_{y,1})/(\hat{q}_{x,1}\hat{p}_{y,1})$,

  (a) If $\hat{\theta}_1 \leq 1$, reject arm x and stop the trial.
  (b) If $\hat{\theta}_1 \geq \theta_a$, accept arm x and stop the trial.
  (c) If $1 < \hat{\theta}_1 < \theta_a$, proceed to the second stage.

Table 8.11 Minimax and optimal two-stage designs with both interim futility and superiority tests for Fisher's exact test with $(\alpha^*, 1 - \beta^*) = (.1, .8)$

			Minimax Two-Stage Design					Optimal Two-Stage Design				
P_y	P_x	θ	n	α	$1-\beta$	EN_0	EN_1	(n,n_1)	α	$1-\beta$	EN_0	EN_1
.05	.15	3.353	(94, 61)	.0503	.8000	80.28	79.30	(97, 50)	.0528	.8010	77.89	76.97
	.2	4.750	(52, 49)	.0315	.8007	50.78	50.57	(54, 27)	.0345	.8010	44.02	42.76
	.25	6.333	(34, 25)	.0219	.8015	30.73	30.29	(35, 20)	.0213	.8064	29.83	28.98
.1	.25	3.000	(68, 42)	.0593	.8005	56.90	55.65	(71, 34)	.0618	.8025	55.51	54.49
	.3	3.857	(43, 25)	.0509	.8014	35.72	35.33	(45, 21)	.0528	.8012	35.51	34.18
.15	.3	2.429	(80, 54)	.0683	.8000	68.40	67.97	(84, 40)	.0734	.8007	64.76	64.38
	.35	3.051	(50, 30)	.0623	.8012	41.45	41.20	(51, 25)	.0654	.8007	40.06	39.71
.2	.35	2.154	(91, 60)	.0737	.8003	76.91	76.75	(95, 47)	.0773	.8002	73.47	72.97
	.4	2.667	(56, 34)	.0708	.8007	46.33	44.24	(59, 25)	.0733	.8001	44.40	44.06
.25	.4	2.000	(99, 67)	.0773	.8005	84.27	84.03	(103, 54)	.0801	.8008	80.67	80.05
	.45	2.455	(59, 40)	.0693	.8046	50.48	50.36	(62, 30)	.0750	.8013	47.90	47.67
.3	.45	1.909	(105, 93)	.0772	.8000	99.38	98.65	(112, 54)	.0835	.8021	85.43	84.76
	.5	2.333	(60, 52)	.0695	.8001	56.34	56.05	(66, 31)	.0793	.8008	50.43	49.49
.35	.5	1.857	(110, 67)	.0804	.8022	90.05	89.79	(113, 60)	.0834	.8015	88.52	88.38
	.55	2.270	(65, 35)	.0774	.8016	51.50	51.37	(67, 31)	.0810	.8001	50.91	50.00
.4	.55	1.833	(110, 74)	.0805	.8001	93.20	92.90	(119, 58)	.0881	.8008	90.80	87.47
	.6	2.250	(65, 35)	.0789	.8002	51.46	51.36	(67, 32)	.0851	.8011	51.27	49.74
.45	.6	1.833	(110, 74)	.0838	.8001	93.18	92.90	(119, 58)	.0911	.8008	90.77	87.47
	.65	2.270	(65, 35)	.0815	.8016	51.43	51.37	(67, 31)	.0868	.8001	50.83	50.00
.5	.65	1.857	(110, 67)	.0846	.8023	89.98	89.79	(113, 61)	.0855	.8013	88.87	88.25
	.7	2.333	(60, 52)	.0724	.8001	56.31	56.05	(66, 31)	.0867	.8008	50.27	49.49
.55	.7	1.909	(105, 93)	.0737	.8000	99.35	98.65	(112, 54)	.0853	.8021	85.23	84.76
	.75	2.455	(59, 40)	.0739	.8046	50.35	50.36	(62, 30)	.0809	.8013	47.65	47.67
.6	.75	2.000	(99, 67)	.0802	.8005	84.12	84.03	(103, 54)	.0855	.8008	80.42	80.05
	.8	2.667	(56, 34)	.0827	.8007	46.08	44.24	(60, 26)	.0860	.8048	44.91	44.18
.65	.8	2.154	(91, 60)	.0805	.8003	76.68	76.75	(95, 47)	.0862	.8002	73.07	72.97
	.85	3.051	(50, 30)	.0761	.8012	41.08	41.20	(51, 25)	.0821	.8007	39.53	39.71
.7	.85	2.429	(80, 54)	.0797	.8000	68.09	67.97	(84, 40)	.0863	.8007	64.14	64.38
	.9	3.857	(43, 25)	.0774	.8014	35.10	35.33	(45, 20)	.0795	.8013	34.21	34.57
.75	.9	3.000	(68, 42)	.0813	.8005	56.31	55.65	(71, 34)	.0837	.8025	54.56	54.49
	.95	6.333	(34, 32)	.0633	.8001	33.12	33.04	(35, 20)	.0759	.8064	28.59	28.98
.8	.95	4.750	(52, 49)	.0658	.8007	50.65	50.57	(54, 27)	.0672	.8010	42.33	42.76
.85	.95	3.353	(94, 61)	.0792	.8000	79.17	79.30	(97, 50)	.0789	.8010	76.13	76.97

Table 8.12 Minimax and optimal two-stage designs with both interim futility and superiority tests for Fisher's exact test with $(\alpha^*, 1 - \beta^*) = (.1, .85)$

p_y	p_x	θ	Minimax Two-Stage Design					Optimal Two-Stage Design				
			n	α	$1-\beta$	EN_0	EN_1	(n,n_1)	α	$1-\beta$	EN_0	EN_1
.05	.15	3.353	(109, 70)	.0544	.8507	92.56	91.93	(114, 51)	.0575	.8501	88.33	86.27
	.2	4.750	(61, 34)	.0376	.8541	50.60	49.31	(63, 27)	.0406	.8506	49.70	48.01
	.25	6.333	(39, 25)	.0254	.8527	33.91	33.24	(40, 21)	.0245	.8531	33.36	31.66
.1	.25	3.000	(79, 43)	.0637	.8502	63.60	61.27	(84, 36)	.0668	.8509	63.80	60.70
	.3	3.857	(50, 25)	.0542	.8504	39.89	39.35	(53, 21)	.0564	.8521	40.34	38.57
.15	.3	2.429	(94, 58)	.0727	.8503	77.87	75.34	(101, 42)	.0760	.8504	75.11	72.74
	.35	3.051	(58, 35)	.0637	.8525	48.04	47.78	(61, 27)	.0682	.8504	46.60	44.40
.2	.35	2.154	(107, 67)	.0751	.8514	88.72	88.37	(115, 49)	.0805	.8514	85.33	82.84
	.4	2.667	(64, 40)	.0689	.8519	53.34	53.15	(67, 31)	.0729	.8505	51.28	50.14
.25	.4	2.000	(117, 77)	.0783	.8500	98.48	96.81	(124, 54)	.0825	.8516	92.10	91.22
	.45	2.455	(70, 43)	.0737	.8502	57.84	56.19	(74, 32)	.0783	.8500	55.42	53.33
.3	.45	1.909	(122, 80)	.0781	.8509	102.44	102.32	(136, 56)	.0858	.8502	99.29	96.49
	.5	2.333	(72, 46)	.0737	.8505	60.18	59.61	(75, 36)	.0780	.8501	57.50	56.53
.35	.5	1.857	(130, 78)	.0821	.8504	105.74	103.24	(135, 62)	.0852	.8501	101.24	99.44
	.55	2.270	(73, 45)	.0751	.8520	60.23	60.13	(82, 32)	.0836	.8529	59.61	57.34
.4	.55	1.833	(131, 76)	.0827	.8501	105.31	103.77	(146, 54)	.0887	.8518	103.60	102.68
	.6	2.250	(73, 45)	.0798	.8508	60.20	60.12	(82, 32)	.0862	.8514	59.54	57.34
.45	.6	1.833	(131, 76)	.0857	.8500	105.29	103.77	(146, 54)	.0916	.8518	103.54	102.68
	.65	2.270	(73, 45)	.0833	.8520	60.18	60.13	(82, 32)	.0893	.8529	59.50	57.34
.5	.65	1.857	(130, 78)	.0867	.8504	105.66	103.24	(135, 62)	.0887	.8501	101.11	99.44
	.7	2.333	(72, 46)	.0833	.8505	60.08	59.61	(75, 36)	.0817	.8502	57.33	56.53
.55	.7	1.909	(122, 80)	.0783	.8509	102.33	102.32	(136, 56)	.0889	.8500	99.02	96.49
	.75	2.455	(70, 43)	.0831	.8502	57.66	56.19	(74, 32)	.0831	.8516	55.10	53.33
.6	.75	2.000	(117, 78)	.0846	.8502	98.77	96.91	(124, 54)	.0875	.8505	91.74	91.22
	.8	2.667	(64, 40)	.0731	.8519	53.09	53.15	(67, 31)	.0839	.8514	50.85	50.14
.65	.8	2.154	(107, 67)	.0800	.8514	88.44	88.37	(115, 49)	.0884	.8514	84.78	82.84
	.85	3.051	(58, 35)	.0774	.8525	47.65	47.78	(61, 27)	.0854	.8504	45.93	44.40
.7	.85	2.429	(94, 58)	.0823	.8503	77.45	75.34	(101, 42)	.0886	.8504	74.30	72.74
	.9	3.857	(50, 25)	.0787	.8504	39.03	39.35	(53, 21)	.0805	.8522	39.14	38.57
.75	.9	3.000	(79, 43)	.0838	.8502	62.79	61.27	(84, 36)	.0789	.8509	62.60	60.70
	.95	6.333	(39, 26)	.0715	.8512	33.33	33.21	(40, 20)	.0770	.8522	31.45	31.97
.8	.95	4.750	(61, 34)	.0784	.8541	49.13	49.31	(63, 27)	.0684	.8506	47.44	48.01
.85	.95	3.353	(109, 70)	.0779	.8507	91.34	91.93	(114, 51)	.0797	.8501	85.99	86.27

Table 8.13   Minimax and optimal two-stage designs with both interim futility and superiority tests for Fisher's exact test with $(\alpha^*, 1-\beta^*) = (.1, .9)$.

p_y	p_x	θ	Minimax Two-Stage Design					Optimal Two-Stage Design				
			n	α	$1-\beta$	EN_0	EN_1	(n, n_1)	α	$1-\beta$	EN_0	EN_1
.05	.15	3.353	(130, 70)	.0599	.9000	104.71	103.73	(132, 65)	.0610	.9000	103.96	98.87
	.2	4.750	(71, 40)	.0416	.9006	58.76	57.84	(72, 36)	.0432	.9012	58.01	54.77
	.25	6.333	(46, 30)	.0290	.9010	39.97	39.29	(48, 24)	.0311	.9037	39.35	34.94
.1	.25	3.000	(93, 54)	.0653	.9001	76.01	75.17	(97, 44)	.0676	.9005	74.29	69.98
	.3	3.857	(59, 32)	.0558	.9002	47.77	45.88	(61, 28)	.0589	.9029	47.47	44.08
.15	.3	2.429	(112, 69)	.0717	.9001	92.55	91.03	(119, 52)	.0770	.9009	89.18	83.57
	.35	3.051	(69, 38)	.0665	.9003	55.49	53.13	(71, 33)	.0683	.9003	54.62	51.51
.2	.35	2.154	(128, 78)	.0769	.9003	105.00	102.23	(136, 59)	.0811	.9007	101.04	95.18
	.4	2.667	(77, 48)	.0702	.9003	63.98	62.18	(82, 34)	.0764	.9005	60.90	56.34
.25	.4	2.000	(139, 100)	.0779	.9002	120.77	120.65	(148, 65)	.0834	.9000	109.85	104.82
	.45	2.455	(81, 58)	.0718	.9000	70.48	69.27	(88, 39)	.0787	.9018	66.05	61.95
.3	.45	1.909	(147, 94)	.0800	.9004	122.18	121.72	(162, 66)	.0865	.9002	117.63	111.07
	.5	2.333	(88, 49)	.0787	.9001	70.21	67.42	(93, 39)	.0815	.9016	68.66	64.32
.35	.5	1.857	(157, 93)	.0839	.9000	126.96	123.19	(166, 71)	.0865	.9004	121.83	117.37
	.55	2.270	(90, 45)	.0772	.9003	69.48	69.31	(96, 35)	.0822	.9002	68.54	68.28
.4	.55	1.833	(159, 85)	.0837	.9004	124.31	120.74	(169, 72)	.0872	.9003	123.79	118.38
	.6	2.250	(90, 47)	.0808	.9007	70.30	68.74	(90, 47)	.0808	.9007	70.30	68.74
.45	.6	1.833	(159, 85)	.0870	.9004	124.27	120.74	(169, 72)	.0879	.9003	123.74	118.38
	.65	2.270	(90, 45)	.0831	.9003	69.40	69.31	(96, 35)	.0877	.9002	68.41	68.28
.5	.65	1.857	(157, 93)	.0847	.9000	126.87	123.19	(166, 71)	.0870	.9004	121.67	117.37
	.7	2.333	(88, 49)	.0841	.9001	70.07	67.42	(93, 39)	.0827	.9016	68.43	64.32
.55	.7	1.909	(147, 94)	.0836	.9004	122.05	121.72	(162, 66)	.0875	.9003	117.34	111.07
	.75	2.455	(81, 58)	.0711	.9000	70.35	69.27	(88, 39)	.0875	.9018	65.72	61.95
.6	.75	2.000	(139, 101)	.0805	.9002	121.09	120.77	(148, 65)	.0869	.9000	109.46	104.82
	.8	2.667	(77, 48)	.0802	.9003	63.70	62.18	(82, 34)	.0876	.9005	60.36	56.34
.65	.8	2.154	(128, 78)	.0827	.9003	104.67	102.23	(136, 58)	.0881	.9005	100.02	95.61
	.85	3.051	(69, 38)	.0791	.9003	54.98	53.13	(71, 32)	.0832	.9004	53.53	51.92
.7	.85	2.429	(112, 69)	.0807	.9001	92.09	91.03	(119, 52)	.0881	.9009	88.36	83.57
	.9	3.857	(59, 32)	.0785	.9002	46.97	45.88	(61, 28)	.0841	.9029	46.41	44.08
.75	.9	3.000	(93, 54)	.0790	.9001	75.23	75.17	(97, 44)	.0861	.9005	73.10	69.98
	.95	6.333	(46, 31)	.0703	.9012	39.38	39.25	(48, 23)	.0741	.9042	37.20	35.24
.8	.95	4.750	(71, 40)	.0761	.9006	57.23	57.84	(72, 35)	.0811	.9011	55.71	55.13
.85	.95	3.353	(130, 70)	.0807	.9000	102.84	103.73	(132, 65)	.0842	.9000	101.79	98.87

Table 8.14 Minimax and optimal two-stage designs with both interim futility and superiority tests for Fisher's exact test with $(\alpha^*, 1 - \beta^*) = (.15, .8)$

p_y	p_x	θ	Minimax Two-Stage Design					Optimal Two-Stage Design				
			n	α	$1-\beta$	EN_0	EN_1	(n,n_1)	α	$1-\beta$	EN_0	EN_1
.05	.15	3.353	(78, 43)	.0855	.8005	64.04	61.77	(78, 43)	.0855	.8005	64.04	61.77
	.2	4.750	(44, 27)	.0625	.8048	37.72	36.92	(45, 22)	.0645	.8033	36.88	34.57
	.25	6.333	(29, 15)	.0473	.8075	24.57	23.60	(29, 15)	.0473	.8075	24.57	23.60
.1	.25	3.000	(55, 40)	.0881	.8000	48.62	48.42	(57, 31)	.0957	.8010	46.22	43.52
	.3	3.857	(36, 20)	.0793	.8047	29.72	29.32	(37, 16)	.0848	.8007	29.03	27.69
.15	.3	2.429	(65, 47)	.1027	.8017	57.04	56.81	(67, 34)	.1086	.8001	52.74	52.05
	.35	3.051	(41, 25)	.0920	.8022	34.27	34.05	(42, 20)	.0958	.8015	32.96	32.61
.2	.35	2.154	(73, 49)	.1102	.8003	62.21	61.30	(79, 36)	.1199	.8003	60.03	57.91
	.4	2.667	(45, 27)	.1053	.8007	37.22	36.18	(47, 21)	.1101	.8002	36.00	35.00
.25	.4	2.000	(81, 51)	.1192	.8000	67.37	65.57	(84, 40)	.1218	.8001	64.26	64.04
	.45	2.455	(47, 30)	.1035	.8001	39.51	39.39	(49, 26)	.1109	.8004	38.97	38.25
.3	.45	1.909	(84, 55)	.1170	.8004	70.70	70.03	(92, 41)	.1274	.8004	68.95	68.04
	.5	2.333	(52, 32)	.1140	.8007	43.09	42.14	(56, 21)	.1226	.8020	40.84	39.71
.35	.5	1.857	(86, 60)	.1196	.8034	73.99	73.92	(95, 45)	.1298	.8005	72.20	68.82
	.55	2.270	(53, 31)	.1115	.8013	43.16	42.61	(57, 20)	.1260	.8008	40.93	40.73
.4	.55	1.833	(86, 60)	.1262	.8010	73.96	73.91	(96, 45)	.1336	.8015	72.68	69.31
	.6	2.250	(53, 31)	.1131	.8000	43.13	42.61	(55, 29)	.1227	.8025	43.38	41.08
.45	.6	1.833	(86, 60)	.1301	.8010	73.95	73.91	(96, 45)	.1375	.8015	72.65	69.31
	.65	2.270	(53, 31)	.1162	.8013	43.12	42.61	(57, 20)	.1345	.8008	40.83	40.73
.5	.65	1.857	(86, 61)	.1315	.8037	74.40	74.10	(95, 45)	.1380	.8005	72.10	68.82
	.7	2.333	(52, 32)	.1163	.8007	42.99	42.14	(56, 21)	.1330	.8020	40.64	39.71
.55	.7	1.909	(84, 55)	.1292	.8004	70.61	70.03	(92, 41)	.1296	.8004	68.75	68.04
	.75	2.455	(47, 30)	.1084	.8001	39.38	39.39	(49, 26)	.1202	.8004	38.77	38.25
.6	.75	2.000	(81, 51)	.1259	.8000	67.21	65.57	(84, 41)	.1297	.8009	64.43	63.86
	.8	2.667	(45, 27)	.1207	.8007	36.99	36.18	(47, 21)	.1229	.8002	35.62	35.00
.65	.8	2.154	(73, 49)	.1193	.8003	62.01	61.30	(79, 36)	.1327	.8003	59.61	57.91
	.85	3.051	(41, 25)	.1144	.8022	33.94	34.05	(42, 20)	.1224	.8015	32.45	32.61
.7	.85	2.429	(65, 47)	.1158	.8017	56.81	56.81	(67, 34)	.1265	.8001	52.24	52.05
	.9	3.857	(36, 20)	.1139	.8047	29.10	29.32	(37, 16)	.1257	.8007	28.11	27.69
.75	.9	3.000	(55, 40)	.1199	.8003	48.27	46.63	(57, 31)	.1272	.8010	45.52	43.52
	.95	6.333	(29, 16)	.1152	.8081	23.56	23.41	(29, 16)	.1152	.8081	23.56	23.41
.8	.95	4.750	(44, 27)	.1134	.8048	36.65	36.92	(45, 20)	.1141	.8053	34.47	35.17
.85	.95	3.353	(78, 43)	.1236	.8005	62.61	61.77	(78, 43)	.1236	.8005	62.61	61.77

Table 8.15 Minimax and optimal two-stage designs with both interim futility and superiority tests for Fisher's exact test with $(\alpha^*, 1 - \beta^*) = (.15, .85)$

			Minimax Two-Stage Design					Optimal Two-Stage Design				
p_y	p_x	θ	n	α	$1-\beta$	EN_0	EN_1	(n,n_1)	α	$1-\beta$	EN_0	EN_1
.05	.15	3.353	(91,50)	.0877	.8505	74.33	73.52	(94,43)	.0914	.8502	73.66	70.35
	.2	4.750	(51,27)	.0682	.8529	42.13	41.00	(53,23)	.0705	.8515	42.29	38.54
	.25	6.333	(33,16)	.0516	.8512	27.51	25.69	(33,16)	.0516	.8512	27.51	25.69
.1	.25	3.000	(65,39)	.0966	.8500	53.98	50.94	(68,32)	.1020	.8500	53.03	48.62
	.3	3.857	(41,25)	.0823	.8507	34.53	34.18	(45,17)	.0927	.8525	34.27	31.54
.15	.3	2.429	(78,46)	.1096	.8504	63.87	60.70	(82,37)	.1136	.8505	62.43	59.23
	.35	3.051	(48,29)	.0985	.8503	39.90	37.77	(50,22)	.1047	.8507	38.37	36.36
.2	.35	2.154	(88,56)	.1139	.8502	73.51	72.24	(91,46)	.1201	.8502	70.84	66.75
	.4	2.667	(52,35)	.1002	.8501	44.51	44.37	(54,28)	.1092	.8504	42.73	40.63
.25	.4	2.000	(94,62)	.1153	.8500	79.32	78.45	(104,44)	.1268	.8501	76.94	73.35
	.45	2.455	(58,32)	.1137	.8500	46.50	45.20	(60,29)	.1181	.8508	46.37	43.37
.3	.45	1.909	(103,65)	.1241	.8502	85.45	83.25	(107,53)	.1278	.8500	82.28	77.94
	.5	2.333	(60,31)	.1140	.8509	47.10	46.32	(63,28)	.1203	.8520	47.53	44.99
.35	.5	1.857	(105,66)	.1213	.8501	86.92	84.33	(111,51)	.1288	.8510	83.48	80.16
	.55	2.270	(60,37)	.1140	.8502	49.62	48.65	(65,26)	.1238	.8512	47.75	46.68
.4	.55	1.833	(106,65)	.1257	.8503	86.96	84.70	(113,49)	.1329	.8504	83.63	81.65
	.6	2.250	(60,39)	.1206	.8507	50.47	48.86	(66,26)	.1304	.8524	48.25	47.20
.45	.6	1.833	(106,65)	.1296	.8503	86.94	84.70	(113,49)	.1370	.8503	83.59	81.65
	.65	2.270	(60,37)	.1237	.8502	49.57	48.65	(65,26)	.1333	.8512	47.66	46.68
.5	.65	1.857	(105,66)	.1302	.8501	86.85	84.33	(111,51)	.1387	.8510	83.36	80.16
	.7	2.333	(60,31)	.1270	.8509	46.96	46.32	(63,28)	.1355	.8520	47.36	44.99
.55	.7	1.909	(103,65)	.1265	.8502	85.33	83.25	(107,53)	.1362	.8501	82.10	77.94
	.75	2.455	(58,32)	.1266	.8500	46.30	45.20	(60,29)	.1324	.8508	46.13	43.37
.6	.75	2.000	(94,62)	.1217	.8500	79.17	78.45	(104,44)	.1336	.8501	76.60	73.35
	.8	2.667	(52,36)	.1064	.8504	44.77	44.47	(54,28)	.1211	.8504	42.41	40.63
.65	.8	2.154	(88,56)	.1257	.8502	73.26	72.24	(92,42)	.1290	.8507	69.28	67.93
	.85	3.051	(48,29)	.1207	.8503	39.54	37.77	(50,21)	.1230	.8507	37.36	36.73
.7	.85	2.429	(78,46)	.1244	.8504	63.45	60.70	(82,37)	.1303	.8505	61.77	59.23
	.9	3.857	(41,25)	.1090	.8507	33.98	34.18	(45,17)	.1272	.8525	33.08	31.54
.75	.9	3.000	(65,39)	.1236	.8500	53.35	50.94	(68,32)	.1308	.8500	52.07	48.62
	.95	6.333	(33,16)	.1195	.8512	25.88	25.69	(33,16)	.1195	.8512	25.88	25.69
.8	.95	4.750	(51,27)	.1159	.8529	40.63	41.00	(53,23)	.1114	.8515	40.21	38.54
.85	.95	3.353	(91,50)	.1207	.8505	72.80	73.52	(94,43)	.1271	.8502	71.58	70.35

Table 8.16 Minimax and optimal two-stage designs with both interim futility and superiority tests for Fisher's exact test with $(\alpha^*, 1 - \beta^*) = (.15, .9)$

			Minimax Two-Stage Design					Optimal Two-Stage Design				
p_y	p_x	θ	n	α	$1-\beta$	EN_0	EN_1	(n,n_1)	α	$1-\beta$	EN_0	EN_1
.05	.15	3.353	(110, 63)	.0919	.9001	90.40	87.90	(118, 46)	.0983	.9001	89.04	81.46
	.2	4.750	(60, 34)	.0737	.9005	49.99	48.74	(61, 29)	.0750	.9013	49.01	46.03
	.25	6.333	(40, 20)	.0585	.9001	33.10	31.97	(41, 19)	.0612	.9054	33.52	28.91
.1	.25	3.000	(78, 53)	.0963	.9005	67.12	64.36	(82, 36)	.1032	.9005	62.64	59.67
	.3	3.857	(50, 25)	.0864	.9009	39.89	39.35	(51, 23)	.0905	.9014	39.79	36.61
.15	.3	2.429	(93, 60)	.1083	.9005	78.19	77.96	(98, 46)	.1148	.9002	75.04	69.88
	.35	3.051	(57, 36)	.1004	.9001	47.89	47.18	(64, 24)	.1101	.9028	47.24	42.31
.2	.35	2.154	(105, 71)	.1153	.9001	89.42	87.58	(118, 46)	.1247	.9002	85.74	79.20
	.4	2.667	(65, 37)	.1095	.9000	52.62	51.23	(69, 29)	.1159	.9017	51.62	47.50
.25	.4	2.000	(117, 79)	.1210	.9001	99.39	97.04	(127, 52)	.1272	.9001	92.89	87.48
	.45	2.455	(68, 40)	.1107	.9006	55.44	55.27	(73, 32)	.1166	.9001	54.86	52.82
.3	.45	1.909	(121, 80)	.1188	.9004	101.91	101.79	(133, 58)	.1290	.9001	98.53	94.21
	.5	2.333	(75, 44)	.1201	.9005	60.94	58.59	(77, 34)	.1219	.9009	57.76	54.07
.35	.5	1.857	(131, 92)	.1250	.9001	112.70	110.74	(140, 58)	.1303	.9002	102.18	97.61
	.55	2.270	(77, 39)	.1203	.9004	59.79	56.83	(80, 32)	.1224	.9014	58.50	56.33
.4	.55	1.833	(132, 99)	.1178	.9000	116.45	114.79	(140, 66)	.1296	.9007	105.62	100.79
	.6	2.250	(77, 43)	.1151	.9003	61.49	59.60	(81, 31)	.1268	.9011	58.58	57.38
.45	.6	1.833	(132, 99)	.1204	.9000	116.44	114.79	(140, 66)	.1288	.9007	105.58	100.79
	.65	2.270	(77, 39)	.1233	.9004	59.72	56.83	(80, 32)	.1307	.9014	58.40	56.33
.5	.65	1.857	(131, 92)	.1213	.9001	112.65	110.74	(139, 60)	.1345	.9001	102.37	96.42
	.7	2.333	(75, 44)	.1168	.9005	60.81	58.59	(77, 34)	.1296	.9009	57.57	54.07
.55	.7	1.909	(121, 80)	.1266	.9004	101.80	101.79	(133, 58)	.1331	.9001	98.29	94.21
	.75	2.455	(68, 40)	.1185	.9006	55.25	55.27	(73, 32)	.1232	.9001	54.55	52.82
.6	.75	2.000	(117, 79)	.1300	.9001	99.23	97.04	(127, 52)	.1308	.9001	92.49	87.48
	.8	2.667	(65, 37)	.1220	.9000	52.32	51.23	(69, 29)	.1259	.9017	51.13	47.50
.65	.8	2.154	(105, 71)	.1183	.9001	89.19	87.58	(118, 46)	.1331	.9002	85.13	79.20
	.85	3.051	(57, 36)	.1098	.9001	47.53	47.18	(64, 24)	.1297	.9028	46.40	42.31
.7	.85	2.429	(93, 60)	.1193	.9005	77.81	77.96	(98, 46)	.1292	.9002	74.36	69.88
	.9	3.857	(50, 25)	.1173	.9009	39.03	39.35	(51, 22)	.1228	.9006	38.40	36.99
.75	.9	3.000	(78, 53)	.1189	.9005	66.62	64.36	(81, 40)	.1281	.9004	62.61	58.11
	.95	6.333	(40, 20)	.1105	.9001	31.45	31.97	(41, 18)	.1212	.9053	31.26	29.23
.8	.95	4.750	(60, 34)	.1136	.9005	48.57	48.74	(61, 28)	.1204	.9008	46.70	46.40
.85	.95	3.353	(110, 63)	.1201	.9001	88.84	87.90	(118, 46)	.1243	.9001	86.20	81.46

Table 8.17 Minimax and optimal two-stage designs with both interim futility and superiority tests for Fisher's exact test with $(\alpha^*, 1-\beta^*) = (.2, .8)$.

p_y	p_x	θ	Minimax Two-Stage Design					Optimal Two-Stage Design				
			n	α	$1-\beta$	EN_0	EN_1	(n,n_1)	α	$1-\beta$	EN_0	EN_1
.05	.15	3.353	(65, 46)	.1107	.8001	57.36	55.36	(66, 36)	.1201	.8004	54.34	50.75
	.2	4.750	(37, 20)	.0804	.8028	31.14	30.31	(40, 17)	.0884	.8022	32.43	28.50
	.25	6.333	(25, 15)	.0485	.8069	21.84	21.14	(26, 12)	.0522	.8066	21.93	19.48
.1	.25	3.000	(46, 29)	.1230	.8000	39.00	37.90	(48, 24)	.1326	.8006	38.34	35.68
	.3	3.857	(30, 16)	.1097	.8002	24.69	23.79	(30, 16)	.1097	.8002	24.69	23.79
.15	.3	2.429	(54, 37)	.1400	.8003	46.61	45.40	(56, 28)	.1470	.8012	44.10	43.09
	.35	3.051	(34, 21)	.1243	.8012	28.63	28.05	(35, 16)	.1331	.8004	27.39	26.43
.2	.35	2.154	(62, 36)	.1554	.8001	50.53	49.25	(65, 31)	.1618	.8001	50.15	47.37
	.4	2.667	(38, 23)	.1400	.8009	31.60	30.26	(40, 19)	.1540	.8010	31.20	28.53
.25	.4	2.000	(66, 42)	.1539	.8000	55.21	54.41	(70, 34)	.1625	.8008	54.01	53.44
	.45	2.455	(40, 22)	.1457	.8001	32.25	31.17	(40, 22)	.1457	.8001	32.25	31.17
.3	.45	1.909	(68, 48)	.1563	.8001	58.89	58.47	(74, 34)	.1669	.8017	56.11	55.53
	.5	2.333	(40, 29)	.1453	.8000	35.13	34.10	(43, 20)	.1577	.8010	33.08	32.91
.35	.5	1.857	(69, 54)	.1644	.8019	62.10	61.94	(80, 38)	.1725	.8003	61.01	58.12
	.55	2.270	(41, 30)	.1510	.8009	36.09	36.04	(46, 24)	.1624	.8027	36.32	34.14
.4	.55	1.833	(70, 54)	.1727	.8018	62.63	62.47	(81, 38)	.1721	.8003	61.50	58.60
	.6	2.250	(41, 31)	.1579	.8002	36.52	36.28	(46, 24)	.1616	.8008	36.29	34.14
.45	.6	1.833	(70, 54)	.1753	.8018	62.62	62.47	(81, 38)	.1746	.8003	61.47	58.60
	.65	2.270	(41, 30)	.1617	.8009	36.07	36.04	(46, 24)	.1626	.8027	36.27	34.14
.5	.65	1.857	(69, 54)	.1763	.8019	62.07	61.94	(79, 40)	.1767	.8007	61.23	57.64
	.7	2.333	(40, 29)	.1678	.8000	35.07	34.10	(43, 20)	.1670	.8010	32.94	32.91
.55	.7	1.909	(68, 48)	.1663	.8001	58.82	58.47	(74, 34)	.1749	.8017	55.94	55.53
	.75	2.455	(40, 22)	.1656	.8001	32.08	31.17	(40, 22)	.1656	.8001	32.08	31.17
.6	.75	2.000	(66, 42)	.1719	.8000	55.06	54.41	(70, 34)	.1758	.8008	53.77	53.44
	.8	2.667	(38, 23)	.1634	.8009	31.40	30.26	(40, 19)	.1772	.8010	30.88	28.53
.65	.8	2.154	(62, 36)	.1658	.8001	50.28	49.25	(65, 31)	.1741	.8001	49.80	47.37
	.85	3.051	(34, 21)	.1483	.8012	28.33	28.05	(35, 16)	.1613	.8004	26.90	26.43
.7	.85	2.429	(54, 37)	.1581	.8003	46.36	45.40	(56, 28)	.1657	.8012	43.62	43.09
	.9	3.857	(30, 16)	.1559	.8002	24.07	23.79	(33, 11)	.1696	.8035	24.03	23.51
.75	.9	3.000	(46, 29)	.1575	.8000	38.53	37.90	(48, 24)	.1717	.8006	37.59	35.68
	.95	6.333	(25, 16)	.1415	.8058	21.23	21.13	(26, 11)	.1612	.8075	19.97	19.78
.8	.95	4.750	(37, 20)	.1531	.8028	29.84	30.31	(40, 16)	.1501	.8048	30.12	28.80
.85	.95	3.353	(65, 46)	.1554	.8001	56.61	55.36	(67, 32)	.1661	.8007	51.95	51.57

Table 8.18 Minimax and optimal two-stage designs with both interim futility and superiority tests for Fisher's exact test with $(\alpha^*, 1-\beta^*) = (.2, .85)$

			Minimax Two-Stage Design					Optimal Two-Stage Design				
p_y	p_x	θ	n	α	$1-\beta$	EN_0	EN_1	(n, n_1)	α	$1-\beta$	EN_0	EN_1
.05	.15	3.353	(78, 47)	.1197	.8503	65.49	61.83	(81, 37)	.1231	.8506	63.83	57.94
	.2	4.750	(43, 25)	.0925	.8502	36.45	33.35	(43, 25)	.0925	.8502	36.45	33.35
	.25	6.333	(29, 15)	.0600	.8518	24.57	23.60	(31, 14)	.0666	.8520	25.75	21.52
.1	.25	3.000	(56, 30)	.1333	.8502	45.26	43.05	(60, 24)	.1418	.8506	45.51	41.52
	.3	3.857	(35, 20)	.1104	.8527	29.11	28.74	(36, 16)	.1179	.8502	28.41	27.13
.15	.3	2.429	(65, 40)	.1434	.8511	54.07	53.85	(70, 30)	.1543	.8508	52.90	49.99
	.35	3.051	(42, 21)	.1355	.8510	33.32	32.39	(44, 18)	.1427	.8514	33.44	30.55
.2	.35	2.154	(74, 43)	.1546	.8501	60.17	58.62	(77, 39)	.1611	.8506	60.15	56.59
	.4	2.667	(45, 25)	.1406	.8506	36.41	36.21	(46, 22)	.1462	.8513	35.81	34.26
.25	.4	2.000	(78, 55)	.1559	.8502	67.51	66.94	(88, 39)	.1701	.8505	66.05	61.74
	.45	2.455	(46, 30)	.1422	.8502	38.95	38.83	(52, 23)	.1601	.8516	39.47	37.04
.3	.45	1.909	(87, 51)	.1653	.8501	70.55	68.49	(88, 46)	.1663	.8505	68.90	65.46
	.5	2.333	(52, 29)	.1592	.8504	41.81	39.67	(55, 22)	.1624	.8507	40.66	38.79
.35	.5	1.857	(89, 52)	.1658	.8508	72.01	69.54	(94, 40)	.1706	.8504	69.52	69.34
	.55	2.270	(54, 28)	.1611	.8511	42.45	40.62	(57, 21)	.1645	.8506	41.31	40.21
.4	.55	1.833	(89, 59)	.1654	.8504	75.12	73.16	(90, 51)	.1711	.8501	72.07	69.95
	.6	2.250	(54, 29)	.1611	.8513	42.83	40.61	(58, 21)	.1706	.8507	41.81	40.74
.45	.6	1.833	(89, 59)	.1694	.8504	75.11	73.16	(90, 51)	.1750	.8501	72.04	69.95
	.65	2.270	(54, 28)	.1617	.8511	42.39	40.62	(57, 21)	.1736	.8506	41.21	40.21
.5	.65	1.857	(88, 60)	.1698	.8500	75.02	72.91	(94, 41)	.1794	.8516	69.83	69.06
	.7	2.333	(52, 29)	.1602	.8504	41.70	39.67	(55, 22)	.1738	.8507	40.47	38.79
.55	.7	1.909	(87, 51)	.1716	.8501	70.43	68.49	(88, 46)	.1754	.8505	68.75	65.46
	.75	2.455	(46, 30)	.1573	.8502	38.82	38.83	(52, 23)	.1710	.8516	39.21	37.04
.6	.75	2.000	(78, 55)	.1540	.8502	67.39	66.94	(88, 39)	.1786	.8505	65.75	61.74
	.8	2.667	(44, 30)	.1613	.8500	37.73	36.16	(46, 22)	.1607	.8513	35.47	34.26
.65	.8	2.154	(74, 43)	.1673	.8501	59.89	58.62	(77, 39)	.1730	.8506	59.79	56.59
	.85	3.051	(42, 21)	.1633	.8510	32.85	32.39	(44, 18)	.1736	.8514	32.80	30.55
.7	.85	2.429	(65, 40)	.1571	.8511	53.71	53.85	(70, 30)	.1735	.8508	52.24	49.99
	.9	3.857	(35, 20)	.1442	.8527	28.53	28.74	(36, 16)	.1588	.8502	27.53	27.13
.75	.9	3.000	(56, 30)	.1641	.8502	44.54	43.05	(60, 24)	.1752	.8506	44.39	41.52
	.95	6.333	(29, 16)	.1497	.8527	23.56	23.41	(31, 13)	.1453	.8569	23.62	21.76
.8	.95	4.750	(43, 25)	.1603	.8502	35.27	33.35	(44, 20)	.1576	.8512	33.89	34.56
.85	.95	3.353	(78, 47)	.1626	.8503	64.29	61.83	(81, 37)	.1725	.8506	61.87	57.94

Table 8.19 Minimax and optimal two-stage designs with both interim futility and superiority tests for Fisher's exact test with $(\alpha^*, 1 - \beta^*) = (.2, .9)$

			Minimax Two-Stage Design					Optimal Two-Stage Design				
P_y	P_x	θ	n	α	$1-\beta$	EN_0	EN_1	(n, n_1)	α	$1-\beta$	EN_0	EN_1
.05	.15	3.353	(95, 58)	.1227	.9000	79.70	75.32	(97, 48)	.1260	.9005	77.18	70.78
	.2	4.750	(52, 27)	.1029	.9018	42.76	41.59	(53, 25)	.1071	.9004	42.82	37.99
	.25	6.333	(35, 16)	.0755	.9014	28.86	26.84	(35, 17)	.0756	.9030	29.07	26.51
.1	.25	3.000	(67, 45)	.1371	.9001	57.55	55.41	(71, 32)	.1427	.9005	54.78	50.00
	.3	3.857	(43, 25)	.1173	.9011	35.72	35.33	(46, 19)	.1275	.9017	35.47	31.18
.15	.3	2.429	(81, 52)	.1521	.9004	68.09	65.66	(86, 39)	.1580	.9011	65.48	60.68
	.35	3.051	(50, 28)	.1388	.9002	40.65	38.70	(52, 23)	.1424	.9011	39.90	37.06
.2	.35	2.154	(91, 55)	.1550	.9001	74.71	73.74	(97, 45)	.1636	.9000	73.73	69.70
	.4	2.667	(55, 32)	.1443	.9001	44.93	43.71	(61, 24)	.1580	.9006	45.17	40.98
.25	.4	2.000	(99, 81)	.1554	.9000	90.65	90.41	(109, 46)	.1690	.9000	80.52	75.14
	.45	2.455	(61, 36)	.1548	.9004	49.86	49.19	(63, 29)	.1595	.9007	48.05	44.76
.3	.45	1.909	(102, 79)	.1603	.9000	91.30	89.93	(106, 58)	.1665	.9002	83.94	81.18
	.5	2.333	(62, 44)	.1456	.9004	53.83	52.47	(68, 30)	.1645	.9015	51.13	46.85
.35	.5	1.857	(112, 63)	.1722	.9003	89.32	87.59	(120, 52)	.1766	.9003	88.78	84.24
	.55	2.270	(63, 43)	.1525	.9003	53.90	52.77	(65, 33)	.1605	.9005	50.64	48.57
.4	.55	1.833	(114, 62)	.1718	.9002	89.90	88.66	(114, 62)	.1718	.9002	89.90	88.66
	.6	2.250	(63, 47)	.1582	.9002	55.67	55.09	(65, 34)	.1679	.9008	51.03	48.48
.45	.6	1.833	(114, 62)	.1744	.9002	89.87	88.66	(114, 62)	.1744	.9002	89.87	88.66
	.65	2.270	(63, 43)	.1624	.9003	53.86	52.77	(65, 33)	.1708	.9005	50.57	48.57
.5	.65	1.857	(112, 63)	.1747	.9003	89.24	87.59	(120, 52)	.1774	.9003	88.65	84.24
	.7	2.333	(62, 44)	.1623	.9004	53.76	52.47	(68, 30)	.1723	.9015	50.95	46.85
.55	.7	1.909	(102, 79)	.1765	.9001	91.23	89.93	(106, 58)	.1674	.9002	83.78	81.18
	.75	2.455	(61, 36)	.1595	.9004	49.68	49.19	(63, 29)	.1638	.9007	47.78	44.76
.6	.75	2.000	(99, 80)	.1728	.9000	90.11	88.83	(110, 45)	.1738	.9003	80.28	75.92
	.8	2.667	(55, 32)	.1508	.9001	44.67	43.71	(61, 24)	.1738	.9006	44.66	40.98
.65	.8	2.154	(91, 55)	.1606	.9001	74.43	73.74	(97, 45)	.1757	.9000	73.29	69.70
	.85	3.051	(50, 28)	.1613	.9002	40.23	38.70	(52, 23)	.1633	.9011	39.28	37.06
.7	.85	2.429	(81, 52)	.1654	.9004	67.74	65.66	(86, 39)	.1730	.9011	64.81	60.68
	.9	3.857	(43, 25)	.1509	.9011	35.10	35.33	(46, 19)	.1710	.9017	34.40	31.18
.75	.9	3.000	(67, 45)	.1526	.9001	57.07	55.41	(71, 32)	.1702	.9005	53.74	50.00
	.95	6.333	(35, 16)	.1557	.9014	27.04	26.84	(38, 12)	.1537	.9024	27.44	25.89
.8	.95	4.750	(52, 27)	.1535	.9018	41.20	41.59	(53, 25)	.1670	.9004	40.98	37.99
.85	.95	3.353	(95, 58)	.1612	.9000	78.42	75.32	(97, 48)	.1690	.9005	75.30	70.78

- *Stage 2*: Accrue an additional m_2 patients to arm x and n_2 patients to arm y, and observe X_2 and Y_2. For $\hat{p}_x = X/m$, $\hat{p}_y = Y/n$, $\hat{q}_k = 1 - \hat{p}_k$, and $\hat{\theta} = (\hat{p}_x \hat{q}_y)/(\hat{q}_x \hat{p}_y)$,

  (a) Accept arm x for further investigation if $\hat{\theta} \geq a$.
  (b) Otherwise, reject arm x.

Given $Z_l = z_l$, X_l has probability mass function

$$f_l(x_l|z_l, \theta) = \frac{\binom{m_l}{x_l}\binom{n_l}{z_l - x_l}\theta^{x_l}}{\sum_{i=m_{l-}}^{m_{l+}} \binom{m_l}{i}\binom{n_l}{z_l - i}\theta^i}$$

for $m_{l-} \leq x_l \leq m_{l+}$, where $m_{l-} = \max(0, z_l - n_l)$ and $m_{l+} = \min(z_l, m_l)$. Let $\hat{\theta}_1 = \{x_1(n_1 - y_1)\}/\{y_1(m_1 - x_1)\}$ and $\hat{\theta} = \{x(n - y)\}/\{y(m - x)\}$ denote the estimates of θ after stage 1 and 2, respectively. Note that $\hat{\theta}_1 = \hat{\theta}_1(x_1)$ is a function of x_1 given z_1, and $\hat{\theta} = \hat{\theta}(x_1, x_2)$ is a function of (x_1, x_2) given (z_1, z_2). Given the type I error rate α^* and (m_1, m_2, z_1, z_2), we find a satisfying $\alpha(z_1, z_2) \leq \alpha^*$, where

$$\begin{aligned}
\alpha(z_1, z_2) &= P\{\hat{\theta}_1(X_1) \geq \theta_a | z_1, H_0\} + P\{1 < \hat{\theta}_1(X_1) < \theta_a, \hat{\theta}(X_1, X_2) \geq a | z_1, z_2, H_0\} \\
&= \sum_{x_1 = m_{1-}}^{m_{1+}} I\{\hat{\theta}_1(x_1) \geq \theta_a\} f_1(x_1 | z_1, 1) \\
&\quad + \sum_{x_1 = m_{1-}}^{m_{1+}} \sum_{x_2 = m_{2-}}^{m_{2+}} I\{1 < \hat{\theta}_1(x_1) < \theta_a, \hat{\theta}(x_1, x_2) \geq a\} f_1(x_1 | z_1, 1) f_2(x_2 | z_2, 1).
\end{aligned}$$

The conditional power of the two-stage design is calculated by

$$\begin{aligned}
1 - \beta(z_1, z_2) &= P\{\hat{\theta}_1(X_1) \geq \theta_a | z_1, H_a\} + P\{1 < \hat{\theta}_1(X_1) \\
&\quad < \theta_a, \hat{\theta}(X_1, X_2) \geq a | z_1, z_2, H_a\} \\
&= \sum_{x_1 = m_{1-}}^{m_{1+}} I\{\hat{\theta}_1(x_1) \geq \theta_a\} f_1(x_1 | z_1, \theta_a) + \sum_{x_1 = m_{1-}}^{m_{1+}} \sum_{x_2 = m_{2-}}^{m_{2+}} I\{1 < \hat{\theta}_1(x_1) \\
&\quad < \theta_a, \hat{\theta}(x_1, x_2) \geq a\} f_1(x_1 | z_1, \theta_a) f_2(x_2 | z_2, \theta_a).
\end{aligned}$$

Noting that Z_l is sum of two independent binomial random variables, X_l and Y_l, its probability mass function is give as

$$g_l(z_l) = \sum_{x_l = m_{l-}}^{m_{l+}} \binom{m_l}{x_l} p_x^{x_l} q_x^{m_l - x_l} \binom{n_l}{z_l - x_l} p_y^{z_l - x_l} q_y^{n_l - z_l + x_l}$$

for $z_l = 0, \ldots, m_l + n_l$. Under $H_0 : \theta = 1$, $g_l(z_l)$ is expressed as

$$g_{0l}(z_l) = \sum_{x_l=m_{l-}}^{m_{l+}} \binom{m_l}{x_l} \binom{n_l}{z_l - x_l} p_y^{z_l} q_y^{m_l + n_l - z_l}.$$

Hence, the marginal type I error rate and power of above two-stage design are calculated by

$$\alpha = \mathrm{E}\{\alpha(Z_1, Z_2)\} = \sum_{z_1=0}^{m_1+n_1} \sum_{z_2=0}^{m_2+n_2} \alpha(z_1, z_2) g_{01}(z_1) g_{02}(z_2)$$

and

$$1 - \beta = \mathrm{E}\{1 - \beta(Z_1, Z_2)\} = \sum_{z_1=0}^{m_1+n_1} \sum_{z_2=0}^{m_2+n_2} \{1 - \alpha(z_1, z_2)\} g_1(z_1) g_2(z_2),$$

respectively. Since $\alpha(z_1, z_2) \le \alpha^*$ for all (z_1, z_2), we have $\alpha \le \alpha^*$.

For a specified a type I error rate α^* and a power $1 - \beta^*$, we want to select a two-stage design satisfying $\alpha \le \alpha^*$ and $1 - \beta \le 1 - \beta^*$. When H_h ($h = 0, a$) is true, the probability of early termination and the expected sample size for arm x are calculated as

$$\mathrm{PET}_h = 1 - \mathrm{P}\{1 < \hat{\theta}_1(X_1) < \theta_a | z_1, H_h\}$$

and

$$\mathrm{EN}_h = m_1 \times \mathrm{PET}_h + m \times (1 - \mathrm{PET}_h),$$

respectively. Let $\mathrm{EN} = (\mathrm{EN}_0 + \mathrm{EN}_a)/2$ denote the average sample size for arm x. Among the two-stage designs satisfying the $(\alpha^*, 1 - \beta^*)$-restriction, the *optimal design* is defined as the one with the smallest EN.

The *minimax design* is defined as the one with the smallest m (or $m + n$) among the two-stage designs satisfying the $(\alpha^*, 1 - \beta^*)$-restriction.

8.3.2   Conditional P-Value

When a randomized phase II trial is completed, we usually report whether to accept or reject the experimental therapy, but not how significant the evidence supporting the decision was. Toward this effort, we propose to calculate a p-value conditioning on the total number of responders from each stage. If the study is stopped after stage 1, we calculate a p-value using the standard Fisher's exact test. If the study is continued to the second stage to observe (n_1, n_2, z_1, z_2) and (x_1, x_2), then a conditional p-value given (n_1, n_2, z_1, z_2) is calculated by

$$
\begin{aligned}
\text{p-value} &= P\{\hat{\theta}_1(X_1) \geq \theta_a | z_1, H_0\} + P\{1 < \hat{\theta}_1(X_1) < \theta_a, \hat{\theta}(X_1, X_2) \\
&\qquad \geq \hat{\theta}(x_1, x_2) | z_1, z_2, H_0\} \\
&= \sum_{i_1 = m_{1-}}^{m_{1+}} I\{\hat{\theta}_1(i_1) \geq \theta_a\} f_1(i_1 | z_1, 1) \\
&\quad + \sum_{i_1 = m_{1-}}^{m_{1+}} \sum_{i_2 = m_{2-}}^{m_{2+}} I\{1 < \hat{\theta}_1(i_1) < \theta_a, \hat{\theta}(i_1, i_2) \geq \hat{\theta}\} f_1(i_1 | z_1, 1) f_2(i_2 | z_2, 1),
\end{aligned}
$$

where $\hat{\theta} = \{x(n-y)\}/\{y(m-x)\}$.

This p-value calculation can be applied to the two-stage randomized phase II trial with an interim futility test only or with both futility and superiority tests. Often, the realized sample size may be different from the planned one due to various reasons. In this case, a p-value method can be very useful.

8.4 Discussions

A two-sample exact binomial test involves a nuisance parameter p_0, the common response rate for two arms under H_0. In order to remove the nuisance parameter in testing, we considered controlling the maximal type I error rate over $p_0 \in (0, 1)$ in Chapter 7, while we consider the Fisher's exact test by conditioning the null distribution of the test statistic on the sufficient statistic of p_0 in this chapter.

We compare the performance of our Fisher's test with that of binomial test with the strict type I error control. Figure 8.1 displays the type I error rate and power in the range of $0 < p_y < 1 - \Delta$ for single-stage designs with $n = 60$ per arm, $\Delta = p_x - p_y = 0.15$ or 0.2 under H_1, and $\alpha = 0.1, 0.15$, or 0.2 under $H_0 : p_x = p_y$. The solid lines are for Fisher's test, and the dotted lines are for binomial; the lower two lines represent type I error rate, and the upper two lines represent power. As is well known, Fisher's test controls the type I error rate conservatively over the range of p_y. The conservativeness gets slightly stronger with small p_y values close to 0. Binomial test controls the type I error rate accurately around $p_y = 0.5$, but becomes more conservative for p_y values far from 0.5, especially with small p_y values. For $\alpha = 0.1$, Fisher's test and binomial test have similar power around $0.2 \leq p_y \leq 0.4$ except that the binomial test is slightly more powerful for $p_y \approx 0.4$. Otherwise, Fisher's test is more powerful. The difference in power between the two methods becomes larger with $\Delta = 0.15$. We observe similar trends overall, but the difference in

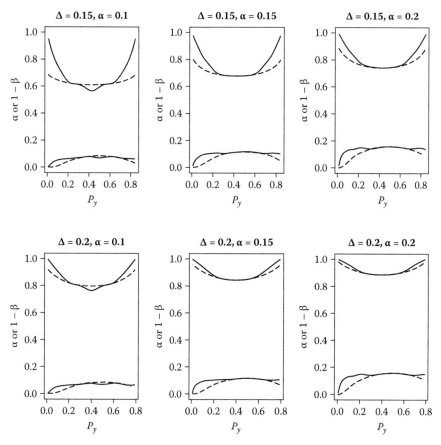

Figure 8.1 Single-stage designs with $n = 60$ per arm: Type I error rate and power for Fisher's test (solid lines) and binomial test (dotted lines).

power becomes smaller with $\Delta = 0.2$, especially when combined with a large $\alpha(= 0.2)$.

Figure 8.2 displays the type I error rate and power of two-stage designs with a futility test for $n_1 = n_2 = 30$ per arm. We observe that compared to binomial test, Fisher's test controls the type I error more accurately in most range of p_y values. If $\alpha = 0.1$, Fisher's test is more powerful than the binomial test over the whole range of p_y values. But with a larger α, such as 0.15 or 0.2, the binomial test is slightly more powerful for $p_y \approx 0.4$. As in the single-stage design case, the difference in power diminishes as Δ and α increase. Roughly speaking, Fisher exact test is recommended for single-stage trials over the binomial test, while the former is recommended over the latter only when the response rate of the control is lower than 30% or higher than 60%. But more accurate recommendation between the two tests under a design set can be made by comparing the sample sizes of the optimal designs for these tests.

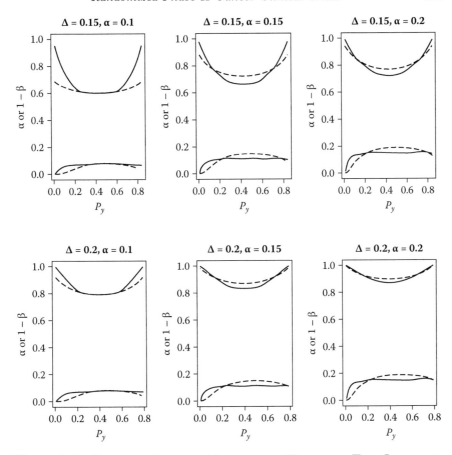

Figure 8.2 Two-stage designs with $n_1 = n_2 = 30$ per arm: Type I error rate and power for Fisher's test (solid lines) and binomial test (dotted lines).

References

Fisher, R.A. (1935). The logic of inductive inference (with discussion). *Journal of Royal Statistical Society*, 98, 39–82.

Jung, S.H., Lee, T.Y., Kim, K.M., and George, S. (2004). Admissible two-stage designs for phase II cancer clinical trials. *Statistics in Medicine*, 23, 561–569.

Simon, R. (1989). Optimal two-stage designs for phase II clinical trials. *Controlled Clinical Trials*, 10, 1–10.

Chapter 9

Randomized Phase II Trials with Heterogeneous Patient Populations: Stratified Fisher's Exact Test

Suppose that we want to compare the response rates between an experimental arm and a control arm. Often in a between-arm comparison, the characteristics of study patients may be heterogeneous. In this case, the heterogeneity is characterized by some known predictors, and a stratified method is applied to the final analysis. When the distribution of the stratification factors is identical between two arms, unstratified testing ignoring the population heterogeneity controls the type I error rate but loses statistical efficiency. If the distribution of the predictors is different between two arms, however, unstratified testing does not maintain the type I error rate accurately, which can be more serious than losing statistical efficiency. In order to balance the distribution of the factors, we usually randomize the patients by stratifying for the important predictors.

In this chapter, we consider randomized phase II clinical trials based on stratified Fisher's (1935) exact test for a binary endpoint. We investigate single-stage and two-stage designs for each test statistic.

9.1 Single-Stage Stratified Fisher's Exact Test

In this section, we consider single-stage randomized phase II trials. Suppose that there are J strata with different response rates. Let N denote the total sample size, and n_j the sample size in stratum j ($\sum_{j=1}^{J} n_j = N$). Among n_j patients in stratum $j (= 1, \ldots, J)$, m_{1j} are allocated to arm 1 (experimental) and m_{2j} to arm 2 (control), that is, $m_{1j} + m_{2j} = n_j$. For stratum j, arm $k (= 1, 2)$ has a response rate p_{kj}. Let $q_{kj} = 1 - p_{kj}$ and $\theta_j = p_{1j} q_{2j}/(q_{1j} p_{2j})$ denote the odds ratio in stratum j. Suppose that we want to test

$$H_0 : \theta_1 = \cdots = \theta_J = 1$$

against

$$H_1 : \theta_j \geq 1 \text{ for } j = 1, \ldots, J \text{ and } \theta_j > 1 \text{ for some } j = 1, \ldots, J.$$

For stratum $j(=1,\ldots,J)$, let x_j and y_j denote the numbers of responders for arms 1 and 2, respectively, and $z_j = x_j + y_j$ denote the total number of responders from the two arms. The frequency data in stratum j can be described as in Table 9.1.

Table 9.1 Frequency data of 2×2 table for stratum $j(=1,\ldots,J)$

Response	Arm		
	Experimental	Control	Total
Yes	x_j	y_j	z_j
No	$m_{1j} - x_j$	$m_{2j} - y_j$	$n_j - z_j$
Total	m_{1j}	m_{2j}	n_j

9.1.1 Statistical Testing

We reject H_0 in favor of H_1 if $S = \sum_{j=1}^{J} x_{1j}$ is large. Under H_0, conditioning on the margin totals (z_j, m_{1j}, n_j), x_j has the hypergeometric distribution

$$f_0(x_j | z_j, m_{1j}, n_j) = \frac{\binom{m_{1j}}{x_j}\binom{m_{2j}}{z_j - x_j}}{\sum_{i=m_{j-}}^{m_{j+}} \binom{m_j}{i}\binom{m_j}{z_j - i}}$$

for $m_{j-} \leq x_j \leq m_{j+}$, where $m_{j-} = \max(0, z_j - m_{2j})$ and $m_{j+} = \min(z_j, m_{1j})$. Let $\boldsymbol{z} = (z_1, \ldots, z_J)$, $\boldsymbol{m} = (m_{11}, \ldots, m_{1J})$, and $\boldsymbol{n} = (n_1, \ldots, n_J)$. Given $(\boldsymbol{z}, \boldsymbol{m}, \boldsymbol{n})$, the conditional p-value for an observed value of $s = \sum_{j=1}^{J} x_j$, pv = pv$(s|\boldsymbol{z}, \boldsymbol{m}, \boldsymbol{n})$, is obtained by

$$\text{pv} = P(S \geq s | \boldsymbol{z}, \boldsymbol{m}, \boldsymbol{n})$$

$$= \sum_{i_1 = m_{1-}}^{m_{1+}} \cdots \sum_{i_J = m_{J-}}^{m_{J+}} I\left(\sum_{j=1}^{J} i_j \geq s\right) \prod_{j=1}^{J} f_0(i_j | z_j, m_{1j}, n_j).$$

Given the type I error rate α^*, we reject H_0 if pv $< \alpha^*$.

Note that Mante–Haenszel (1959) test rejects H_0 in favor of H_1 for a large value of S, and its p-value is calculated using the standardized test statistic

$$W = \frac{S - E}{\sqrt{V}},$$

which is asymptotically $N(0,1)$ under H_0, where $E = \sum_{j=1}^{J} E_j$, $V = \sum_{j=1}^{J} V_j$, $E_j = z_j m_{1j}/n_j$, and $V_j = z_j m_{1j} m_{2j}(n_j - z_j)/\{n_j^2(n_j - 1)\}$. Westfall, Zaykin, and Young (2002) propose a permutation procedure for a stratified Mantel–Haenszel test, which permutes the two-sample binary data within each stratum in the context of multiple testing. Their permutation maintains the margin totals for 2×2 tables, $\{(z_j, m_{1j}, n_j), 1 \leq j \leq J\}$, and E_j and V_j depend on the margin totals only, so that the permutation-based Mantel–Haenszel test will be identical to our stratified Fisher's exact test if they go through all the possible $\prod_{j=1}^{J}(m_{j+} - m_{j-} + 1)$ permutations. In order to save computing time, a permutation test often randomly selects partial permutations to approximate the exact p-value. In this case, the resulting p-value approximated from partial permutations will be varying, depending on the selected seed number for random number generation or the number of permutations, while the exact method always provides a constant exact p-value for a given data set.

Example 9.1
Li et al. (1979) are interested in whether thymosin (experimental), compared to placebo (control), has any effect in the treatment of bronchogenic carcinoma patients receiving radiotherapy. Table 9.2 summarizes the data for three strata. The one-sided p-value to test if the experimental arm has a higher treatment effect is 0.1563 by the stratified Fisher's exact test.

Table 9.2 Response to thymosin in bronchogenic carcinoma patients (T = thymosin, P = placebo)

	Stratum 1			Stratum 2			Stratum 3		
	T	P	Total	T	P	Total	T	P	Total
Success	10	12	22	9	11	20	8	7	15
Failure	1	1	2	0	1	1	0	3	3
Total	11	13	24	9	12	21	8	10	18

9.1.2 Power and Sample Size Calculation

Jung et al. (2007) propose a sample size calculation method for the Mantel–Haenszel test. In this section, we derive a sample size formula for the stratified Fisher's exact test by specifying the values of the same input parameters as those for Mantel–Haenszel test by Jung et al. (2007). The following are input parameters to be specified for a sample size calculation.

Input Parameters

- Type I and II error rate and power: $(\alpha^*, 1 - \beta^*)$
- Response rates for arm 2 (control): $(p_{21}, \dots, p_{2J})$
- Odds ratios: $(\theta_1, \dots, \theta_J)$ under H_1, where $\theta_j > 0$. Note that, given p_{2j} and θ_j, we have $p_{1j} = \theta_j p_{2j}/(q_{2j} + \theta_j p_{2j})$ for stratum $j(= 1, \dots, J)$.

- Prevalence for each stratum: $(\eta_1, \dots, \eta_J)$, where $\eta_j = E(n_j/N)$. Note that $\eta_j > 0$ and $\sum_{j=1}^{J} \eta_j = 1$.
- Allocation proportion for arm 1 (experimental) within each stratum, $\gamma = m_{1j}/n_j$, with $0 < \gamma < 1$.

In a randomized phase II trial with the total sample size N prespecified at the design stage, $\{(x_j, z_j, n_j), 1 \leq j \leq J\}$ are random variables with following marginal and conditional probability mass functions that are indexed by the above input parameters. Note that given n_j, $m_{1j} = \gamma n_j$ and $m_{2j} = (1 - \gamma)n_j$ are fixed at the design stage, although they may be considered to be random at the data analysis.

Distribution Functions

- Conditional distribution of x_j given (z_j, n_j):

$$f_j(x_j|z_j, n_j) = \frac{\binom{m_{1j}}{x_j}\binom{m_{2j}}{z_j - x_j}\theta_j^{x_j}}{\sum_{i=m_{j-}}^{m_{j+}}\binom{m_{1j}}{i}\binom{m_{2j}}{z_j - i}\theta_j^{i}}$$

  for $m_{j-} \leq x_j \leq m_{j+}$, where $m_{j-} = \max(0, z_j - m_{2j})$, $m_{j+} = \min(z_j, m_{1j})$, and $j = 1, \dots, J$. Under H_0, this is simplified to $f_0(x_j|z_j, n_j) = f_0(x_j|z_j, m_{1j}, n_j)$.

- Conditional distribution of z_j given n_j:
  Given n_j, $x_j \sim B(m_{1j}, p_{1j})$ and $y_j \sim B(m_{2j}, p_{2j})$ are independent, so that the conditional probability mass function of $z_j = x_j + y_j$ is expressed as

$$g_j(z_j|n_j) = \sum_{x=m_{j-}}^{m_{j+}}\binom{m_{1j}}{x}p_{1j}^x q_{1j}^{m_{1j}-x}\binom{m_{2j}}{z_j - x}p_{2j}^{z_j - x}q_{2j}^{m_{2j}-z_j+x}$$

  for $z_j = 0, 1, \dots, n_j$ and $j = 1, \dots, J$, where $q_{kj} = 1 - p_{kj}$ and $B(m, p)$ denote the binomial distribution with number of trials m and success probability p. Under H_0, this is simplified to

$$g_{0j}(z_j|n_j) = p_{2j}^{z_j} q_{2j}^{n_j - z_j} \sum_{x=m_{j-}}^{m_{j+}}\binom{m_{1j}}{x}\binom{m_{2j}}{z_j - x}.$$

  Note that $\binom{0}{0}p^0(1 - p)^0 = 1$ for $p \in (0, 1)$.

- Conditional distribution of $(n_1, \dots, n_J)$ given N is multinomial with probability mass function

$$l_N(n_1, \dots, n_J) = \frac{N!}{\prod_{j=1}^{J} n_j!} \prod_{j=1}^{J} \eta_j^{n_j}$$

  for $0 \leq n_1 \leq N, \dots, 0 \leq n_J \leq N$ and $\sum_{j=1}^{J} n_j = N$.

We first derive the power function for a given sample size N using these distribution functions. Let $z = (z_1, \ldots, z_J)$ and $n = (n_1, \ldots, n_J)$. Given (z, n) and type I error rate α^*, the critical value $a_{\alpha^*} = a_{\alpha^*}(z, n)$ is the smallest integer a satisfying

$$P(S \geq a | z, n, H_0) = \sum_{i_1=m_{1-}}^{m_{1+}} \cdots \sum_{i_J=m_{J-}}^{m_{J+}} I\left(\sum_{j=1}^{J} i_j \geq a\right) \prod_{j=1}^{J} f_0(i_j | z_j, n_j) \leq \alpha^*.$$

Note that $s \geq a_{\alpha^*}(z, n)$ if and only if $\mathrm{pv}(s | z, m, n) \leq \alpha^*$. We call $\alpha(z, n) = P(S \geq a_{\alpha^*} | z, n, H_0)$ the conditional type I error rate given (z, n). Similarly, the conditional power $1 - \beta(z, n)$ given (z, n) is obtained by

$$P(S \geq a_{\alpha^*} | z, n, H_1) = \sum_{i_1=m_{1-}}^{m_{1+}} \cdots \sum_{i_J=m_{J-}}^{m_{J+}} I\left(\sum_{j=1}^{J} i_j \geq a_{\alpha^*}\right) \prod_{j=1}^{J} f_j(i_j | z_j, n_j).$$

For a chosen N, the marginal type I error rate and power are given as

$$\alpha_N \equiv E\{\alpha(z, n) | H_0\} = E^n[E^z\{\alpha(z, n) | n, H_0\} | n]$$

$$= \sum_{n \in \mathcal{D}_N} \sum_{z_1=m_{1-}}^{m_{1+}} \cdots \sum_{z_J=m_{J-}}^{m_{J+}} \alpha(z_1, \ldots, z_J; n_1, \ldots, n_J)$$

$$\times \left\{\prod_{j=1}^{J} g_{0j}(z_j | n_j)\right\} l_N(n_1, \ldots, n_J)$$

and

$$1 - \beta_N \equiv E\{1 - \beta(z, n) | H_1\} = E^n[E^z\{\alpha(z, n) | n, H_1\} | n]$$

$$= \sum_{n \in \mathcal{D}_N} \sum_{z_1=m_{1-}}^{m_{1+}} \cdots \sum_{z_J=m_{J-}}^{m_{J+}} \{1 - \beta(z_1, \ldots, z_J; n_1, \ldots, n_J)\}$$

$$\times \left\{\prod_{j=1}^{J} g_j(z_j | n_j)\right\} l_N(n_1, \ldots, n_J),$$

respectively, where $\mathcal{D}_N = \{(n_1, \ldots, n_J) : 0 \leq n_1 \leq N, \ldots, 0 \leq n_J \leq N, \sum_{j=1}^{J} n_j = N\}$ and $E^z(\cdot)$ denotes the expected value with respect to a random vector z.

Since $\alpha(z, n) \leq \alpha^*$ for all (z, n), we have $\alpha_N \leq \alpha^*$. Given power $1 - \beta^*$, the required sample size is chosen by the smallest integer N satisfying $1 - \beta_N \geq 1 - \beta^*$. In other words, while the statistical testing controls the conditional type I error $\alpha(z, n)$ below α^*, the sample size is determined to guarantee a specified level of marginal power. In summary, a sample size is calculated as follows.

Sample Size Calculation

(A) Specify input parameters: J, $(\alpha^*, 1 - \beta^*)$, $(p_{21}, \ldots, p_{2J})$, $(\theta_1, \ldots, \theta_J)$, $(\eta_1, \ldots, \eta_J)$, γ.

(B) Starting from the sample size for Mantel–Haenszel test N_{MH}, do the following by increasing N by 1,

    (B1) For $j = 1, \ldots, J$, $z_j \in [0, n_j]$, $n_j \in [0, N]$, and $\sum_{j=1}^{J} n_j = N$,

        (i) Find $a_{\alpha^*} = a_{\alpha^*}(z, n)$.

        (ii) Calculate $1 - \beta(z, n) = P(S \geq a_{\alpha^*} | z, n, H_1)$.

    (B2) Calculate $1 - \beta_N = E\{1 - \beta(z, n) | H_1\}$.

(C) Stop (B) if $1 - \beta_N \geq 1 - \beta^*$. This N is the required sample size.

9.1.3 Numerical Studies

We want to compare the small sample performance of the stratified Fisher's test and Mantel–Haenszel tests using simulations. In order to consider unequal allocations among strata, let $y_j = n_j/N$. We generate $B = 10,000$ simulation samples of size $N = 25$, 50, or 75 with $J = 2$ strata under $\eta_1 = 0.25$, 0.5, or 0.75; $(\gamma_1, \gamma_2) = (1/4, 3/4)$, $(1/2, 1/2)$, or $(3/4, 1/4)$; $p_{21} = 0.1$, $p_{22} = 0.3$, or 0.7; $(\theta_1, \theta_2) = (1, 1)$, $(5, 10)$, $(7.5, 7.5)$, or $(10, 5)$. The stratified Fisher's test, standard (unstratified) Fisher's test, and Mantel–Haenszel test are applied to each simulation sample, and the empirical power for each test is calculated as the proportion of simulation samples rejecting H_0 with one-sided $\alpha^* = 0.05$. The exact type I error rate and power for the stratified Fisher's test can be calculated by using the methods in Section 9.1.2, but through simulations we want to compare the performance of the these testing methods applied to the same data sets. We consider large odds ratios to investigate the performance of Fisher's tests and the Mantel–Haenszel test with small sample sizes.

Table 9.3 summarizes the simulation results. With 10,000 simulations and $\alpha^* = 0.05$, the 95% confidence limits for the empirical type I error rate are 0.05 ± 0.004. Because of the discreteness of the exact tests and the conservative control of the conditional type I error at all possible outcomes, the stratified Fisher's test is always conservative as expected, especially with a small sample size ($N = 25$). The unstratified test has a similar type I error rate to stratified Fisher's test when allocation proportions are identical between two strata (i.e., $\gamma_1 = \gamma_2$). However, if more patients are allocated in the stratum with higher response rates (that is, $\gamma_1 = 1/4$ and $\gamma_2 = 3/4$), then the unstratified Fisher's test becomes anticonservative. On the other hand, if more patients are allocated to the stratum with smaller response rates (that is, $\gamma_1 = 3/4$ and $\gamma_2 = 1/4$), then the unstratified Fisher's test becomes very conservative. In this sense, testing ignoring the strata can be biased unless the allocation proportions are identical across strata. With $N = 25$ or 50, the

Mantel–Haenszel test is anticonservative with $p_{22} = 0.7$ (that is, when two strata have very different response rates) or with $\eta_1 = 0.75$ (that is, when a small number of subjects are allocated to the stratum with large response probabilities). The anticonservativeness diminishes as N increases but is still of some issue with $\eta_1 = 0.75$ and $N = 75$.

When allocation proportions are equal across the strata, ignoring the strata results in a slight loss of statistical power. The stratified Fisher's test is less powerful than the Mantel–Haenszel test, but the difference in power decreases in N. For all three testing methods, the power increases when more patients are allocated to the stratum with the larger odds ratio, e.g., $\theta_1 < \theta_2$ and $\eta_1 < 1/2$.

Table 9.4 reports the sample sizes for the Mantel–Haenszel test and stratified Fisher's test. Also reported are sample sizes for the stratified Fisher's test by fixing (m, n) or only n at their expected values. The design parameters are set at one-sided $\alpha^* = 0.05$; $1 - \beta^* = 0.9$; $J = 2$ strata; $\gamma = 0.25, 0.5,$ or 0.75; $(\eta_1, \eta_2) = (0.25, 0.25), (0.25, 0.75), (0.5, 0.5), (0.75, 0.25),$ or $(0.75, 0.75)$; $(p_{21}, p_{22}) = (0.1, 0.3)$; $(\theta_1, \theta_2) = (5, 10), (7.5, 7.5),$ or $(10, 5)$. For the stratified Fisher's test, fixing (m, n) at their expected values reduces N, while fixing only n requires almost the same N compared to the case with random (m, n). The sample sizes are minimized with a balanced allocation, that is, $\gamma = 1/2$. We also observe that the cases of (η_1, η_2), $(1 - \eta_1, \eta_2)$, $(\eta_1, 1 - \eta_2)$, and $(1 - \eta_1, 1 - \eta_2)$ require similar sample sizes. That is, when the allocation between two arms is unbalanced, the required sample size does not much depend on whether the larger arm is control or experimental across the different strata.

Under each setting, the sample size for the stratified Fisher's test is about 30% larger than that of the Mantel–Haenszel test. This difference results from the conservative type I error and power control of the stratified Fisher's test. For example, from Table 9.3, with $(\gamma, \eta_1, \eta_2, p_{21}, p_{22}) = (0.5, 0.25, 0.75, 0.1, 0.3)$, the stratified Fisher's test controls the type I error at 0.0230 with $N = 75$ and has a power of 0.9042 at $(\theta_1, \theta_2) = (5, 10)$. Under this design setting, the stratified Fisher's test requires a sample size of size of $N = 75$ with $(\alpha^*, 1 - \beta^*) = (0.05, 0.9)$ from Table 9.4. For the Mantel–Haenszel test, the required sample size with $(\alpha^*, 1 - \beta^*) = (0.0230, 0.9042)$ under the same design setting is $N = 73$, which is close to $N = 75$ required for the stratified Fisher's test. In other words, the conservativeness of the Fisher test results from the discreteness of the exact testing distributions. The Mantel–Haenszel test approximates this exact distribution when the sample size is large. Crans and Schuster (2008) propose to conduct Fisher's test with a larger type I error $\alpha^* = \alpha + \epsilon$ $(\epsilon > 0)$ so that the maximal marginal type I error rate within the whole range $[0, 1]$ of the response probability under H_0 becomes close to the intended α level.

Suppose that we want to design a study similar to that of Li et al. (1979). Since this is a balanced randomization study, we fix (n_1, n_2, n_3) at $(N/3, N/3, N/3)$ and (m_1, m_2, m_3) at $(N/6, N/6, N/6)$. We further assume that

Table 9.3 Empirical power of stratified Fisher's test/unstratified Fisher's test/Mantel–Haenszel test with one-sided $\alpha^* = 0.05$, $J = 2$ strata, and $p_{21} = 0.1$

γ	(η_1, η_2)	p_{22}	$(\theta_1, \theta_2) = (1, 1)$	$(5, 10)$	$(7.5, 7.5)$	$(10, 5)$
(a) $N = 25$						
.25	(1/4, 3/4)	.3	.0094/.0354/.0370	.4812/.7864/.6809	.4305/.7230/.6332	.3470/.5989/.5387
		.7	.0149/.1785/.0572	.2464/.7160/.5062	.2556/.7143/.5011	.2395/.6782/.4642
	(1/2, 1/2)	.3	.0179/.0176/.0522	.6164/.5878/.7595	.5764/.5762/.7179	.4668/.4855/.6261
		.7	.0161/.0189/.0493	.2608/.2398/.5003	.2909/.2693/.5202	.2803/.2671/.4854
	(3/4, 1/4)	.3	.0171/.0055/.0599	.4447/.2817/.6448	.4061/.3229/.6053	.3354/.3220/.5223
		.7	.0059/.0007/.0314	.0847/.0211/.2523	.1073/.0354/.2934	.1192/.0435/.3024
.5	(1/4, 3/4)	.3	.0101/.0560/.0476	.3750/.7984/.5898	.4091/.7852/.6219	.3862/.7073/.5919
		.7	.0157/.2987/.0668	.2285/.8140/.4737	.2847/.8356/.5371	.3156/.8318/.5563
	(1/2, 1/2)	.3	.0118/.0120/.0455	.4852/.4608/.6653	.5366/.5253/.6958	.5055/.5131/.6689
		.7	.0164/.0210/.0507	.2564/.2177/.4796	.3441/.2914/.5603	.3980/.3447/.6036
	(3/4, 1/4)	.3	.0130/.0032/.0542	.3260/.1740/.5389	.3627/.2698/.5717	.3467/.3266/.5583
		.7	.0052/.0001/.0255	.0951/.0146/.2684	.1547/.0308/.3673	.2019/.0511/.4286
.75	(1/4, 3/4)	.3	.0096/.0380/.0564	.2830/.6508/.5041	.3815/.6876/.5959	.4382/.6830/.6485
		.7	.0125/.2124/.0669	.2238/.6819/.4463	.3325/.7500/.5620	.4054/.7967/.6364
	(1/2, 1/2)	.3	.0104/.0106/.0425	.3572/.3681/.5478	.4739/.4814/.6543	.5553/.5570/.7143
		.7	.0097/.0166/.0478	.2514/.2274/.4532	.3981/.3510/.5950	.5014/.4460/.6863
	(3/4, 1/4)	.3	.0033/.0009/.0321	.1904/.1315/.3921	.2896/.2468/.5013	.3479/.3443/.5649
		.7	.0019/.0004/.0162	.0999/.0258/.2703	.1980/.0592/.4100	.2937/.1077/.5202
(b) $N = 50$						
.25	(1/4, 3/4)	.3	.0188/.0808/.0419	.8271/.9837/.9073	.7918/.9713/.8816	.6851/.9156/.7950
		.7	.0228/.3873/.0525	.5607/.9696/.7422	.5702/.9702/.7431	.5318/.9555/.7115
	(1/2, 1/2)	.3	.0287/.0272/.0540	.9343/.9174/.9657	.9064/.8958/.9463	.8343/.8353/.8983
		.7	.0219/.0278/.0460	.6610/.5045/.7930	.6856/.5609/.8058	.6426/.5581/.7657
	(3/4, 1/4)	.3	.0248/.0051/.0546	.8273/.5754/.9048	.7890/.6340/.8734	.6789/.6166/.7898
		.7	.0170/.0002/.0473	.4361/.0335/.6240	.4653/.0614/.6427	.4568/.0870/.6180

Table 9.3 Empirical power of stratified Fisher's test/unstratified Fisher's test/Mantel–Haenszel test with one-sided $\alpha^* = 0.05$, $J = 2$ strata, and $p_{21} = 0.1$ (continued)

γ	(η_1, η_2)	p_{22}	$(\theta_1, \theta_2) = (1, 1)$	$(5, 10)$	$(7.5, 7.5)$	$(10, 5)$
.5	(1/4, 3/4)	.3	.0192/.1345/.0522	.7341/.9864/.8457	.7670/.9848/.8652	.7416/.9670/.8373
		.7	.0229/.6002/.0586	.5288/.9872/.7099	.6113/.9911/.7734	.6658/.9930/.8047
	(1/2, 1/2)	.3	.0208/.0212/.0498	.8547/.8247/.9174	.8818/.8670/.9344	.8610/.8560/.9173
		.7	.0243/.0289/.0527	.6250/.4701/.7606	.7359/.5956/.8400	.7785/.6685/.8656
	(3/4, 1/4)	.3	.0199/.0014/.0507	.7192/.3740/.8281	.7542/.5538/.8476	.7333/.6580/.8377
		.7	.0142/.0000/.0413	.4254/.0163/.5971	.5495/.0442/.7021	.6067/.0854/.7388
.75	(1/4, 3/4)	.3	.0181/.1024/.0550	.6018/.9394/.7492	.7407/.9580/.8486	.7877/.9579/.8821
		.7	.0197/.4640/.0624	.4961/.9534/.6698	.6632/.9773/.8036	.7632/.9863/.8708
	(1/2, 1/2)	.3	.0208/.0211/.0525	.7304/.7025/.8277	.8521/.8385/.9153	.8978/.8935/.9425
		.7	.0206/.0250/.0521	.6033/.4931/.7383	.7891/.6826/.8764	.8757/.7958/.9325
	(3/4, 1/4)	.3	.0142/.0016/.0458	.5771/.3242/.7119	.7015/.5407/.8109	.7597/.6874/.8567
		.7	.0083/.0000/.0321	.4141/.0343/.5740	.6104/.1125/.7415	.7184/.2060/.8282

(c) $N = 75$

γ	(η_1, η_2)	p_{22}	$(\theta_1, \theta_2) = (1, 1)$	$(5, 10)$	$(7.5, 7.5)$	$(10, 5)$
.25	(1/4, 3/4)	.3	.0250/.1274/.0474	.9552/.9995/.9779	.9335/.9980/.9639	.8760/.9887/.9250
		.7	.0279/.5583/.0554	.7572/.9975/.8654	.7694/.9969/.8714	.7293/.9949/.8366
	(1/2, 1/2)	.3	.0262/.0279/.0472	.9917/.9872/.9961	.9844/.9806/.9919	.9561/.9538/.9726
		.7	.0291/.0316/.0519	.8660/.7010/.9223	.8730/.7500/.9236	.8442/.7538/.8998
	(3/4, 1/4)	.3	.0249/.0028/.0559	.9545/.7684/.9761	.9339/.8248/.9646	.8701/.8162/.9197
		.7	.0235/.0001/.0467	.7096/.0394/.8142	.7305/.0862/.8230	.7008/.1235/.7999
.5	(1/4, 3/4)	.3	.0230/.1274/.0472	.9042/.9993/.9472	.9214/.9995/.9586	.9059/.9976/.9490
		.7	.0266/.7866/.0547	.7246/.9999/.8375	.8066/.9996/.8946	.8395/.9999/.9145
	(1/2, 1/2)	.3	.0245/.0258/.0498	.9660/.9506/.9818	.9768/.9694/.9873	.9686/.9661/.9812
		.7	.0280/.0307/.0544	.8388/.6587/.9044	.9096/.7792/.9496	.9294/.8395/.9611
	(3/4, 1/4)	.3	.0234/.0013/.0487	.8984/.5448/.9407	.9153/.7408/.9519	.9025/.8300/.9408
		.7	.0212/.0000/.0477	.6646/.0130/.7738	.7788/.0473/.8618	.8244/.1121/.8891
.75	(1/4, 3/4)	.3	.0238/.1521/.0543	.8057/.9919/.8838	.9024/.9964/.9468	.9277/.9967/.9627
		.7	.0238/.6531/.0567	.6984/.9953/.8135	.8531/.9983/.9209	.9172/.9990/.9576
	(1/2, 1/2)	.3	.0236/.0237/.0491	.9092/.8914/.9491	.9672/.9591/.9837	.9830/.9786/.9907
		.7	.0249/.0317/.0527	.8070/.6657/.8778	.9352/.8521/.9631	.9751/.9312/.9873
	(3/4, 1/4)	.3	.0193/.0016/.0469	.7965/.4821/.8670	.8917/.7363/.9323	.9260/.8699/.9581
		.7	.0171/.0000/.0413	.6444/.0400/.7582	.8299/.1583/.8996	.9038/.3032/.9475

Table 9.4   Sample size for Mantel–Haenszel test/stratified Fisher's test with (m, n) fixed/stratified Fisher's test with n fixed/stratified Fisher's test under $J = 2$ strata, $(p_{21}, p_{22}) = (0.1, 0.3)$, one-sided $\alpha^* = 0.05$, and $1 - \beta^* = 0.9$

		(θ_1, θ_2)		
γ	(η_1, η_2)	**(5, 10)**	**(7.5, 7.5)**	**(10, 5)**
0.25	(0.25, 0.25)	46/59/61/61	51/64/66/66	65/80/82/82
	(0.25, 0.75)	45/53/60/61	50/62/66/66	65/79/82/82
	(0.5, 0.5)	36/43/45/45	39/48/49/49	50/59/62/62
	(0.75, 0.25)	46/59/61/61	51/64/66/67	65/80/83/83
	(0.75, 0.75)	46/53/60/61	51/60/66/66	65/76/83/83
0.5	(0.25, 0.25)	58/72/75/76	55/72/72/71	58/72/75/75
	(0.25, 0.75)	58/65/75/75	54/65/70/71	58/72/75/75
	(0.5, 0.5)	45/53/56/54	43/50/53/53	45/54/56/56
	(0.75, 0.25)	59/72/75/76	56/66/71/71	59/72/76/78
	(0.75, 0.75)	59/69/75/76	55/63/71/71	59/68/76/76
0.75	(0.25, 0.25)	78/96/97/98	59/75/76/76	52/64/67/67
	(0.25, 0.75)	77/89/97/97	59/69/76/76	52/64/67/67
	(0.5, 0.5)	61/70/73/73	47/55/57/57	41/49/51/51
	(0.75, 0.25)	80/96/98/99	61/75/77/77	53/65/69/69
	(0.75, 0.75)	80/85/98/99	61/69/77/77	53/62/69/69

$(p_{21}, p_{22}, p_{23}) = (0.9, 0.75, 0.6)$, and $(\theta_1, \theta_2, \theta_3) = (1, 30, 30)$. (The estimates from Table 9.2 are $\hat{\theta}_1 = 0.833$ and $\hat{\theta}_2 = \hat{\theta}_3 = \infty$.) In order to control the one-sided conditional type I error at $\alpha^* = 0.1$ and the marginal power at $1 - \beta^* = 0.9$, we need $N = 83$. Under the design, this sample size provides marginal $\alpha_N = 0.0625$ and power $1 - \beta_N = 0.9087$.

9.1.4   Discussions

Numerous testing methods have been proposed to test on two binomial proportions adjusting for the stratum effect based on different assumptions. For example, the Cochran (1954) test assumes common odds ratios across strata, and Gart (1985) assumes common relative risks. The Mantel–Haenszel test makes no assumption about the parameters. These methods are based on large sample theories, so that their testing results may be distorted with a small sample size or sparse data.

In this chapter, we propose to use an exact test extending Fisher's test to the analysis of many 2×2 tables together with its sample size calculation method for designing and analyzing randomized phase II trials with heterogeneous patient populations. This test does not make any assumptions of large sample size or equal parameter values across strata, so that it does not require checking any assumptions before testing. The power and sample sizes are compared between the exact test and the Mantel–Haenszel test using simulations and the proposed sample size formulas. While the type I error rate for the Mantel–Haenszel test can be anticonservative with a small sample size or sparse data, the exact test always controls the type I error rate below a specified level. When the effect size is so large that the required sample size is small (say, about $N = 70$ or smaller), the exact test needs about 20% to 30% larger sample size than the Mantel–Haenszel test. However, because of the small sample sizes, the increase in sample size in this case is not very large in absolute number (say, 10 to 20), so that for robustness of the testing results, we propose to use the exact test by slightly increasing the sample size rather than obtaining a biased result with an asymptotic test.

If $J \geq 3$, the sample size calculation for the stratified Fisher's test requires a long computing time. We found, in calculating the marginal type I error rate and power, that fixing the sizes of strata $(n_1, \ldots, n_J)$ at their expected numbers provides very accurate sample sizes for the stratified Fisher's test even when $(n_1, \ldots, n_J)$ are random, while drastically saving the computing time.

9.2   Two-Stage Designs with an Interim Futility Test

In this section, we consider two-stage randomized phase II clinical trials, so that we can stop the trial early when the experimental arm is shown to be inefficacious compared to the control. At stage $l(= 1, 2)$, N_l patients are randomized between two arms stratified for J strata. Let $N = N_1 + N_2$ denote the maximal sample size, and, for stage l, n_{lj} the sample size in stratum j ($\sum_{j=1}^{J} n_{lj} = N_l$). Among n_{lj} patients in stratum $j(= 1, \ldots, J)$, m_{1lj} are allocated to arm 1 (experimental) and m_{2lj} to arm 2 (control). For stratum j during stage l, let x_{lj} and y_{lj} denote the numbers of responders for arms 1 and 2, respectively, and $z_{lj} = x_{lj} + y_{lj}$ the total number of responders from the two arms. The frequency data in stratum j at stage l can be described as in Table 9.5.

Table 9.5   Frequencies (and response probabilities) of stratum $j(= 1, \ldots, J)$ at stage $l(= 1, 2)$

		Arm 1	Arm 2	Total
Response	Yes	$x_{lj}\ (p_{1j})$	$y_{lj}\ (p_{2j})$	z_{lj}
	No	$m_{1lj} - x_{lj}\ (q_{1j})$	$m_{2lj} - y_{lj}\ (q_{2j})$	$n_{lj} - z_{lj}$
	Total	m_{1lj}	m_{2lj}	n_{lj}

In a two-stage randomized phase II trial with stage l sample size N_l prespecified, $\{(x_{lj}, z_{lj}, n_{lj}), 1 \leq j \leq J\}$ are random variables with the following marginal and conditional probability mass functions. Note that given n_{lj},

$m_{1lj} = \gamma n_{lj}$, and $m_{2lj} = (1 - \gamma)n_{lj}$ are fixed at the design stage, although they may be random at the data analysis.

Distribution Functions

- Conditional distribution of x_{lj} given (z_{lj}, n_{lj}):

$$f_j(x_{lj}|z_{lj}, n_{lj}) = \frac{\binom{m_{1lj}}{x_{lj}}\binom{m_{2lj}}{z_{lj}-x_{lj}}\theta_j^{x_{lj}}}{\sum_{i=m_{lj-}}^{m_{lj+}}\binom{m_{1lj}}{i}\binom{m_{2lj}}{z_{lj}-i}\theta_j^{i}}$$

for $m_{lj-} \leq x_{lj} \leq m_{lj+}$, where $m_{lj-} = \max(0, z_{lj} - m_{2lj})$, $m_{lj+} = \min(z_{lj}, m_{1lj})$, and $j = 1, \ldots, J$. Under H_0, this is simplified to

$$f_0(x_{lj}|z_{lj}, n_{lj}) = \frac{\binom{m_{1lj}}{x_{lj}}\binom{m_{2lj}}{z_{lj}-x_{lj}}}{\sum_{i=m_{lj-}}^{m_{lj+}}\binom{m_{1lj}}{i}\binom{m_{2lj}}{z_{lj}-i}}.$$

- Conditional distribution of z_{lj} given n_{lj}:
  Given n_{lj}, $x_{1lj} \sim B(m_{1lj}, p_{1j})$ and $y_{lj} \sim B(m_{2lj}, p_{2j})$ are independent, so that the conditional probability mass function of $z_{lj} = x_{lj} + y_{lj}$ is expressed as

$$g_j(z_{lj}|m_{1lj}, n_{lj}) = \sum_{x=m_{lj-}}^{m_{lj+}} \binom{m_{1lj}}{x} p_{1j}^x q_{1j}^{m_{1lj}-x} \binom{m_{2lj}}{z_{lj}-x} p_{2j}^{z_{lj}-x} q_{2j}^{m_{2kj}-z_{lj}+x}$$

for $z_{lj} = 0, 1, \ldots, n_{lj}$ and $j = 1, \ldots, J$. Under H_0, this is simplified to

$$g_{0j}(z_{lj}|n_{lj}) = p_{2j}^{z_{lj}} q_{2j}^{n_{lj}-z_{lj}} \sum_{x=m_{lj-}}^{m_{lj+}} \binom{m_{1lj}}{x} \binom{m_{2lj}}{z_{lj}-x}.$$

- We assume that, within each stratum, patients are randomized to arm 1 with probability γ, that is, $m_{1lj}/n_{lj} = \gamma$.

- Let η_j denote the prevalence of stratum j ($\sum_{j=1}^{J} \eta_j = 1$). At stage l, the conditional distribution of $(n_{l1}, \ldots, n_{lJ})$ given the stage l sample size $N_l = \sum_{j=1}^{J} n_{lj}$ is multinomial with probability mass function

$$h(n_{l1}, \ldots, n_{lJ}|N_l) = \frac{N_l!}{\prod_{j=1}^{J} n_{lj}!} \prod_{j=1}^{J} \eta_j^{n_{lj}}$$

for $0 \leq n_{l1} \leq N_l, \ldots, 0 \leq n_{lJ} \leq N_l$ and $\sum_{j=1}^{J} n_{lj} = N_l$.

Let $S_l = \sum_{j=1}^{J} x_{lj}$ and $S = S_1 + S_2$. A two-stage randomized phase II trial with a futility rejection value a_1 and the second-stage rejection value a are chosen conditional on $\{(z_{lj}, n_{lj}), l = 1, 2, j = 1, \ldots, J\}$ is conducted as follows.

Stage 1: Recruit N_1 patients, of which $N_{11} = \gamma N_1$ are randomized to arm 1 and $N_{21} = (1-\gamma)N_1$ are randomized to arm 2; observe $\{(x_{1j}, z_{1j}), j = 1, \ldots, J\}$ together with $(n_{1j}, j = 1, \ldots, J)$.

    a. Given $\{(z_{1j}, n_{1j}), j = 1, \ldots, J\}$, find a stopping value a_1.
    b. If $S_1 \geq a_1$, proceed to stage 2.
    c. Otherwise, reject the experimental therapy (arm 1) and stop the trial.

Stage 2: Recruit N_2 patients, of which $N_{12} = \gamma N_2$ patients are randomized to arm 1 and $N_{22} = (1 - \gamma)N_2$ patients are randomized to arm 2; observe $\{(x_{2j}, z_{2j}), j = 1, \ldots, J\}$ together with $(n_{2j}, j = 1, \ldots, J)$.

    a. Given $\{(z_{lj}, n_{lj}), l = 1, 2; j = 1, \ldots, J\}$, find a rejection value a.
    b. Accept the experimental arm for further investigation if $S \geq a$.

Given the type I error rate α^*, we have to determine critical values (a_1, a) conditioning on $\{(z_{lj}, n_{lj}), l = 1, 2, j = 1, \ldots, J\}$.

9.2.1   How to Choose (a_1, a)

In this section, we assume that (N_1, N_2) are given. After stage 1, we determine a rejection value a_1 for S_1 conditioning on the observed values of $\{(z_{1j}, n_{1j}), j = 1, \ldots, J\}$. We may consider following approaches:

(I) We may wish to stop the trial if the experimental arm has a smaller number of responders than the expected number of responders under H_0. In this case, we choose $a_1 = [\sum_{j=1}^{J} z_{1j} m_{11j}/n_{1j}]$, where $[c]$ denotes the largest integer not exceeding c.

(II) Based on type II error rate spending: For a chosen $\beta_1(< \beta^*)$, we choose the smallest integer a_1 satisfying

$$P\{S_1 < a_1|(z_{1j}, n_{1j}, \theta_j), j = 1, \ldots, J\} \leq \beta_1,$$

where the conditional probability in the left-hand side is calculated by

$$\sum_{i_{11}=m_{11-}}^{m_{11+}} \cdots \sum_{i_{1J}=m_{1J-}}^{m_{1J+}} I\left(\sum_{j=1}^{J} i_{1j} < a_1\right) \prod_{j=1}^{J} f_j(i_{1j}|z_{1j}, n_{1j}).$$

(III) Probability of early termination (PET): One may want to choose a_1 so that the conditional PET under H_0 is at least a prespecified level ψ by choosing

$$P[S_1 < a_1|\{(z_{1j}, n_{1j}), j = 1, \ldots, J\}, H_0] \geq \psi,$$

where the conditional probability in the left-hand side is calculated by the largest integer a_1 satisfying

$$\sum_{i_{11}=m_{11-}}^{m_{11+}} \cdots \sum_{i_{1J}=m_{1J-}}^{m_{1J+}} I\left(\sum_{j=1}^{J} i_{1j} < a_1\right) \prod_{j=1}^{J} f_0(i_{1j}|z_{1j}, n_{1j}).$$

Suppose that a_1 is chosen by one of these methods. Then, the rejection value for stage 2, a, is chosen so that the conditional type I error rate is controlled at or below a specified level α^*, that is, a is the smallest integer satisfying $\alpha(z, n) \leq \alpha^*$, where

$$\alpha(z, n) = P(S_1 \geq a_1 S \geq a | z, n, H_0)$$

$$= \sum_{i_{11}=m_{11-}}^{m_{11+}} \cdots \sum_{i_{1J}=m_{1J-}}^{m_{1J+}} \sum_{i_{21}=m_{21-}}^{m_{21+}} \cdots \sum_{i_{2J}=m_{2J-}}^{m_{2J+}} I\left(\sum_{j=1}^{J} i_{1j} \geq a_1, \sum_{l=1}^{2}\sum_{j=1}^{J} i_{lj} \geq a\right)$$

$$\times \prod_{l=1}^{2}\prod_{j=1}^{J} f_0(i_{lj} | z_{lj}, n_{lj}).$$

For chosen (a_1, a), the conditional power is calculated by

$$1 - \beta = P(S_1 \geq a_1 S \geq a | z, n, H_1)$$

$$= \sum_{i_{11}=m_{11-}}^{m_{11+}} \cdots \sum_{i_{1J}=m_{1J-}}^{m_{1J+}} \sum_{i_{21}=m_{21-}}^{m_{21+}} \cdots \sum_{i_{2J}=m_{2J-}}^{m_{2J+}} I\left(\sum_{j=1}^{J} i_{1j} \geq a_1, \sum_{k=1}^{2}\sum_{j=1}^{J} i_{kj} \geq a\right)$$

$$\times \prod_{l=1}^{2}\prod_{j=1}^{J} f_j(i_{lj} | z_{lj}, n_{lj}).$$

9.2.2   Two-Stage Designs for Stratified Fisher's Exact Test

To design a randomized phase II trial based on the Fisher test, we need to specify design parameters: (i) $(\alpha^*, 1 - \beta^*)$; (ii) response rates under H_1, $\{(p_{1j}, p_{2j}), j = 1, \ldots, J\}$; (iii) allocation proportions, $\gamma = N_{k1}/N_k$; prevalence of each cluster, $\eta_j = n_{kj}/N_k$ for $j = 1, \ldots, J$.

With values of these design parameters specified, we calculate sample size (N_1, N_2) as follows:

- Given N,
  For $N_1 = 1, \ldots, N - 1$ and $N_2 = N - N_1$, calculate

  1. For $n_{lj} = 0, \ldots, N_l$ and $\sum_{j=1}^{J} n_{lj} = N_l$,
     (i) For $z_{lj} = 0, 1, \ldots, n_{lj}$,
        – Find (a_1, a) to control the conditional type I error rate $\alpha(z, n)$ below α^*.
        – For the chosen (a_1, a), calculate the conditional power $1 - \beta$ (z, n).
     (ii) Calculate the conditional power

     $$1 - \beta(n) = \sum_{z_{11}=0}^{n_{11}} \cdots \sum_{z_{1J}=0}^{n_{1J}} \sum_{z_{21}=0}^{n_{21}} \cdots \sum_{z_{2J}=0}^{n_{2J}} \{1 - \beta(z, n)\} \prod_{l=1}^{2}\prod_{j=1}^{J} g_j(z_{lj} | n_{lj}),$$

     where m_{1lj} is the round-off value of γn_{lj}.

2. Calculate the marginal power

$$1 - \beta = \sum_{(n_{11},\ldots,n_{1J}) \in C_1} \sum_{(n_{21},\ldots,n_{2J}) \in C_2} \{1 - \beta(n)\} \prod_{l=1}^{2} h(n_{l1},\ldots,n_{lJ}|N_l),$$

where $C_l = \{(n_{l1},\ldots,n_{lJ}) : 0 \le n_{l1} \le N_l, \ldots, 0 \le n_{lJ} \le N_l, \sum_{j=1}^{J} n_{lj} = N_l\}$ for $l = 1, 2$.

3. If $1 - \beta \ge 1 - \beta^*$, save (N_1, N) as a candidate design, and repeat the above procedure with $N_1 = N_1 + 1$

- Repeat the above procedure with $N = N + 1$.

For a design (N_1, N_2) satisfying the $(\alpha^*, 1 - \beta^*)$-condition, the conditional probability of early termination under H_0 is calculated as

$$\text{PET}_0(z_{11}, \ldots, z_{1J}, n_{11}, \ldots, n_{1J}) = P(S_1 < a_1 | z_{11}, \ldots, z_{1J}, n_{11}, \ldots, n_{1J}).$$

Recall that a_1 may be a function of $(z_{11}, \ldots, z_{1J}, n_{11}, \ldots, n_{1J})$. But to simplify the computing time, we propose to choose option (i), that is, $a_1 = [\sum_{j=1}^{J} z_{1j} m_{11j}/n_{1j}]$. By taking the expectation of the conditional probability of early termination with respect to $(z_{11}, \ldots, z_{1J}, n_{11}, \ldots, n_{1J})$, we obtain the marginal probability of early termination under H_0, PET_0. Among those (N_1, N_2) satisfying the $(\alpha^*, 1 - \beta^*)$-condition, the Simon-type (1989) minimax and the optimal designs can be chosen as follows:

Minimax design chooses (N_1, N_2) with the smallest maximal sample size $N(= N_1 + N_2)$.

Optimal design chooses (N_1, N_2) with the smallest marginal expected sample size EN under H_0, where

$$\text{EN} = N_1 \times \text{PET}_0 + N \times (1 - \text{PET}_0).$$

For a chosen two-stage design (N_1, N_2), we can calculate the marginal type I error rate α by taking expectation of the conditional type I error rate $\alpha(z_{11}, \ldots, z_{1J}, n_{11}, \ldots, n_{1J})$ with respect to $(z_{11}, \ldots, z_{1J}, n_{11}, \ldots, n_{1J})$.

9.2.3   Conditional P-Value

When a study is completed, one may want to calculate a p-value to see how significant the outcome is. If the a trial is terminated after stage 1, then we calculate a p-value using the Fisher exact test for a single-stage design. Suppose that the study is completed after the second stage with observations x together with marginal totals (z, m, n). For the observed test statistics $s_l = \sum_{j=1}^{J} x_{1lj}$ and $s = s_1 + s_2$, let a_1 denote the rejection value for stage 1 that is chosen by one of the rules proposed in Section 9.2.1 with $s_1 \ge a_1$. Then, the conditional p-value is calculated as

$$\text{p-value} = P(S_1 \geq a_1, S \geq s | \boldsymbol{z}, \boldsymbol{m}, \boldsymbol{n}, H_0)$$

$$= \sum_{i_{11}=m_{11-}}^{m_{11+}} \cdots \sum_{i_{1J}=m_{1J-}}^{m_{1J+}} \sum_{i_{21}=m_{21-}}^{m_{21+}} \cdots \sum_{i_{2J}=m_{2J-}}^{m_{2J+}} I\left(\sum_{j=1}^{J} i_{1j} \geq a_1, \sum_{l=1}^{2}\sum_{j=1}^{J} i_{lj} \geq a\right)$$

$$\times \prod_{l=1}^{2}\prod_{j=1}^{J} f_0(i_{lj}|z_{lj}, m_{lj}, n_{lj})$$

for $m_{lj-} = \max(0, z_{lj} - m_{2lj})$ and $m_{lj+} = \min(z_{lj}, m_{1lj})$.

References

Cochran, W.C. (1954). Some methods of strengthening the common χ^2 tests. *Biometrics*, 10, 417–451.

Crans, G.G. and Schuster, J.J. (2008). How conservative is Fisher's exact test? A quantitave evaluation of the two-sample comparative binomial trial. *Statistics in Medicine*, 27, 3598–3611.

Fisher, R.A. (1935). The logic of inductive inference (with discussion). *Journal of Royal Statistical Society*, 98, 39–82.

Gart, J.J. (1985). Approximate tests and interval estimation of the common relative risk in the combination of 2×2 tables. *Biometrika*, 72, 673–677.

Jung, S.H., Chow, S.C., and Chi, E.M. (2007). A note on sample size calculation based on propensity analysis in nonrandomized trials. *Journal of Biopharmaceutical Statistics*, 17, 35–41.

Li, S.H., Simon, R.M., and Gart, J.J. (1979). Small sample properties of the Mantel–Haenszel test. *Biometrika*, 66, 181–183.

Mantel, N. and Haenszel, W. (1959). Statistical aspects of the analysis of data from retrospective studies of disease. *Journal of the National Cancer Institute*, 22, 719–748.

Simon, R. (1989). Optimal two-stage designs for phase II clinical trials. *Controlled Clinical Trials*, 10, 1–10.

Westfall, P.H., Zaykin, D.V., and Young, S.S. (2002). *Multiple tests for genetic effects in association studies*. Methods in Molecular Biology, vol. 184 Biostatistical Methods, pp. 143–168. Stephen Looney, Ed., Humana Press, Toloway, NJ.

Chapter 10

Randomized Phase II Clinical Trials Based on Survival Endpoints: Two-Sample Log-Rank Test

While binary endpoints, such as overall response, are popularly used as the primary outcome of phase II cancer clinical trials, we sometimes use time to an event, such as time to progression or recurrence, as the primary outcome as well. When the study endpoint is time to an event, the maximum likelihood estimator (MLE) for exponential survival distributions may be used to compare survival distributions among treatment arms. Sample size calculation methods for test statistics based on the MLE of exponential distributions have been proposed by Pasternack and Gilbert (1971), George and Desu (1973), and Lachin (1981). Rubinstein et al. (1981) propose to use the sample size formula derived for the MLE test for the log-rank test by showing that this formula provides a reasonable power for the log-rank test through simulations. Their simulations are limited to balanced designs only.

Because of their robustness, nonparametric rank tests are generally preferred to parametric MLE tests in survival analysis. The log-rank test (Peto and Peto, 1972) has been widely used for testing the equality of two survival distributions in the presence of censoring. The asymptotic normality of the log-rank test can be found in Andersen et al. (1982) and Fleming and Harrington (1991). Numerous methods have been proposed for sample size estimation, including Lakatos (1977), Schoenfeld (1983), and Yateman and Skene (1992). In this chapter, we discuss design of randomized phase II clinical trials with a survival endpoint to be analyzed by the log-rank test.

10.1 Two-Sample Log-Rank Test

10.1.1 Test Statistic

In this chapter, we assume that arm 1 is a control arm and arm 2 is an experimental arm. Suppose that n_k patients are randomized to arm k $(k = 1, 2)$ and the survival times from the n_k patients are independent and identically distributed with cumulative hazard function $\Lambda_k(t)$ and hazard function $\lambda_k(t) = \partial\Lambda_k(t)/\partial t$. Under the proportional hazards assumption, $\Delta = \lambda_1(t)/\lambda_2(t)$ denotes the hazard ratio. We want to test $H_0 : \Delta = 1$ against $H_1 : \Delta > 1$.

Let T_{ki} denote the survival time for patient i in arm k ($1 \le i \le n_k; k = 1, 2$). Then we usually observe (X_{ki}, δ_{ki}), where X_{ki} is the minimum of T_{ki} and censoring time C_{ki} and δ_{ki} is an event indicator taking 1 if the patient had an event and 0 otherwise. Within each arm, the censoring times are independent of the survival times. Let $N_k(t) = \sum_{i=1}^{n_k} \delta_{ki} I(X_{ki} \le t)$ and $Y_k(t) = \sum_{i=1}^{n_k} I(X_{ki} \ge t)$ denote the death and the at-risk processes for arm k, respectively. Let $N(t) = N_1(t) + N_2(t)$ and $Y(t) = Y_1(t) + Y_2(t)$. Then, the log-rank test statistic is given as

$$W = \frac{1}{\sqrt{n}} \int_0^\infty \frac{Y_1(t)Y_2(t)}{Y(t)} \{d\hat{\Lambda}_1(t) - d\hat{\Lambda}_2(t)\},$$

where $\hat{\Lambda}_k(t) = \int_0^t Y_k(s)^{-1} dN_k(s)$ is the Nelson–Aalen (Nelson, 1969; Aalen, 1978) estimator of $\Lambda_k(t)$. Under H_0, $W/\hat{\sigma}$ is asymptotically standard normal with

$$\hat{\sigma}^2 = \frac{1}{n} \int_0^\infty \frac{Y_1(t)Y_2(t)}{Y(t)^2} dN(t)$$

see, for example, Fleming and Harrington (1991). Hence, we reject H_0, in favor of H_1, if $W/\hat{\sigma} > z_{1-\alpha}$ with one-sided type I error rate α.

10.1.2   Sample Size Calculation

Let $p_k = n_k/n$ ($p_1 + p_2 = 1$) denote the allocation proportion for arm k. We assume that patients are accrued with a constant accrual rate, r, during an accrual period and followed during an additional follow-up period b after the last patient is entered. Let $S_k(t) = \exp\{-\Lambda_k(t)\} = P(T_{ki} \ge t)$ denote the survivor function for arm k, and $G(t) = P(C_{ki} \ge t)$ denote the survivor function of the censoring distribution which is common between two arms.

The following results are based on Theorem 4.1. Note that $Y_k(t)/n$ uniformly converges to $p_k G(t) S_k(t)$. Under H_1, $\hat{\sigma}^2$ converges to

$$\sigma_0^2 = p_1^2 p_2 \int_0^\infty \frac{G(t) S_1(t)^2 S_2(t)}{\{p_1 S_1(t) + p_2 S_2(t)\}^2} d\Lambda_1(t)$$

$$+ p_1 p_2^2 \int_0^\infty \frac{G(t) S_1(t) S_2(t)^2}{\{p_1 S_1(t) + p_2 S_2(t)\}^2} d\Lambda_2(t)$$

and the variance of W is given as

$$\sigma_1^2 = p_1 p_2^2 \int_0^\infty \frac{G(t) S_1(t) S_2(t)^2}{\{p_1 S_1(t) + p_2 S_2(t)\}^2} d\Lambda_1(t)$$

$$+ p_1^2 p_2 \int_0^\infty \frac{G(t) S_1(t)^2 S_2(t)}{\{p_1 S_1(t) + p_2 S_2(t)\}^2} d\Lambda_2(t).$$

Furthermore, under H_1, we can show that $E(W) = \sqrt{n}\omega$, where

$$\omega = p_1 p_2 \int_0^\infty \frac{G(t)S_1(t)S_2(t)}{p_1 S_1(t) + p_2 S_2(t)} \{d\Lambda_1(t) - d\Lambda_2(t)\}.$$

Hence, given n, the power is given as

$$1 - \beta = P\left(\frac{W}{\hat{\sigma}} \geq z_{1-\alpha}|H_1\right)$$

$$= P\left(\frac{W - \sqrt{n}\omega}{\sigma_1} \geq \frac{\sigma_0}{\sigma_1}z_{1-\alpha} - \frac{\sqrt{n}\omega}{\sigma_1}\Big|H_1\right)$$

$$= \bar{\Phi}\left(\frac{\sigma_0}{\sigma_1}z_{1-\alpha} - \frac{\sqrt{n}\omega}{\sigma_1}\right),$$

where $\bar{\Phi}(\cdot) = 1 - \Phi(\cdot)$ and $\Phi(\cdot)$ is the cumulative distribution function of the standard normal distribution. Given power $1 - \beta$, the required sample size is given as

$$n = \left(\frac{\sigma_0 z_{1-\alpha} + \sigma_1 z_{1-\beta}}{\omega}\right)^2. \tag{10.1}$$

Note that this formula is derived without a parametric assumption for survival distributions or a nearby alternative assumption hypothesis.

By modifying George and Desu's (1973) formula, Rubinstein et al. (1981) propose to approximate the sample size for the log-rank test by that of the exponential MLE test, that is,

$$\left(\frac{\log \Delta_1}{z_{1-\alpha} + z_{1-\beta}}\right)^2 = D_1^{-1} + D_2^{-1} \tag{10.2}$$

under a balanced allocation ($p_1 = p_2 = 1/2$), where Δ_1 denotes the hazard ratio under H_1 and D_k denotes the number of events from arm k.

Using a nearby alternative hypothesis approximation (that is, $\Delta_1 \approx 1$), Schoenfeld (1983) derives the total number of events,

$$D = \frac{(z_{1-\alpha} + z_{1-\beta})^2}{p_1 p_2 (\log \Delta_1)^2} \tag{10.3}$$

required for the log-rank test.

Noting that for $\Delta_1 \approx 1$ or $S_1(t) \approx S_2(t)$, we have $\log \Delta_1 \approx \Delta_1 - 1$ and the probability of an event for arm k is

$$d_k = P(T_k \leq C) \approx -\int_0^\infty G(t)dS_k(t),$$

we can show that our formula (10.1) can be approximated by the latter two formulas (10.2) and (10.3) under the balanced allocation.

10.1.2.1   Under Exponential Survival and Uniform Censoring Distributions

Suppose that patients are accrued at a constant rate during accrual period a and all patients are followed for an additional follow-up period b after completion of accrual. Then, $C_{ki} \sim U(b, a+b)$ with survivor function $G(t) = 1$ if $t \le b$; $= 1 - (t-b)/a$ if $b < t \le a+b$; $= 0$ if $t > a+b$. Furthermore, suppose that the survival times have an exponential distribution with hazard rate λ_k for arm $k(= 1, 2)$. Then, we have $S_k(t) = \exp(-\lambda_k t)$ and $\Lambda_k(t) = \lambda_k t$.

Under these distributional assumptions, we have

$$
\sigma_0^2 = p_1^2 p_2 \lambda_1 \left\{ \int_0^{a+b} \frac{e^{-(2\lambda_1+\lambda_2)t}}{(p_1 e^{-\lambda_1 t} + p_2 e^{-\lambda_2 t})^2} dt - \frac{1}{a} \int_b^{a+b} \frac{(t-b)e^{-(2\lambda_1+\lambda_2)t}}{(p_1 e^{-\lambda_1 t} + p_2 e^{-\lambda_2 t})^2} dt \right\}
$$
$$
+ p_1 p_2^2 \lambda_2 \left\{ \int_0^{a+b} \frac{e^{-(\lambda_1+2\lambda_2)t}}{(p_1 e^{-\lambda_1 t} + p_2 e^{-\lambda_2 t})^2} dt - \frac{1}{a} \int_b^{a+b} \frac{(t-b)e^{-(\lambda_1+2\lambda_2)t}}{(p_1 e^{-\lambda_1 t} + p_2 e^{-\lambda_2 t})^2} dt \right\}
$$
(10.4)

$$
\sigma_1^2 = p_1 p_2^2 \lambda_1 \left\{ \int_0^{a+b} \frac{e^{-(\lambda_1+2\lambda_2)t}}{(p_1 e^{-\lambda_1 t} + p_2 e^{-\lambda_2 t})^2} dt - \frac{1}{a} \int_b^{a+b} \frac{(t-b)e^{-(\lambda_1+2\lambda_2)t}}{(p_1 e^{-\lambda_1 t} + p_2 e^{-\lambda_2 t})^2} dt \right\}
$$
$$
+ p_1^2 p_2 \lambda_2 \left\{ \int_0^{a+b} \frac{e^{-(2\lambda_1+\lambda_2)t}}{(p_1 e^{-\lambda_1 t} + p_2 e^{-\lambda_2 t})^2} dt - \frac{1}{a} \int_b^{a+b} \frac{(t-b)e^{-(2\lambda_1+\lambda_2)t}}{(p_1 e^{-\lambda_1 t} + p_2 e^{-\lambda_2 t})^2} dt \right\}
$$
(10.5)

and

$$
\omega = p_1 p_2 (\lambda_1 - \lambda_2) \left\{ \int_0^{a+b} \frac{e^{-(\lambda_1+\lambda_2)t}}{p_1 e^{-\lambda_1 t} + p_2 e^{-\lambda_2 t}} dt - \frac{1}{a} \int_b^{a+b} \frac{(t-b)e^{-(\lambda_1+\lambda_2)t}}{p_1 e^{-\lambda_1 t} + p_2 e^{-\lambda_2 t}} dt \right\}.
$$
(10.6)

We calculate these integrals using a numerical method. By plugging these in (10.1), we can calculate the sample size for given input values of $(\alpha, 1-\beta, \lambda_1, \lambda_2, a, b, p_1)$.

The required number of events at the analysis is calculated by $D = n(p_1 d_1 + p_2 d_2)$, where

$$
d_k = - \int_0^\infty G(t) dS_k(t) = 1 - \frac{e^{-b\lambda_k}}{a\lambda_k}(1 - e^{-a\lambda_k}).
$$

10.1.2.2   When Accrual Rate Is Specified Instead of Accrual Period

Now, we consider a sample size calculation when the accrual rate r is given instead of the accrual period a. Given $(\alpha, 1-\beta, \lambda_1, \lambda_2, r, b, p_1)$, $\sigma_1^2 = \sigma_1^2(a)$, $\sigma_2^2 = \sigma_2^2(a)$, and $\omega = \omega(a)$ are functions of a from (10.4)–(10.6). Also, under a constant accrual rate assumption, we have $n = a \times r$ approximately. So, by replacing n with $a \times r$ in (10.1), we obtain an equation on a,

$$a \times r = \left\{ \frac{\sigma_0(a)z_{1-\alpha} + \sigma_1(a)z_{1-\beta}}{\omega(a)} \right\}^2.$$

We solve this equation using a numerical method, such as the bisection method. Let a^* denote the solution to this equation. Then, the required sample size is obtained as $n = a^* \times r$.

Example 10.1
Suppose that the control arm is known to have 20% of 1-year progression-free survival (PFS). We want to show that the experimental arm is expected to increase 1-year PFS to 40%. Assuming an exponential PFS model, the annual hazard rates for the two arms are $\lambda_1 = 1.609$ and $\lambda_2 = 0.916$ with a hazard ratio of $\Delta_1 = 1.756$. Assuming a monthly accrual of 5 patients ($r = 60$ per year) and $b = 1$ year of additional follow-up period, the required sample size for the log-rank test with 1-sided $\alpha = 10\%$ and 90% of power with balanced allocation ($p_1 = p_2 = 1/2$) is given as $n = 102$ (51 per arm), requiring an accrual period of about 20 months ($a = 102/5$). In the final analysis, we expect $D = 89$ events (48 and 41 for arms 1 and 2, respectively) under H_1.

10.2   Two-Stage Log-Rank Test

Multistage clinical trial design for the two-sample log-rank has been widely investigated, for example, Slud and Wei (1982) and Tsiatis (1982). For randomized phase II trials, two-stage design will be most appropriate due to its small size and relatively short study period compared to large-scale phase III trials. With a survival endpoint, it is important to find a reasonable interim analysis time point. If it is scheduled for an early stage of a study, we may not have enough number of events for a reasonable probability to stop the study early in case of futility or superiority of the experimental therapy. On the other hand, if it is scheduled for a late stage of the study, we may have most of the planned patient accrual already so that the interim analysis may not be able to save resources even when the analysis result indicates to stop the trial. This is likely to happen for a phase II trial with a fast patient accrual. If this is the case, we may consider the single-stage design that was discussed in the previous section.

10.2.1   Statistical Testing

We conduct an interim analysis at time τ that may be determined in terms of the number of events or calendar time. We assume that τ is smaller than the planned accrual period a, so that we can save the number of patients if the experimental therapy does not show efficacy compared to the control.

For patient $i(= 1, \dots, n_k)$ in arm k, let T_{ki} denote the survival time with survivor distribution $S_k(t)$ and cumulative hazard function $\Lambda_k(t)$, and e_{ki} denote the entering time $(0 \leq e_{ki} \leq a)$. C_{ki} denotes the censoring time at the final analysis with survivor function $P(C_{ki} \geq t) = G(t)$ that is defined by the accrual and missing trends and additional follow-up period. The censoring time at the interim analysis is denoted as $\tilde{C}_{ki} = \max\{\min(\tau - e_{ki}, C_{ki}), 0\}$. For a patient who is accrued during stage 1 (that is, $e_{ki} < \tau$), $\tilde{C}_{ki}$ has a survivor function $G_1(t) = P\{\min(\tau - e_{ki}, C_{ki}) \geq t\}$. We observe $(\tilde{X}_{ki}, \tilde{\delta}_{ki})$ at the interim analysis and (X_{ki}, δ_{ki}) at the final analysis, where $\tilde{X}_{ki} = \min(T_{ki}, \tilde{C}_{ki})$, $\tilde{\delta}_{ki} = I(T_{ki} \leq \tilde{C}_{ki})$, $X_{ki} = \min(T_{ki}, C_{ki})$, and $\delta_{ki} = I(T_{ki} \leq C_{ki})$. We define at-risk processes $\tilde{Y}_{ki}(t) = I(\tilde{X}_{ki} \geq t)$ and $Y_{ki}(t) = I(X_{ki} \geq t)$, and event processes $\tilde{N}_{ki}(t) = \tilde{\delta}_{ki} I(\tilde{X}_{ki} \leq t)$ and $N_{ki}(t) = \delta_{ki} I(X_{ki} \leq t)$. Define $\tilde{Y}_k(t) = \sum_{i=1}^{n_k} \tilde{Y}_{ki}(t)$, $\tilde{Y}(t) = \tilde{Y}_1(t) + \tilde{Y}_2(t)$, $Y_k(t) = \sum_{i=1}^{n_k} Y_{ki}(t)$, $Y(t) = Y_1(t) + Y_2(t)$, $\tilde{N}_k(t) = \sum_{i=1}^{n_k} \tilde{N}_{ki}(t)$, $\tilde{N}(t) = \tilde{N}_1(t) + \tilde{N}_2(t)$, $N_k(t) = \sum_{i=1}^{n_k} N_{ki}(t)$, and $N(t) = N_1(t) + N_2(t)$.

Let $\tilde{n} = \sum_{i=1}^{n} I(e_{ki} \leq T)$ denote the number of patients who are entered before the interim analysis ($\tilde{n} < n$). Test statistics at the interim and final analyses are calculated as

$$W_1 = \frac{1}{\sqrt{\tilde{n}}} \int_0^\infty \frac{\tilde{Y}_1(t)\tilde{Y}_2(t)}{\tilde{Y}(t)} \{d\tilde{\Lambda}_1(t) - d\tilde{\Lambda}_2(t)\}$$

and

$$W = \frac{1}{\sqrt{n}} \int_0^\infty \frac{Y_1(t)Y_2(t)}{Y(t)} \{d\hat{\Lambda}_1(t) - d\hat{\Lambda}_2(t)\},$$

respectively. Here, $\tilde{\Lambda}_k(t) = \int_0^t \tilde{Y}_k(s)^{-1} d\tilde{N}_k(s)$ and $\hat{\Lambda}_k(t) = \int_0^t Y_k(s)^{-1} dN_k(s)$ are the Nelson–Aalen (Nelson, 1969; Aalen, 1978) estimate of $\Lambda_k(t)$ from the data at the interim analysis and the final analysis, respectively.

For large sample sizes at the interim and final analyses, the null distribution of (W_1, W) is approximately bivariate normal with means 0, variances and covariance that can be approximated by

$$\text{var}(W_1) = \hat{\sigma}_1^2 = \frac{1}{\tilde{n}} \int_0^\infty \frac{\tilde{Y}_1(t)\tilde{Y}_2(t)}{\tilde{Y}(t)^2} d\tilde{N}(t),$$

$$\text{var}(W) = \hat{\sigma}^2 = \frac{1}{n} \int_0^\infty \frac{Y_1(t)Y_2(t)}{Y(t)^2} dN(t),$$

and $\text{cov}(W) = \hat{\sigma}_1^2$, respectively; see, for example, Tsiatis (1982).

For the patients who enter the study after τ (that is, $e_{ki} > \tau$), their survival times are censored at time 0 at the interim analysis (that is, $\tilde{X}_{ki} = 0$ and $\tilde{\delta}_{ki} = 0$), so that they make no contributions to W_1 and $\hat{\sigma}_1^2$. A two-stage trial using the log-rank test is conducted as follows. In this chapter, we consider two-stage designs with an interim analysis using the futility test only, but an extension to those with both futility and superiority is straightforward:

- *Design stage*: Specify α and an interim analysis time and an early stopping value c_1.
- *Stage 1*: If $W_1/\hat{\sigma}_1 < c_1$, then reject the experimental therapy (arm 2) and stop the trial. Otherwise, proceed to stage 2.
- *Stage 2*: If $W/\hat{\sigma} \geq c$, then accept the experimental therapy. Here, critical value c satisfies

$$\alpha = P\left(\frac{W_1}{\hat{\sigma}_1} \geq c_1, \frac{W}{\hat{\sigma}} \geq c \Big| H_0\right),$$

which can be approximated by

$$\alpha = \int_c^{\infty} \phi(z)\bar{\Phi}\left(\frac{c_1 - \hat{\rho}z}{\sqrt{1 - \hat{\rho}^2}}\right) dz,$$

where $\hat{\rho} = \sqrt{\hat{\sigma}_1/\hat{\sigma}}$, and $\phi(\cdot)$ and $\bar{\Phi}(\cdot)$ are the probability density function and the survivor function of $N(0, 1)$ distribution, respectively.

Wieand, Schroeder, and O'Fallon (1994) propose a two-stage design with an interim futility test when 50% of the events that are expected at the final analysis are observed. They assume that the accrual period is long enough, compared to the median survival time, so that the interim analysis can be conducted during accrual period. They propose an early termination when the estimated hazard rate for the experimental arm is larger than that of the control arm. This is approximately equivalent to using $c_1 = 0$ in our two-stage design. Readers may read Pampallona and Tsiatis (1994) and Lachin (2005) about general group sequential futility testing methods.

10.2.2 Sample Size Calculation

Let $p_k = n_k/n$ $(p_1 + p_2 = 1)$ denote the allocation proportion for arm k. At first, we derive a power function given τ and c_1 together with accrual period a, follow-up period b, $\Lambda_k(t)$ for $k = 1, 2$ under H_1, and $(\alpha, 1 - \beta)$. An interim analysis time τ may be determined in terms of calendar time or observed number of events, but at the design stage, we assume that it is determined as a calendar time. If we want to specify it in terms of the number of events, we can convert it to a calendar time based on the expected accrual rate and specified survival distributions at the design stage. We choose a value for c_1 depending on how aggressively we want to screen out an inefficacious experimental therapy at the interim analysis.

The power function is given as

$$1 - \beta = P\left(\frac{W_1}{\hat{\sigma}_1} \geq c_1, \frac{W}{\hat{\sigma}} \geq c \Big| H_1\right).$$

In order to derive a power function, we have to calculate c for a specified type I error rate α, that is,

$$\alpha = P\left(\frac{W_1}{\hat{\sigma}_1} \geq c_1, \frac{W}{\hat{\sigma}} \geq c \,\middle|\, H_0\right),$$

although it may be recalculated at the final analysis using the collected survival data. Hence, for a power calculation, we need to derive the limits of $\hat{\sigma}_1^2$ and $\hat{\sigma}^2$ under both H_0 and H_1, and $E(W_1)$, $E(W)$, $\text{var}(W_1)$, and $\text{var}(W)$ under H_1. By the independent increment of the log-rank test statistic, the correlation coefficient of W_1 and W is $\sqrt{\text{var}(W_1)/\text{var}(W)}$ under both H_0 and H_1.

We derive the following asymptotic results using Theorem 4.1. Under H_0, we have $E(W_1) = E(W) = 0$. Furthermore, for large n, we can show that $\hat{\sigma}_1^2$ and $\hat{\sigma}^2$ converge

$$v_1 = -p_1 p_2 \int_0^\infty G_1(t) dS_2(t)$$

and

$$v = -p_1 p_2 \int_0^\infty G(t) dS_2(t),$$

respectively, under H_0. Note also that $\text{var}(W_1) = v_1$ and $\text{var}(W_1) = v$ under H_0. Hence, by independent increment of the log-rank statistic, $\text{corr}(W_1, W)$ is $\rho_0 = \sqrt{v_1/v}$ under H_0. We need this asymptotic result under H_0 to calculate c.

Under H_1, we have $E(W_1) = \sqrt{\tilde{n}}\omega_1$ and $E(W) = \sqrt{n}\omega$, where

$$\omega_1 = p_1 p_2 \int_0^\infty \frac{G_1(t) S_1(t) S_2(t)}{p_1 S_1(t) + p_2 S_2(t)} \{d\Lambda_1(t) - d\Lambda_2(t)\}$$

and

$$\omega = p_1 p_2 \int_0^\infty \frac{G(t) S_1(t) S_2(t)}{p_1 S_1(t) + p_2 S_2(t)} \{d\Lambda_1(t) - d\Lambda_2(t)\}.$$

Furthermore, $\hat{\sigma}_1^2$ and $\hat{\sigma}^2$ converge to

$$\sigma_{01}^2 = p_1^2 p_2 \int_0^\infty \frac{G_1(t) S_1(t)^2 S_2(t)}{\{p_1 S_1(t) + p_2 S_2(t)\}^2} d\Lambda_1(t)$$

$$+ p_1 p_2^2 \int_0^\infty \frac{G_1(t) S_1(t) S_2(t)^2}{\{p_1 S_1(t) + p_2 S_2(t)\}^2} d\Lambda_2(t)$$

and

$$\sigma_0^2 = p_1^2 p_2 \int_0^\infty \frac{G(t) S_1(t)^2 S_2(t)}{\{p_1 S_1(t) + p_2 S_2(t)\}^2} d\Lambda_1(t)$$

$$+ p_1 p_2^2 \int_0^\infty \frac{G(t) S_1(t) S_2(t)^2}{\{p_1 S_1(t) + p_2 S_2(t)\}^2} d\Lambda_2(t),$$

respectively. The variances of W_1 and W are given as

$$\sigma_{11}^2 = p_1 p_2^2 \int_0^\infty \frac{G_1(t) S_1(t) S_2(t)^2}{\{p_1 S_1(t) + p_2 S_2(t)\}^2} d\Lambda_1(t)$$

$$+ p_1^2 p_2 \int_0^\infty \frac{G_1(t) S_1(t)^2 S_2(t)}{\{p_1 S_1(t) + p_2 S_2(t)\}^2} d\Lambda_2(t)$$

and

$$\sigma_1^2 = p_1 p_2^2 \int_0^\infty \frac{G(t) S_1(t) S_2(t)^2}{\{p_1 S_1(t) + p_2 S_2(t)\}^2} d\Lambda_1(t)$$

$$+ p_1^2 p_2 \int_0^\infty \frac{G(t) S_1(t)^2 S_2(t)}{\{p_1 S_1(t) + p_2 S_2(t)\}^2} d\Lambda_2(t),$$

respectively, under H_1. By independent increment of the log-rank statistic, $\mathrm{corr}(W_1, W)$ is given as $\rho_1 = \sigma_{11}/\sigma_1$.

In summary, $(W_1/\hat{\sigma}_1, W/\hat{\sigma})$ is asymptotically distributed as $N(0, \Sigma_0)$ under H_0 and $N(\mu, \Sigma_1)$ under H_1, where

$$\mu = \begin{pmatrix} \sqrt{\bar{n}}\omega_1/\sigma_{11} \\ \sqrt{n}\omega/\sigma_1 \end{pmatrix}, \quad \Sigma_0 = \begin{pmatrix} 1 & \rho_0 \\ \rho_0 & 1 \end{pmatrix}, \quad \Sigma_1 = \begin{pmatrix} \sigma_{11}^2/\sigma_{01}^2 & \rho_1\sigma_{11}\sigma_1/\sigma_{01}\sigma_0 \\ \rho_1\sigma_{11}\sigma_1/\sigma_{01}\sigma_0 & \sigma_1^2/\sigma_0^2 \end{pmatrix}.$$

If (X, Y) is a bivariate normal random vector with means μ_x and μ_y, variances σ_x^2 and σ_y^2, and correlation coefficient ρ, then it is well known that the conditional distribution of X given $Y = y$ is normal with mean $\mu_x + (\rho\sigma_x/\sigma_y)(y - \mu_y)$ and variance $\sigma_x^2(1 - \rho^2)$. This result simplifies the calculation of type I error rate and power below. For example, given design parameters $(\alpha, 1 - \beta, p_1, r, b, \Lambda_1(t), \Lambda_2(t), \tau, c_1)$, $(X, Y) = (W_1/\hat{\sigma}_1, W/\hat{\sigma})$ is asymptotically $N(0, \Sigma_0)$ under H_0. So, in this case, $Y \sim N(0, 1)$ and the conditional distribution of X given $Y = y$ is $N(\rho_0 y, 1 - \rho_0^2)$. Note that c satisfies

$$\alpha = P(X \geq c_1, Y \geq c) = \int_c^\infty \int_{c_1}^\infty f(x, y) dx\, dy = \int_c^\infty \left\{ \int_{c_1}^\infty f(x|y) dx \right\} f(y) dy,$$

where $f(x, y)$, $f(y)$, and $f(x|y)$ denote the probability density functions of (X, Y), Y, and $X|Y = y$, respectively. Here, $f(y) = \phi(y)$ and

$$\int_c^\infty f(x|y) dx = \bar{\Phi}\left(\frac{c_1 - \rho_0 y}{\sqrt{1 - \rho_0^2}} \right),$$

so that we obtain c by solving the equation

$$\alpha = \int_c^\infty \phi(y) \bar{\Phi}\left(\frac{c_1 - \rho_0 y}{\sqrt{1 - \rho_0^2}} \right) dy.$$

If the interim analysis time and the stopping value are reasonably chosen, the power of a two-stage design is not much lower than that of the corresponding single-stage design. So, when searching for the required accrual period (or sample size) of a two-stage design, we may start from that of the corresponding single-stage design. Assuming an accrual pattern with a constant accrual rate, the design procedure of a two-stage design can be summarized as follows:

- Given $(\alpha, 1 - \beta, p_1, r, b, \Lambda_1(t), \Lambda_2(t))$, calculate the sample size n and accrual period a_0 required for a single-stage design.
- Determine an interim analysis time τ during the accrual period a_0 of the chosen single-stage design (that is, $\tau < a_0$) and the stopping value c_1 at the interim analysis.
- Then the accrual period required for a two-stage design is obtained around a_0 as follows:

(A) At $a = a_0$ (note that $\tilde{n} = r\tau$ and $n = ra_0$),
  – Obtain c by solving equation

$$\alpha = \int_c^\infty \phi(z)\bar{\Phi}\left(\frac{c_1 - \rho_0 z}{\sqrt{1 - \rho_0^2}}\right) dz.$$

  – Given $(\tilde{n}, n, c_1, c, \alpha)$, calculate

$$\text{power} = \int_{\bar{c}}^\infty \phi(z)\bar{\Phi}\left(\frac{\bar{c}_1 - \rho_1 z}{\sqrt{1 - \rho_1^2}}\right) dz,$$

where

$$\bar{c}_1 = \frac{\sigma_{01}}{\sigma_{11}}\left(c_1 - \frac{\omega_1\sqrt{\tilde{n}}}{\sigma_{01}}\right) \text{ and } \bar{c} = \frac{\sigma_0}{\sigma_1}\left(c - \frac{\omega\sqrt{n}}{\sigma_0}\right).$$

(B) If the power is smaller than $1 - \beta$, increase a slightly, and repeat (A) until the power is close enough to $1 - \beta$. We may change the interim analysis time τ at this step too.

At the design stage, we may want to calculate the stopping probabilities under H_0 and under H_1

$$\text{PET}_0 = P(W_1/\hat{\sigma}_1 \leq c_1|H_0) = \Phi(c_1)$$

and

$$\text{PET}_1 = P(W_1/\hat{\sigma}_1 \leq c_1|H_1) = \Phi(\bar{c}_1).$$

While PET_0 should not be too small in order for an interim futility test to be of worth, PET_1 should not be too large to avoid early rejection of an efficacious therapy with immature data.

10.2.2.1 Under Uniform Accrual and Exponential Survival Models

Suppose that the survival distributions are exponential with hazard rates λ_1 and λ_2 in arms 1 and 2, respectively. If patients are accrued at a constant rate during period a and followed for an additional period of b, and the interim analysis takes place before completion of accrual (that is, $\tau < a$), then the censoring distribution at the interim analysis is $U(0, \tau)$ and that after the second stage is $U(b, a+b)$ with survivor functions

$$
G_1(t) = \begin{cases} 1 & \text{if } t \le 0 \\ 1 - t/\tau & \text{if } 0 < t \le \tau \\ 0 & \text{if } t > \tau \end{cases}
$$

and

$$
G(t) = \begin{cases} 1 & \text{if } t \le b \\ 1 - (t-b)/a & \text{if } b < t \le a+b, \\ 0 & \text{if } t > a+b \end{cases}
$$

respectively. Since $\tau < a$, $G_1(t)$ is free of a. Note that we only assume administrative censoring. If loss to follow-up is expected, then we may incorporate it in the calculation if its distribution is given, or we may increase the final sample size by the expected proportion of loss to follow-up.

Under these distributional assumptions, σ_0^2, σ_1^2, and ω are the same as those in (10.4), (10.5), and (10.6), respectively, and

$$
v_1 = p_1 p_2 \{ 1 - \tfrac{1}{\tau \lambda_1}(1 - e^{-\lambda_1 \tau}) \},
$$

$$
v = p_1 p_2 \{ 1 - \tfrac{1}{a \lambda_1} e^{-b \lambda_1}(1 - e^{-\lambda_1 a}) \},
$$

$$
\sigma_{01}^2 = \frac{p_1^2 p_2 \lambda_1}{\tau} \int_0^\tau \frac{(\tau - t)e^{-(2\lambda_1 + \lambda_2)t}}{(p_1 e^{-\lambda_1 t} + p_2 e^{-\lambda_2 t})^2} dt + \frac{p_1 p_2^2 \lambda_2}{\tau} \int_0^\tau \frac{(\tau - t)e^{-(\lambda_1 + 2\lambda_2)t}}{(p_1 e^{-\lambda_1 t} + p_2 e^{-\lambda_2 t})^2} dt,
$$

$$
\sigma_{11}^2 = \frac{p_1 p_2^2 \lambda_1}{\tau} \int_0^\tau \frac{(\tau - t)e^{-(\lambda_1 + 2\lambda_2)t}}{(p_1 e^{-\lambda_1 t} + p_2 e^{-\lambda_2 t})^2} dt + \frac{p_1^2 p_2 \lambda_2}{\tau} \int_0^\tau \frac{(\tau - t)e^{-(2\lambda_1 + \lambda_2)t}}{(p_1 e^{-\lambda_1 t} + p_2 e^{-\lambda_2 t})^2} dt,
$$

and

$$
\omega_1 = \frac{p_1 p_2 (\lambda_1 - \lambda_2)}{\tau} \int_0^\tau \frac{(\tau - t)e^{-(\lambda_1 + \lambda_2)t}}{p_1 e^{-\lambda_1 t} + p_2 e^{-\lambda_2 t}} dt.
$$

We use a numerical method to calculate these integrals.

Example 10.2

From Example 10.1, a single-stage randomized phase II trial requires $n = 102$ under the design setting $(\alpha, 1 - \beta, \lambda_1, \lambda_2, r, b, p_1) = (0.1, 0.9, 1.609, 0.916, 60, 1, 1/2)$. Under the same design setting, a two-stage trial with an interim analysis at $\tau = 1$ year with $c_1 = -0.5$ requires $n = 106$, which is only slightly larger than that for the single-stage design. At the interim and final analyses, we expect 46 and 93 events, respectively, under H_1. The probabilities of early termination are given as $\text{PET}_0 = 0.31$ and $\text{PET}_1 = 0.03$. From $B = 10,000$ simulations, this two-stage design with $n = 106$ has an empirical type I error of 9.9% and power of 91%, which are very close to the nominal $\alpha = 10\%$ and $1 - \beta = 90\%$, respectively.

10.3 Stratified Two-Sample Log-Rank Test for Single-Stage Designs

Suppose that the patient population consists of J strata defined by some stratification factors. In this case, the randomization of patients will be stratified by the factors so that the two treatment arms have similar patient characteristics in terms of the stratification factors, and the resulting data will be analyzed by the stratified log-rank test. Lakatos (1988) proposed a sample size calculation for the stratified log-rank test using a Markov process method. In this section, we derive a sample size formula using the stochastic integral method for a single-stage design. An extension to two-stage designs can be easily derived as in the previous section for the unstratified two-sample log-rank test.

10.3.1 Test Statistic

Suppose that n_{kj} patients are randomized to arm k $(k = 1, 2)$ from stratum $j (= 1, \ldots, J)$ whose survival times have a cumulative hazard function $\Lambda_{kj}(t)$ and a hazard function $\lambda_{kj}(t) = \partial \Lambda_{kj}(t)/\partial t$. We want to test

$$H_0 : \Lambda_{1j}(t) = \Lambda_{2j}(t) \text{ for all } j = 1, \ldots, J$$

against

$$H_1 : \Lambda_{1j}(t) \geq \Lambda_{2j}(t) \text{ for all } j = 1, \ldots, J$$
$$\text{and with inequality for some } j = 1, \ldots, J.$$

Let T_{kji} and C_{kji} denote the survival and censoring times, respectively, for patient $i (= 1, \ldots, n_{kj})$ from stratum $j (= 1, \ldots, J)$ assigned to arm $k (= 1, 2)$. For $X_{kji} = \min(T_{kji}, C_{kji})$ and $\delta_{kji} = I(T_{kji} \leq C_{kji})$, let $N_{kj}(t) = \sum_{i=1}^{n_{kj}} \delta_{kji} I(X_{kji} \leq t)$ and $Y_{kj}(t) = \sum_{i=1}^{n_{kj}} I(X_{kji} \geq t)$ denote the event and the at-risk processes for arm k and stratum j, respectively. Let $N_j(t) = N_{1j}(t) + N_{2j}(t)$ and $Y_j(t) = Y_{1j}(t) + Y_{2j}(t)$. Then, the stratified log-rank test statistic is given as

$$W = \frac{1}{\sqrt{n}} \sum_{j=1}^{J} \int_0^\infty \frac{Y_{1j}(t) Y_{2j}(t)}{Y_j(t)} \{d\hat{\Lambda}_{1j}(t) - d\hat{\Lambda}_{2j}(t)\},$$

where $n = \sum_{k=1}^{2}\sum_{j=1}^{J} n_{kj}$ and $\hat{\Lambda}_{kj}(t) = \int_0^t Y_{kj}(s)^{-1}dN_{kj}(s)$ are the Nelson–Aalen (Nelson, 1969; Aalen, 1978) estimator of Λ_{kj}. Under H_0, $W/\hat{\sigma}$ is asymptotically standard normal with

$$\hat{\sigma}^2 = \frac{1}{n}\sum_{j=1}^{J}\int_0^\infty \frac{Y_{1j}(t)Y_{2j}(t)}{Y_j(t)^2}dN_j(t),$$

see Schoenfeld and Tsiatis (1987). Hence, we reject H_0, in favor of H_1, if $W/\hat{\sigma} > z_{1-\alpha}$ with one-sided type I error rate α.

10.3.2 Sample Size Calculation

Let $n_j = n_{1j}+n_{2j}$ denote the sample size of stratum j. Suppose that $100p_k\%$ of the patients from each stratum are allocated to arm $k(= 1, 2)$, so that we have $p_k = n_{kj}/n_j$ ($p_1+p_2 = 1$) for stratum j. Let $\gamma_j = n_j/n$ denote the prevalence of stratum j ($\sum_{j=1}^{J}\gamma_j = 1$). We assume that patients are accrued with a constant accrual rate, r, during an accrual period and followed during follow-up period b after the last patient is entered. Let $S_{kj}(t) = \exp\{-\Lambda_{kj}(t)\}$ denote the survivor function of the survival distribution for arm k in stratum j, and $G(t) = P(C_{kji} \geq t)$ denote the survivor function of the common censoring distribution. We assume that the survival and the censoring times are independent for each patient. We derive the following sample size formula using Theorem 4.1.

Under stratified randomization, $Y_{kj}(t)/n$ uniformly converges to $p_k\gamma_j G(t)S_{kj}(t)$. Under H_1, $\hat{\sigma}^2$ converges to

$$\sigma_0^2 = p_1 p_2 \sum_{j=1}^{J}\gamma_j \left[p_1 \int_0^\infty \frac{G(t)S_{1j}(t)^2 S_{2j}(t)}{\{p_1 S_{1j}(t) + p_2 S_{2j}(t)\}^2} d\Lambda_{1j}(t) \right.$$
$$\left. + p_2 \int_0^\infty \frac{G(t)S_{1j}(t)S_{2j}(t)^2}{\{p_1 S_{1j}(t) + p_2 S_{2j}(t)\}^2} d\Lambda_{2j}(t) \right]$$

and the variance of W is given as

$$\sigma_1^2 = p_1 p_2 \sum_{j=1}^{J}\gamma_j \left[p_2 \int_0^\infty \frac{G(t)S_{1j}(t)S_{2j}(t)^2}{\{p_1 S_{1j}(t) + p_2 S_{2j}(t)\}^2} d\Lambda_{1j}(t) \right.$$
$$\left. + p_1 \int_0^\infty \frac{G(t)S_{1j}(t)^2 S_{2j}(t)}{\{p_1 S_{1j}(t) + p_2 S_{2j}(t)\}^2} d\Lambda_{2j}(t) \right].$$

Furthermore, under H_1, the expected value of W is approximated by $\sqrt{n}\omega$, where

$$\omega = p_1 p_2 \sum_{j=1}^{J}\gamma_j \int_0^\infty \frac{G(t)S_{1j}(t)S_{2j}(t)}{p_1 S_{1j}(t) + p_2 S_{2j}(t)}\{d\Lambda_{1j}(t) - d\Lambda_{2j}(t)\}.$$

Hence, given n, the power is given as

$$1 - \beta = P\left(\frac{W}{\hat{\sigma}} \geq z_{1-\alpha}|H_1\right)$$

$$= P\left(\frac{W - \sqrt{n}\omega}{\sigma_1} \geq \frac{\sigma_0}{\sigma_1}z_{1-\alpha} - \frac{\sqrt{n}\omega}{\sigma_1}|H_1\right)$$

$$= \bar{\Phi}\left(\frac{\sigma_0}{\sigma_1}z_{1-\alpha} - \frac{\sqrt{n}\omega}{\sigma_1}\right),$$

where $\bar{\Phi}(\cdot) = 1 - \Phi(\cdot)$ and $\Phi(\cdot)$ is the cumulative distribution function of the standard normal distribution. Hence, the required sample size for power $1 - \beta$ is given as

$$n = \left(\frac{\sigma_0 z_{1-\alpha} + \sigma_1 z_{1-\beta}}{\omega}\right)^2. \tag{10.7}$$

If the patients are expected to be accrued with a constant rate r, we can change the formula (10.7) into an equation on accrual period and solve it with respect to the accrual period a as in the previous sections.

The expected number of events at the analysis is $D = n\sum_{j=1}^{J}\sum_{k=1}^{2}\gamma_j p_k d_{kj}$, where

$$d_{kj} = P(T_{kj} \leq C_{kj}) = -\int_0^{\infty} G(t)dS_{kj}(t).$$

Example 10.3

Suppose that the patient population of a study consists of two strata ($J = 2$) with $\gamma_1 = 40\%$ of high-risk stratum ($j = 1$) and $\gamma_2 = 60\%$ of low-risk stratum ($j = 2$). The control arm ($k = 1$) is known to have $S_{11}(1) = 10\%$ and $S_{12}(1) = 30\%$ of 1-year PFS for strata 1 and 2, respectively. We would be interested in the experimental arm ($k = 2$) if it has at least $S_{21}(1) = 20\%$ and $S_{22}(1) = 50\%$ of 1-year PFS for strata 1 and 2, respectively. Assuming exponential PFS models, the annual hazard rates are given as $\lambda_{11} = 2.30$, $\lambda_{12} = 1.20$, $\lambda_{21} = 1.61$, and $\lambda_{22} = 0.69$, resulting in hazard ratios of $\Delta_1 = \lambda_{11}/\lambda_{21} = 1.43$ and $\Delta_2 = \lambda_{12}/\lambda_{22} = 1.74$ for strata 1 and 2, respectively. Assuming that this study is able to accrue 5 patients per month ($r = 60$ per year) and patients will be followed for an additional $b = 1$ year, the required sample size for the stratified log-rank test with one-sided $\alpha = 10\%$ and $1 - \beta = 90\%$ with balanced allocation ($p_1 = p_2 = 1/2$) is given as $n = 144$ (72 per arm), requiring an accrual period of about 29 months ($a = 144/5$). In the final analysis, we expect about $D = 128$ events under H_1. From $B = 10,000$ simulations, the stratified test with $n = 144$ has an empirical type I error of 10.1% and power of 90%, which are close to the specified $\alpha = 10\%$ and $1 - \beta = 90\%$, respectively.

Although the stratified log-rank test always controls the type I error rate, its power depends on the prevalence of each stratum. For example, suppose that the true prevalence in Example 10.3 is $\gamma_1 = 60\%$ for the high-risk stratum and $\gamma_2 = 40\%$ for the low-risk stratum, instead of $(\gamma_1, \gamma_2) = (40\%, 60\%)$. Assuming that all other design parameter values are unchanged, the required sample size is $n = 163$, compared to $n = 144$ when $(\gamma_1, \gamma_2) = (40\%, 60\%)$. Hence, it is recommended to check the observed prevalence of each stratum in the middle of the study, and recalculate the sample size if the observed prevalence is very different from the specified one at the study design.

References

Aalen, O.O. (1978). Nonparametric inference for a family of counting processes. *Annals of Statistics*, 6, 701–726.

Andersen, P.K., Borgan, O., Gill, R.D., and Kidding, N. (1982). Linear nonparametric tests for comparison of counting processes with application to censored survival data (with discussion). *International Statistical Review*, 50, 219–258.

Fleming, T.R. and Harrington, D.P. (1991). *Counting Processes and Survival Analysis*. Wiley, New York.

George, S.L. and Desu, M.M. (1973). Planning the size and duration of a trial studying the time to some critical event. *Journal of Chronic Disease*, 27, 15–24.

Lachin, J.M. (1981). Introduction to sample size determination and power analysis for clinical trials. *Controlled Clinical Trials*, 2, 93–113.

Lachin, J.M. (2005). A review of methods for futility stopping based on conditional power. *Statistics in Medicine*, 24, 2747–2764.

Lakatos, E. (1977). Sample sizes based on the log-rank statistic in complex clinical trials. *Biometrics*, 64, 156–160.

Lakatos, E. (1988). Sample sizes based on the log-rank statistic in complex clinical trials. *Biometrics*, 44, 229–241.

Nelson, W. (1969). Hazard plotting for incomplete failure data. *Journal of Quality Technology*, 1, 27–52.

Pampallona, S. and Tsiatis, A.A. (1994). Group sequential designs for one-sided and two-sided hypothesis testing with provision for early stopping in favor of the null hypothesis. *Journal of Statistical Planning and Inference*, 42, 19–35.

Pasternack, B.S. and Gilbert, H.S. (1971). Planning the duration of long-term survival time studies designed for accrual by cohorts. *Journal of Chronic Disease*, 24, 13–24.

Peto, R. and Peto, J. (1972). Asymptotically efficient rank invariant test procedures (with discussion). *Journal of the Royal Statistical Society, Series A*, 135, 185–206.

Rubinstein, L., Gail, M., and Santner, T. (1981). Planning the duration of a comparative clinical trial with loss to follow-up and a period of continued observation. *Journal of Chronic Disease*, 27, 15–24.

Schoenfeld, D.A. (1983). Sample size formula for the proportional hazards regression model. *Biometrics*, 39, 499–503.

Schoenfeld, D.A. and Tsiatis, A.A. (1987). A modified log rank test for highly stratified data. *Biometrika*, 74, 167–175.

Slud, E.V. and Wei, L.J. (1982). Two-sample repeated significance tests based on the modified Wilcoxon statistic. *Journal of American Statistical Society*, 77, 862–868.

Tsiatis, A.A. (1982). Repeated significance testing for a general class of statistics used in censored survival analysis. *Journal of American Statistical Society*, 77, 855–861.

Wieand, S., Schroeder, G., and O'Fallon, J.R. (1994). Stopping when the experimental regimen does not appear to help. *Statistics in Medicine*, 13, 1453–1458.

Yateman, N.A. and Skene, A.M. (1992). Sample size for proportional hazards survival studies with arbitrary patient entry and loss to follow-up distributions. *Statistics in Medicine*, 11, 1103–1113.

Chapter 11

Some Flexible Phase II
Clinical Trial Designs

In this chapter, we discuss two statistical methods for design and analysis of some flexible phase II clinical trial designs. These methods are presented in terms of a survival endpoint. However, the concept of the first method, called *generalized log-rank test*, can be extended to any type of endpoints.

11.1   Comparing Survival Distributions under General Hypothesis Testing

We start this section with an example from a single-arm phase II trial that motivated the statistical methods discussed below.

Example 11.1

Chemotherapy ABVD has been a standard regimen for patients with nonbulky stage I and II Hodgkin's lymphoma. In a previous study on 6 cycles of ABVD, each patient had a fluorodeoxyglucose positron-emission tomography (FDG-PET) imaging after 2 cycles of ABVD, for example, Hutchings et al. (2006) and Gallamini et al. (2007). It was found that patients with a negative PET image (group 1) and those with a positive PET image (group 2) had 3-year progression-free survival (PFS) of $S_1(3) = 0.86$ and $S_2(3) = 0.52$, respectively. Assuming an exponential PFS model, these correspond to annual hazard rates of $\lambda_1 = 0.05$ and $\lambda_2 = 0.22$, respectively, and the hazard ratio λ_2/λ_1 is estimated as $\Delta_0 = 4.3$. In a new phase II trial, patients with a negative PET image after 2 cycles of ABVD will be treated by an additional 2 cycles of ABVD, whereas those with a positive PET image after 2 cycles of ABVD will be treated by 2 cycles of a more aggressive chemotherapy called escalated BEACOPP, followed by radiation therapy. By the PET-guided chemotherapy strategy, it is believed that the 3-year PFS of the PET-positive patients can be increased to lower the hazard ratio compared to that of the PET-negative

patients. Note that the group 1 patients will receive the same treatment as
that of the previous study providing the historical data. For the true hazard
ratio Δ, we want to test $H_0 : \Delta \geq \Delta_0$ against $H_1 : \Delta < \Delta_0$ in this study.

11.1.1   Generalized Log-Rank Test

The study of Example 11.1 is conceptually a single-arm trial since we do not
randomize the patients. We will apply the statistical method that will be
discussed in this section to this study. We will also demonstrate the method
with a randomized phase II clinical trial.

In this section, we present the statistical method in terms of a randomized
trial. Let n_k denote the number of patients in arm k and T_{ki} the survival time
for patient i in arm k ($1 \leq i \leq n_k$; $k = 1, 2$). We observe (X_{ki}, δ_{ki}), where X_{ki}
is the minimum of T_{ki} and the censoring time C_{ki}, and δ_{ki} is an event indicator
taking the value 1 if the patient experiences an event and 0 otherwise.

For arm k, $T_{k1}, \ldots, T_{k,n_k}$ are IID with hazard function $\lambda_k(t)$, cumulative hazard function $\Lambda_k(t) = \int_0^t \lambda_k(s)ds$, and survivor function $S_k(t) = \exp(-\Lambda_k(t))$.
Under the proportional hazards assumption, $\Delta = \lambda_2(t)/\lambda_1(t)$ denotes the hazard ratio. From the Cox (1972) regression model using the treatment indicator
as the only covariate, the partial score function $W(\Delta)$ and the information
function $\hat{\sigma}^2(\Delta)$ are given as

$$W(\Delta) = \int_0^\infty \frac{Y_1(t)Y_2(t)}{Y_1(t) + \Delta Y_2(t)}\{\Delta d\hat{\Lambda}_1(t) - d\hat{\Lambda}_2(t)\},$$

and

$$\hat{\sigma}^2(\Delta) = \Delta \int_0^\infty \frac{Y_1(t)Y_2(t)}{\{Y_1(t) + \Delta Y_2(t)\}^2}dN(t),$$

respectively, where $\hat{\Lambda}_k(t) = \int_0^t Y_k^{-1}(t)dN_k(t)$ is the Aalen–Nelson estimator
(Aalen, 1978; Nelson, 1969) for $\Lambda_k(t)$, $Y_k(t) = \sum_{i=1}^{n_k} I(X_{ki} \geq t)$ and $N_k(t) =
\sum_{i=1}^{n_k} \delta_{ki} I(X_{ki} \leq t)$ are the at-risk process and the event process for group k,
respectively, $N(t) = N_1(t) + N_2(t)$, and $I(\cdot)$ is the indicator function. Note
that $W(1)$ is the standard log-rank test statistic (Peto and Peto, 1972). We
call $W(\Delta)$ the generalized log-rank test.

As $n \to \infty$, $W(\Delta_0)/\sigma(\Delta_0)$ converges to the standard normal distribution
under $H_0 : \Delta = \Delta_0$ see, for example, Fleming and Harrington (1991). Since
$W(\Delta)/\hat{\sigma}(\Delta)$ is monotone decreasing in Δ, we reject H_0 in favor of $H_1 : \Delta < \Delta_0$
if $W(\Delta_0)/\hat{\sigma}(\Delta_0) > z_{1-\alpha}$ with one-sided type I error rate α.

The partial maximum likelihood estimate (pMLE) $\hat{\Delta}$ is obtained by solving $W(\Delta) = 0$. The pMLE is a consistent estimator of the true hazard ratio Δ. Furthermore, by the asymptotic linearity, the score-type test statistic $W(\Delta_0)/\hat{\sigma}(\Delta_0)$ is asymptotically equivalent to the Wald-type test statistic
$\hat{\sigma}(\Delta_0)(\hat{\Delta}-\Delta_0)$, so that our sample size formula derived in the following section
is valid for both types of test statistics.

11.1.2 Sample Size Calculation

We want to estimate the sample size $n(= n_1 + n_2)$ under a specific alternative hypothesis that $H_1 : \Delta = \Delta_1(< \Delta_0)$ with a desired power. Jung et al. (2005) propose a sample size formula with $\Delta_0 > 1$ and $\Delta_1 = 1$ for noninferiority trials. We want to extend their formula for general Δ_0 and Δ_1 with $\Delta_1 < \Delta_0$ in this section. Let $p_k = n_k/n$ denote the allocation proportion for arm k.

The asymptotic results in this section are derived under H_1. For arm k, let $f_k(t) = -\partial S_k(t)/\partial t$ denote the probability density function of the survival distribution. Note that $S_2(t) = S_1(t)^{\Delta_1}$ and $f_2(t) = \Delta_1 f_1(t) S_1(t)^{\Delta_1 - 1}$ under H_1. For a censoring variable C, let $G(t) = P(C \geq t)$ denote the survivor function of the censoring distribution which is common to the two arms. By Jung et al. (2005), $\hat{\sigma}^2(\Delta)$ is asymptotically equivalent to $n\sigma^2(\Delta)$, where

$$\sigma^2(\Delta) = \Delta p_1 p_2 \int_0^\infty \frac{G(t)S_1(t)S_2(t)\{p_1 f_1(t) + p_2 f_2(t)\}}{\{p_1 S_1(t) + \Delta p_2 S_2(t)\}^2} dt. \tag{11.1}$$

By the definition of $W(\Delta)$, we have

$$W(\Delta_0) - W(\Delta_1) = n^{-1/2}(\Delta_0 - \Delta_1)$$
$$\times \int_0^\infty \frac{Y_1(t)Y_2(t)}{\{Y_1(t) + \Delta_0 Y_2(t)\}\{Y_1(t) + \Delta_1 Y_2(t)\}} dN(t),$$

which is asymptotically equivalent to $n\omega$, where

$$\omega = (\Delta_0 - \Delta_1) p_1 p_2$$
$$\times \int_0^\infty \frac{G(t)S_1(t)S_2(t)\{p_1 f_1(t) + p_2 f_2(t)\}}{\{p_1 S_1(t) + \Delta_0 p_2 S_2(t)\}\{p_1 S_1(t) + \Delta_1 p_2 S_2(t)\}} dt. \tag{11.2}$$

Note that $S_k(t)$ are the survivor functions of the survival distributions under H_1.

Under H_1, the generalized log-rank statistic can be expressed as

$$\frac{W(\Delta_0)}{\hat{\sigma}(\Delta_0)} = \frac{W(\Delta_1)}{\hat{\sigma}(\Delta_1)} \times \frac{\hat{\sigma}(\Delta_1)}{\hat{\sigma}(\Delta_0)} + \frac{W(\Delta_0) - W(\Delta_1)}{\hat{\sigma}(\Delta_0)},$$

which, from (11.1) and (11.2), can be approximated by

$$\frac{W(\Delta_1)}{\sigma_1} \times \frac{\sigma_1}{\sigma_0} + \frac{\omega\sqrt{n}}{\sigma_0},$$

where $\sigma_h^2 = \sigma^2(\Delta_h)$ for $h = 0, 1$.

Suppose that we want to estimate the sample size for detecting $H_1 : \Delta = \Delta_1$ with a power of $1 - \beta$ by the generalized log-rank test with a one-sided α at $H_0 : \Delta = \Delta_0$, that is,

$$1 - \beta = P\left(\frac{W(\Delta_0)}{\hat{\sigma}(\Delta_0)} > z_{1-\alpha} | H_1\right) \approx P\left(\frac{W(\Delta_1)}{\sigma_1} \times \frac{\sigma_1}{\sigma_0} + \frac{\omega\sqrt{n}}{\sigma_0} > z_{1-\alpha} | H_1\right).$$

Since $W(\Delta_1)/\sigma_1$ is approximately $N(0, 1)$ under H_1, we have

$$-z_{1-\beta} = \left(z_{1-\alpha} - \frac{\omega\sqrt{n}}{\sigma_0}\right)\frac{\sigma_0}{\sigma_1}.$$

Hence, the required sample size is obtained by

$$n = \frac{(\sigma_0 z_{1-\alpha} + \sigma_1 z_{1-\beta})^2}{\omega^2}. \tag{11.3}$$

Note that ω, σ_0^2, and σ_1^2 are functions of the survival distributions $S_1(t)$ and $S_2(t)$ under H_1, and the common censoring distribution $G(t)$. They are calculated using numerical integration methods.

The power of the generalized log-rank test roughly depends on the number of events, rather than the number of patients, so that one may want to calculate the expected number of events at the final data analysis. The number of events D under H_1 is calculated as in the standard log-rank test, that is, $D = n(p_1 d_1 + p_2 d_2)$, where $d_k = 1 + \int_0^\infty S_k(t)dG(t)$ and $S_k(t)$ are the survivor functions of survival distributions specified under H_1, see, for example, Schoenfeld (1983). Note that if the survival distributions are shorter, then the required sample size becomes smaller.

11.1.2.1   Under Uniform Accrual and Exponential Survival Models

In this section, we will illustrate the application of the proposed methods when designing a clinical trial for comparing survival distributions with right censoring as follows.

(A) An exponential distribution can be uniquely specified by a single parameter, such as the hazard rate, the median or the survival probability at a chosen time point. Furthermore, the family of exponential distributions fits real survival data relatively well. So, we often specify the survival distributions using exponential distributions with hazard rates λ_k, that is, $S_k(t) = \exp(-\lambda_k t)$.

(B) When a trial is open, patients are usually uniformly recruited during the accrual period a and additional follow-up period b. In this case, we have

$$G(t) = \begin{cases} 1 & \text{if } t \le b \\ 1 - (t - b)/a & \text{if } b < t \le a + b. \\ 0 & \text{if } t > a + b \end{cases}$$

Under these distributional models, we have

$$\sigma_h^2 = p_1 p_2 \Delta_h \left\{ \int_0^{a+b} \frac{(p_1\lambda_1 e^{-\lambda_1 t} + p_2\lambda_2 e^{-\lambda_2 t})e^{-(\lambda_1+\lambda_2)t}}{(p_1 e^{-\lambda_1 t} + \Delta_h p_2 e^{-\lambda_2 t})^2}dt \right.$$
$$\left. - \frac{1}{a}\int_b^{a+b} \frac{(t - b)(p_1\lambda_1 e^{-\lambda_1 t} + p_2\lambda_2 e^{-\lambda_2 t})e^{-(\lambda_1+\lambda_2)t}}{(p_1 e^{-\lambda_1 t} + \Delta_h p_2 e^{-\lambda_2 t})^2}dt \right\} \tag{11.4}$$

for $h = 0, 1$, and

$$\omega = (\Delta_0 - \Delta_1)p_1 p_2 \left\{ \int_0^{a+b} \frac{(p_1\lambda_1 e^{-\lambda_1 t} + p_2\lambda_2 e^{-\lambda_2 t})e^{-(\lambda_1+\lambda_2)t}}{(p_1 e^{-\lambda_1 t} + \Delta_0 p_2 e^{-\lambda_2 t})(p_1 e^{-\lambda_1 t} + \Delta_1 p_2 e^{-\lambda_2 t})} dt \right.$$

$$\left. - \frac{1}{a} \int_b^{a+b} \frac{(t - b)(p_1\lambda_1 e^{-\lambda_1 t} + p_2\lambda_2 e^{-\lambda_2 t})e^{-(\lambda_1+\lambda_2)t}}{(p_1 e^{-\lambda_1 t} + \Delta_0 p_2 e^{-\lambda_2 t})(p_1 e^{-\lambda_1 t} + \Delta_1 p_2 e^{-\lambda_2 t})} dt \right\}. \quad (11.5)$$

We calculate (11.4) and (11.5) using a numerical integration method. By plugging these in (11.3), we calculate a required sample size for given $(\lambda_1, \Delta_0, \Delta_1, \alpha, 1 - \beta, p_1, a, b)$. Note that the hazard rate for the control arm, λ_1, will be identical under both H_0 and H_1, but that for the experimental arm will be $\lambda_2 = \lambda_1/\Delta_0$ under H_0 and $\lambda_2 = \lambda_1/\Delta_1$ under H_1.

These distributional assumptions can be easily extended to nonexponential survival models and a nonuniform censoring (or accrual) distribution. Furthermore, we assume that there is no loss to follow-up by (B), but it can be easily extended to account for possible loss to follow-up by incorporating it to the censoring distribution, see Jung, Kim, and Chow (2008).

11.1.2.2   When Accrual Rate Is Specified instead of Accrual Period

Suppose that patients are expected to enter the study at a rate of r during the accrual period based on the number of patients treated by the study member sites recently. At the design stage of a new trial, we usually can estimate r from the number of patients recruited to the study center recently, while the accrual period a is unknown. In this case, (B) is replaced by

(B′) Patients are accrued following a Poisson distribution with rate r, and are followed for a period b after the completion of accrual.

With $(\lambda_1, \Delta_0, \Delta_1, \alpha, 1 - \beta, p_1, r, b)$ specified, from (11.4) and (11.5), $\omega = \omega(a)$ and $\sigma_h = \sigma_h(a)$ for $h = 0, 1$ are functions of the unknown a. Hence, under (A) and (B), (11.3) is expressed as

$$n = \frac{\{\sigma_0(a)z_{1-\alpha} + \sigma_1(a)z_{1-\beta}\}^2}{\omega^2(a)}. \quad (11.6)$$

On the other hand, under the Poisson accrual distribution (B′), we have

$$n = a \times r. \quad (11.7)$$

By equating the right-hand sides of (11.6) and (11.7), we obtain an equation on a,

$$a \times r = \frac{\{\sigma_0(a)z_{1-\alpha} + \sigma_1(a)z_{1-\beta}\}^2}{\omega^2(a)}. \quad (11.8)$$

Equation (11.8) is solved using a numerical method, such as the bisection method. Let a^* denote the solution to Equation (11.8). Then, given an accrual rate r instead of an accrual period a, we obtain the sample size by $n = a^* \times r$. The procedure for a sample size calculation may be summarized as follows:

(I) Specify the input variables:

- Type I and II error rates, (α, β)
- Allocation proportions, (p_1, p_2)
- Hazard rate λ_1 for the control arm under exponential survival model, and hazard ratios Δ_0 and Δ_1 under H_0 and H_1, respectively
- Accrual rate r and follow-up period b

(II) Solve

$$a \times r = \frac{\{\sigma_0(a)z_{1-\alpha} + \sigma_1(a)z_{1-\beta}\}^2}{\omega^2(a)}$$

with respect to a using the bisection method.

(III) For the solution $a = a^*$ to the equation in (II), the required sample size is given as $n = a^* \times r$.

11.1.3   Sample Size Calculation under a General Accrual Pattern

In (B$'$), we assume a constant accrual rate over the whole accrual period. Usually in a multicenter trial, however, it takes a while (usually 1 to 2 years) until the study is approved by the institutional review boards of the study centers and the accrual rate is stabilized. Let $u(t)$ for $t \geq 0$ be the function representing the pattern of patient accrual over a time period. For example, if we expect that the accrual will be linearly increasing for the first a_0 years, called the run-in time, and maintain a constant accrual rate of r per year after that, then we have

$$u(t) = \begin{cases} rt & \text{for } 0 \leq t \leq a_0 \\ r & \text{for } t > a_0 \end{cases}. \tag{11.9}$$

This is similar to the piecewise linear accrual pattern considered by Yateman and Skene (1992). Given an accrual period of a and an accrual function $u(t)$, (11.7) is extended to

$$n = \int_0^a u(s)ds. \tag{11.10}$$

The accrual function $u(t)$ is related to the censoring distribution function $G(t)$ as follows. Let E denote the entry time of a patient in the study. The probability density function of E is expressed as

$$\begin{cases} u(t)/\int_0^a u(s)ds & \text{if } 0 \leq t \leq a \\ 0 & \text{otherwise} \end{cases}.$$

Since, for each patient, the censoring time C is related to the entry time E by

$C = a + b - E$, the survivor function of C, $G(t) = P(C \geq t)$, is given as

$$G(t) = P(E \leq a + b - t) = \begin{cases} 1 & \text{if } t \leq b \\ \int_0^{a+b-t} u(s)ds / \int_0^a u(s)ds & \text{if } b < t \leq a + b \\ 0 & \text{if } t > a + b \end{cases}$$

(11.11)

By calculating $\sigma_0^2(a)$, $\sigma_1^2(a)$, and $\omega(a)$ using this $G(t)$ and equating the right-hand sides of (11.3) and (11.10), we obtain an equation on a for a general accrual pattern. Using the solution a^* to this equation, we obtain the required sample as $n = \int_0^{a^*} u(s)ds$.

Combining (11.10) and (11.11), we calculate the probability of observing an event from a patient in arm k by $d_k = 1 - n^{-1} \int_0^\infty S_k(t)u(a + b - t)dt$.

For example, for the piecewise linear accrual pattern of (11.9), we have

$$\int_0^a u(s)ds = \begin{cases} ra^2/2 & \text{if } 0 \leq a \leq a_0 \\ ra_0^2/2 + r(a - a_0) & \text{if } a > a_0 \end{cases}$$

and

$$\int_0^{a+b-t} u(s)ds = \begin{cases} ra_0^2/2 + r(a - a_0) & \text{if } t < b \\ ra_0^2/2 + r(a + b - a_0 - t) & \text{if } b \leq t < a + b - a_0 \\ r(a + b - t)^2/2 & \text{if } a + b - a_0 \leq t < a + b \\ 0 & \text{if } t \geq a + b \end{cases}$$

that are used to calculate $G(t)$ in (11.11).

The sample size calculation procedure for a general accrual pattern can be summarized as follows. Since $n = \int_0^a u(s)ds$, the term $\int_0^a u(s)ds$ is canceled out in the equation of (II) below.

(I) Specify the input variables:

- Type I and II error probabilities (α, β)
- Allocation proportions, p_1, p_2
- Hazard rate λ_1 for the control arm under exponential survival model, and hazard ratios Δ_0 and Δ_1 under H_0 and H_1, respectively
- Accrual pattern $u(t)$, and follow-up period b

(II) Solve

$$1 = \frac{\{\tilde{\sigma}_0(a)z_{1-\alpha} + \tilde{\sigma}_1(a)z_{1-\beta}\}^2}{\tilde{\omega}^2(a)}$$

with respect to a using the bisection method, where

$$\tilde{\sigma}_0^2(a) = \Delta_0 \lambda_1 p_1 p_2 \int_0^{a+b} \frac{\tilde{G}(t)e^{-\lambda_1(1+\Delta_1)t}(p_1 e^{-\lambda_1 t} + \Delta_1 p_2 e^{-\Delta_1 \lambda_1 t})}{(p_1 e^{-\lambda_1 t} + \Delta_0 p_2 e^{-\Delta_1 \lambda_1 t})^2}dt,$$

$$\sigma_1^2(a) = \Delta_1 \lambda_1 p_1 p_2 \int_0^{a+b} \frac{\tilde{G}(t)e^{-\lambda_1(1+\Delta_1)t}}{p_1 e^{-\lambda_1 t} + \Delta_1 p_2 e^{-\Delta_1 \lambda_1 t}}dt,$$

$$\omega(a) = (\Delta_0 - \Delta_1)\lambda_1 p_1 p_2 \int_0^{a+b} \frac{\tilde{G}(t)e^{-\lambda_1(1+\Delta_1)t}}{p_1 e^{-\lambda_1 t} + \Delta_0 p_2 e^{-\Delta_1 \lambda_1 t}}dt,$$

and $\tilde{G}(t) = \int_0^{a+b-t} u(s)ds$.

(III) For the solution $a = a^*$ to the equation in (II), the required sample size is obtained by $n = \int_0^{a^*} u(t)dt$.

This approach to the general accrual trend can be incorporated with any sample size calculation methods for survival data analysis that are discussed in the previous chapters. The following is an example from a randomized phase II trial.

Example 11.2 (A Randomized Phase II Trial)
We consider the example of a randomized phase II trial for patients with locally advanced nasopharyngeal carcinoma. A high-dose (arm 1) chemotherapy A concurrent with radiotherapy is a standard treatment for the patient population. However, the high-dose chemotherapy is not well tolerated by most patients. So, we want to investigate a low-dose (arm 2) concurrent chemotherapy A administered more frequently (weekly vs. every 3 weeks). In arm 2, 1/3 of the arm 1 dose is given weekly, so that the total doses are identical between the two arms if the treatments are given for the whole cycles. It is known that the high-dose chemotherapy has a 3-year progression-free survival (PFS) of $S_1(3) = 0.75$, corresponding to a hazard rate of $\lambda_1 = 0.096$ under an exponential PFS model. In the new randomized phase II trial, we will not be interested in the low-dose chemotherapy if its 3-year PFS is $S_2(3) = 0.65$ or lower, corresponding to $\Delta_0 = 1.4974$, and will be very much interested in it if its 3-year PFS is $S_2(3) = 0.8$ or higher, corresponding to $\Delta_1 = 0.7757$ under an exponential model. Because the weekly low-dose regimen is more tolerable than the high-dose regimen, the patients in arm 2 have a higher chance of receiving the scheduled whole cycles than those in arm 1. So, the cumulative dose in arm 2 will be higher than that in arm 1, and the low-dose regimen will possibly extend the PFS for arm 2 slightly beyond that of arm 1.

Assuming an equal allocation $p_1 = p_2 = 0.5$, an annual accrual rate of $r = 55$ patients and $b = 3$ years of additional follow-up after completion of accrual, we need $n = 138$ patients ($n_k = 69$ per arm) for $1 - \beta = 80\%$ power for detecting $H_1 : \Delta_1 = 0.7757$ by the generalized log-rank test with one-sided $\alpha = 10\%$ for $H_0 : \Delta_0 = 1.4974$. We expect about 42 events (progressions or deaths) at the final data analysis.

In order to validate this sample size, 10,000 samples of size $n = 138$ are generated from the design setting of $(p_1, \lambda_1, \Delta_1, r, b) = (0.5, 0.096, 0.7757, 55, 3)$, and the generalized log-rank test with one-sided $\alpha = 0.1$ is applied to each simulated sample. The empirical power is obtained as 0.7920, which is very close to the nominal $1 - \beta = 0.8$. We also conduct simulations to check the small sample property of the generalized log-rank test by generating 10,000 samples of size $n = 138$ under $H_0 : \Delta_0 = 1.4974$. The empirical type I error rate is 0.0923, which is very close to the nominal $\alpha = 0.1$.

Extending this example, suppose that the accrual is expected to linearly increase for the first year ($a_0 = 1$) and maintain a constant accrual rate of

$r = 55$ per year from the beginning of the second year. Then, we obtain $a^* = 3$ years and $n = 136$. With the slightly longer accrual period (3 years $138/55 = 2.5$ years), this design setting requires a slightly smaller sample size (136 vs. 138) than the setting with a constant accrual rate which was considered above.

Example 11.1 (revisited):
Let's consider the PET-guided Hodgkin's lymphoma trial discussed earlier. Under H_0, we specify $\Delta_0 = 4.3$. By the PET-guided chemotherapy strategy, it is believed that the 3-year PFS of the PET-positive patients can be increased to $S_2(3) = 0.74$, from 0.52, with a corresponding annual hazard ratio of $\lambda_2 = 0.10$, resulting in a hazard ratio of $\Delta_1 = 2.0$. The previous study observed about $p_2 = 20\%$ of PET-positivity. Assuming an annual accrual rate of $r = 60$ patients and $b = 3$ years of additional follow-up after completion of accrual, we need $n = 195$ patients for $1 - \beta = 90\%$ power for detecting $H_1 : \Delta_1 = 2$ by the generalized log-rank test with one-sided $\alpha = 10\%$ for $H_0 : \Delta_0 = 4.3$. Under this specific alternative hypothesis, we expect about 47 events (progressions or deaths) at the data analysis. Since this is not a randomized trial, the resulting allocation proportions may be slightly different from the specified $(p_1, p_2) = (0.8, 0.2)$. If the observed allocation proportions are close to 0.5, the planned sample size has enough power. However, if they are farther from 0.5, we may have to check the statistical power of the study based on the observed proportions, while other design parameters are fixed at the values used when designing the study. In this power checking, we may use the estimated censoring distribution $\hat{G}(t)$ based on the accrual times of patients too.

Simulation studies are conducted to evaluate the calculated sample size under the above design settings of H_0 and H_1, respectively. Using 10,000 simulation samples of size $n = 132$ under each hypothesis, the empirical type I error rate and power are observed as 0.0984 (to be compared to $\alpha = 0.1$) and 0.8749 (to be compared to $1 - \beta = 0.9$), respectively.

We may consider the PET-guided Hodgkin's lymphoma trial as a single-arm phase II trial using the hazard ratio between PET negative group treated with 4 cycles of ABVD and positive group treated with 2 cycles of escalated BEACOPP followed by radiation therapy after 2 cycles of ABVD as the primary endpoint. This study uses the outcome (or the estimated hazard ratio) from a previous study (which treated both PET positive and negative groups by the standard 4 cycles of ABVD) as a historical control. A possible randomized trial with the same study objective is to randomize patients between a control arm treated by 4 cycles of ABVD, regardless of postcycle 2 PET result, and an experimental arm with the PET-guided treatment. The standard log-rank test that is discussed in Chapter 10 can be used to compare the PFS between the two arms in this case.

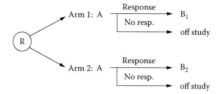

Figure 11.1   A randomized phase II trial design for comparing maintenance therapies.

11.2   Randomized Phase II Trials for Comparing Maintenance Therapies

Suppose that we want to compare the survival distributions between two maintenance therapies combined with a common induction therapy through a randomized phase II clinical trial. In treatment arm 1, patients are treated by an induction therapy A; if they respond, then they proceed to a standard maintenance therapy B_1; otherwise, they are off the study therapy. In treatment arm 2, patients are treated by the same induction therapy A; if they respond, then they proceed to an experimental maintenance therapy B_2; otherwise, they are off the study therapy. The procedure of the trial is described in Figure 11.1. For an intent to treat analysis, all randomized patients are included in the analysis as randomized whether they receive the preassigned maintenance therapy or not.

11.2.1   Two-Sample Log-Rank Test

Suppose that $\tilde{n}_k$ patients are randomized to arm $k(=1,2)$, among which n_k patients respond to induction therapy A and proceed to maintenance therapy B_k, and n_{0k} patients do not respond to induction therapy A and are off the study therapy. Let $n_0 = n_{01} + n_{02}$ denote the total number of nonresponders to induction therapy A, and $n = \tilde{n}_1 + \tilde{n}_2 = n_1 + n_2 + n_0$ the total number of patients. Let T_{0ki} denote the survival time with cumulative hazard function $\Lambda_0(t)$ for patient $i(=1,\ldots,n_{0k})$ in arm k who does not respond to the induction therapy, and T_{ki} denote the survival time with cumulative hazard function $\Lambda_k(t)$ for patient $i(=1,\ldots,n_k)$ in arm k who responds to the induction therapy and receives maintenance therapy B_k. For censoring times C_{0ki} and C_{ki}, we observe from arm k $\{(X_{0ki}, \delta_{0ki}), i = 1, \ldots, n_{0k}; (X_{ki}, \delta_{ki}), i = 1, \ldots, n_{ki}\}$, where $X = \min(T, C)$ and $\delta = I(T \leq C)$. We want to test $H_0 : \Lambda_1(t) = \Lambda_2(t)$ against $H_1 : \Lambda_1(t) > \Lambda_2(t)$.

Let $Y_{ki}(t) = I(X_{ki} \geq t)$, $Y_{0ki}(t) = I(X_{0ki} \geq t)$, $N_{ki}(t) = \delta_{ki}I(X_{ki} \leq t)$, and $N_{0ki}(t) = \delta_{0ki}I(X_{0ki} \geq t)$. Further, let $Y_k(t) = \sum_{i=1}^{n_k} Y_{ki}(t)$, $Y_{0k}(t) = \sum_{i=1}^{n_{0k}} Y_{0ki}(t)$, $N_k(t) = \sum_{i=1}^{n_k} N_{ki}(t)$, $N_{0k}(t) = \sum_{i=1}^{n_{0k}} N_{0ki}(t)$, $Y_0(t) = Y_{01}(t) + Y_{02}(t)$, and $N_0(t) = N_{02}(t) + N_{02}(t)$. The log-rank test statistic based on intent to treat analysis is given as

$$W = \frac{1}{\sqrt{n}} \left[\int_0^\infty \frac{Y_2(t) + Y_{02}(t)}{Y_1(t) + Y_2(t) + Y_0(t)} \{ dN_1(t) + dN_{01}(t) \} \right.$$

$$\left. - \int_0^\infty \frac{Y_1(t) + Y_{01}(t)}{Y_1(t) + Y_2(t) + Y_0(t)} \{ dN_2(t) + dN_{02}(t) \} \right].$$

and its variance estimator under H_0 is

$$\hat{\sigma}^2 = \frac{1}{n} \int_0^\infty \frac{\{ Y_1(t) + Y_{01}(t) \}\{ Y_2(t) + Y_{02}(t) \}}{\{ Y_1(t) + Y_2(t) + Y_0(t) \}^2} \{ dN_1(t) + dN_2(t) + dN_0(t) \}.$$

Under H_0, $W/\hat{\sigma}$ is asymptotically standard normal. Hence, we reject H_0, in favor of H_1, if $W/\hat{\sigma} > z_{1-\alpha}$ with one-sided type I error probability α.

11.2.2 Sample Size Calculation

Let $p_k = \tilde{n}_k/n$ denote the allocation proportion for arm k ($p_1 + p_2 = 1$), and $\gamma = (n_1 + n_2)/n = 1 - n_0/n$ denote the response rate of maintenance therapy A. Note that $n_k/n = \gamma p_k$ and $n_{0k}/n = \bar{\gamma} p_k$, where $\bar{\gamma} = 1 - \gamma$ denotes the probability of nonresponse for A. We assume that patients are accrued with a constant accrual rate, r, during the accrual period and followed during follow-up period b after the last patient is entered. Let $S_k(t) = \exp\{-\Lambda_k(t)\}$ denote the survivor function of the survival distribution for arm k for the patients who respond to induction therapy A and proceed to maintenance therapy B_k, $S_0(t) = \exp\{-\Lambda_0(t)\}$ denote the survivor function for the patients who do not respond to A in either arm, and $G(t)$ denote the survivor function of the common censoring distribution. We derive a sample size formula of the two-sample log-rank test for an intent-to-treat analysis in terms of the following design parameters:

- Type I error probability α and power $1 - \beta$
- Allocation proportions p_1, p_2 ($p_1 + p_2 = 1$)
- Response probability of induction therapy, γ
- $S_0(t) = $ survivor function of nonresponders to the induction therapy
  $S_k(t) = $ survivor function of arm $k (= 1, 2)$ for patients who respond to the induction therapy and receive maintenance therapy B_k
- Accrual rate r (or accrual period a) and additional follow-up period b

Treatment arm k has a mixture survival model with survivor function $\tilde{S}_k(t) = \gamma S_k(t) + \bar{\gamma} S_0(t)$. Let $f_k(t) = -\partial S_k(t)/\partial t$ denote the probability density function for $k = 0, 1, 2$, and $\tilde{f}_k(t) = -\partial \tilde{S}_k(t)/\partial t = \gamma f_k(t) + \bar{\gamma} f_0(t)$ denote the mixture probability density function for arm $k = 1, 2$. Then, the hazard function for arm k is given as

$$\tilde{\lambda}_k(t) = \frac{\gamma f_k(t) + \bar{\gamma} f_0(t)}{\gamma S_k(t) + \bar{\gamma} S_0(t)}.$$

From Section 10.1.2, the required sample size is given as

$$n = \left(\frac{\sigma_0 z_{1-\alpha} + \sigma_1 z_{1-\beta}}{\omega} \right)^2,$$

where

$$\sigma_0^2 = p_1^2 p_2 \int_0^\infty \frac{G(t)\tilde{S}_1(t)^2 \tilde{S}_2(t)\tilde{\lambda}_1(t)}{\{p_1 \tilde{S}_1(t) + p_2 \tilde{S}_2(t)\}^2} dt + p_1 p_2^2 \int_0^\infty \frac{G(t)\tilde{S}_1(t)\tilde{S}_2(t)^2 \tilde{\lambda}_2(t)}{\{p_1 \tilde{S}_1(t) + p_2 \tilde{S}_2(t)\}^2} dt$$

and

$$\sigma_1^2 = p_1 p_2^2 \int_0^\infty \frac{G(t)\tilde{S}_1(t)\tilde{S}_2(t)^2 \tilde{\lambda}_1(t)}{\{p_1 \tilde{S}_1(t) + p_2 \tilde{S}_2(t)\}^2} dt + p_1^2 p_2 \int_0^\infty \frac{G(t)\tilde{S}_1(t)^2 \tilde{S}_2(t)\tilde{\lambda}_2(t)}{\{p_1 \tilde{S}_1(t) + p_2 \tilde{S}_2(t)\}^2} dt.$$

Furthermore, under H_1, we can show that $E(W) = \sqrt{n}\omega$, where

$$\omega = p_1 p_2 \int_0^\infty \frac{G(t)\tilde{S}_1(t)\tilde{S}_2(t)\{\tilde{\lambda}_1(t) - \tilde{\lambda}_2(t)\}}{p_1 \tilde{S}_1(t) + p_2 \tilde{S}_2(t)} dt.$$

The number of events D under H_1 is calculated by $D = n(\bar{\gamma}d_0 + \gamma p_1 d_1 + \gamma p_2 d_2)$, where $d_k = 1 + \int_0^\infty S_k(t) dG(t)$ for $k = 0, 1, 2$.

We can estimate the required sample size as in the previous section assuming exponential survival models and the given accrual rate instead of the accrual period.

Example 11.3

Suppose that patients who do not respond to a common induction therapy A have 10% of 6-month progression-free survival (PFS). Patients who respond to induction therapy A and receive a standard maintenance therapy B_1 are known to have a 6-month PFS of 50%. We will be very interested in an experimental maintenance therapy B_2, combined with induction therapy A, if patients who respond to induction therapy A and receive B_2 have a 6-month PFS of 70% or higher. Assuming an exponential PFS model, the annual hazard rates for the patient groups are $\lambda_0 = 4.605$, $\lambda_1 = 1.386$, and $\lambda_2 = 0.713$. It is expected that this study is able to accrue 5 patients per month ($r = 60$ per year), and we plan to follow the patients for additional $b = 1$ year. Then, the required sample size for the log-rank test with one-sided $\alpha = 10\%$ and 90% of power with balanced allocation ($p_1 = p_2 = 1/2$) is given as $n = 116$ ($\tilde{n}_k = 58$ per arm), requiring an accrual period of about 24 months ($a = 116/5$). At the final analysis, we expect $D = 105$ events (55 and 47 for arms 1 and 2, respectively) under H_1.

References

Aalen, O.O. (1978). Nonparametric inference for a family of counting processes. *Annals of Statistics*, 6, 701–726.

Cox, D.R. (1972). Regression models and life tables (with discussion). *Journal of Royal Statistical Society B*, 34, 187–220.

Fleming, T.R. and Harrington, D.P. (1991). *Counting Processes and Survival Analysis*. Wiley, New York.

Gallamini, A., Hutchings, M., Rigacci, L., Specht, L., Merli, F., Hansen, M., Patti, C., Loft, A., Di Raimondo, F., D'Amore, F., Biggi, A., Vitolo, U., Stelitano, C., Sancetta, R., Trentin, L., Luminari, S., Iannitto, E., Viviani, S., Pierri, I., and Levis, A. (2007). Early interim 2-[18F]fluoro-2-deoxy-D-glucose positron emission tomography is prognostically superior to international prognostic score in advanced-stage Hodgkin's lymphoma: A report from a joint Italian-Danish study. *Journal of Clinical Oncology*, 25 (24), 3746–3752.

Hutchings, M., Loft, A., Hansen, M., Pedersen, L.M., Buhl, T., Jurlander, J., Buus, S., Keiding, S., D'Amore, F., Boesen, A.M., Berthelsen, A.K., and Specht, L. (2006). FDG-PET after two cycles of chemotherapy predicts treatment failure and progression-free survival in Hodgkin lymphoma. *Blood*, 107 (1), 52–59.

Jung, S.H., Kang, S.J., McCall, L., and Blumenstein, B. (2005). Sample size computation for noninferiority log-rank test. *Journal of Biopharmaceutical Statistics*, 15, 957–967.

Jung, S.H., Kim, C., and Chow, S.C. (2008). Sample size calculation for the log-rank tests for multi-arm trials with a control. *Journal of Korean Statistical Society*, 37, 11–22.

Nelson, W. (1969). Hazard plotting for incomplete failure data. *Journal of Quality Technology*, 1, 27–52.

Peto, R. and Peto, J. (1972). Asymptotically efficient rank invariant test procedures (with discussion). *Journal of the Royal Statistical Society, Series A*, 135, 185–206.

Schoenfeld, D.A. (1983). Sample size formula for the proportional hazards regression model. *Biometrics*, 39, 499–503.

Yateman, N.A. and Skene, A.M. (1992). Sample size for proportional hazards survival studies with arbitrary patient entry and loss to follow-up distributions. *Statistics in Medicine*, 11, 1103–1113.

Index

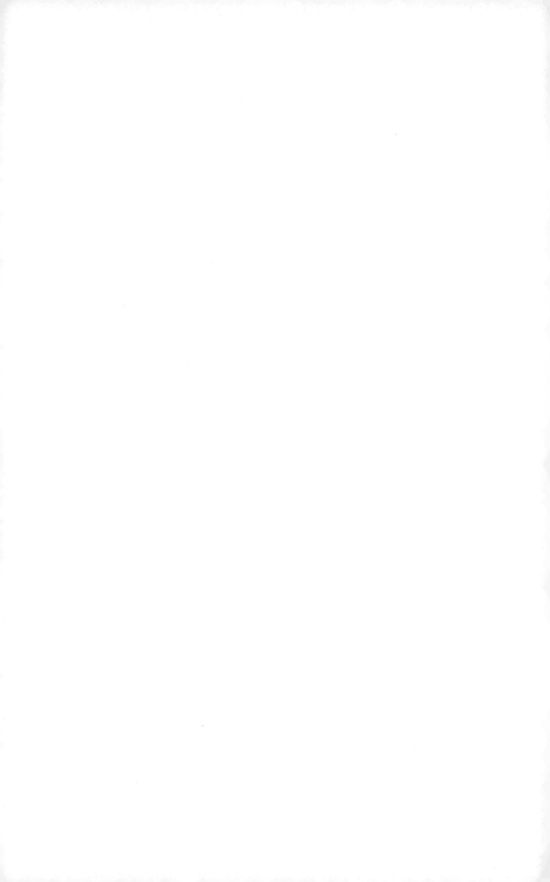

*For Product Safety Concerns and Information please contact
our EU representative GPSR@taylorandfrancis.com Taylor & Francis
Verlag GmbH, Kaufingerstraße 24, 80331 München, Germany*

T - #0171 - 160425 - C0 - 234/156/11 [13] - CB - 9781439871850 - Gloss Lamination